Embedded Systems for Biomedical Applications

This book is an essential guide to the constantly changing environment of embedded systems in healthcare in a world where the convergence of technology and healthcare is becoming increasingly important. It further explains different scenarios corresponding to the latest technologies in the healthcare system for early diagnosis, enhanced treatment, and cure of diseases, including remote patient monitoring, cardiac monitoring, and deep learning for remediation.

- Emphasizes how embedded systems contribute to clinical care by facilitating personalized treatment and informed decision-making for healthcare professionals.
- Highlights the role of embedded systems in tracking treatment progress, enabling healthcare professionals to monitor patient responses and adjust treatment plans accordingly.
- Explores the application of embedded systems in remote patient monitoring, allowing for continuous health monitoring outside traditional healthcare settings.
- Presents the integration of deep learning and telecommunication technology with embedded systems, optimizing their efficiency and utilization in biomedical applications.
- Offers insights into future prospects for advancing biomedical applications through embedded systems, providing a roadmap for further innovation and development in the field.

This reference work is useful for scholars and professionals interested in the applications and optimization of emerging smart technologies in the field of healthcare.

High-Performance Computing for Smart Healthcare: New Developments and Advances

Series Editors

Rishabha Malviya, Galgotias University, India

Balamurugan Balusamy, Shiv Nadar University, India

Sonali Sundram, Galgotias University, India

Forthcoming and Published Titles:

Healthcare-Driven Intelligent Computing Paradigms to Secure Futuristic Smart Cities
Diptendu Sinha Roy, Mir Wajahat Hussain, K. Hemant Kumar Reddy, Deepak Gupta

Embedded Systems for Biomedical Applications
By Rishabha Malviya, Selcan Karakuş, Mukesh Roy

Embedded Systems for Biomedical Applications

Edited by
Rishabha Malviya
Selcan Karakuş
Mukesh Roy

CRC Press
Taylor & Francis Group
Boca Raton London New York

CRC Press is an imprint of the
Taylor & Francis Group, an **informa** business
A CHAPMAN & HALL BOOK

Designed cover image: ShutterStock

First edition published 2025
by CRC Press
2385 NW Executive Center Drive, Suite 320, Boca Raton FL 33431

and by CRC Press
4 Park Square, Milton Park, Abingdon, Oxon, OX14 4RN

CRC Press is an imprint of Taylor & Francis Group, LLC

ISBN: 978-1-032-83191-6 (hbk)
ISBN: 978-1-032-83194-7 (pbk)
ISBN: 978-1-003-50819-9 (ebk)

DOI: 10.1201/9781003508199

Typeset in Times
by SPi Technologies India Pvt Ltd (Straive)

Contents

Editors vii
Contributors ix
Foreword xii
Preface xiii

Chapter 1 Introduction to Embedded Systems in Healthcare: Operational Environments in Healthcare Settings 1

Bhupinder Singh, Rishabha Malviya, Christian Kaunert, and Sathvik Belagodu Sridhar

Chapter 2 Embedded Systems in the Medical Field: Pros and Cons 21

Gizem Karabulut Şevk, Elif Tüzün, and Nuray Beköz Üllen

Chapter 3 Automation of Medical Devices with Embedded Systems 43

Phool Chandra, Shahjad, Neetu Sachan, and Arun Kumar

Chapter 4 Embedded Systems in Developing Imaging Devices 100

Sündüz Alemdar and Nursel Pekel Bayramgil

Chapter 5 Deep Learning of Telecommunication Technology for the Efficient Utilization of Embedded Systems 124

Gulcicek Dere

Chapter 6 Role of Embedded Systems in Diagnosis and Decision-Making for Better Treatment 135

Shristy Verma, Rishabha Malviya, and Sathvik Belagodu Sridhar

Chapter 7 Enhancing Remote Healthcare: Integration of ATOM ECG with eSanjeevani 153

R. Ananthakrishnan, Nitish Naik, Raghav Bansal, Abhinav Cardea, Mukesh Roy, Avval Gupta, Rohit Kumar Kushwaha, Vivek Shahi, and Manish Jawa

Chapter 8 Artificial Intelligence in Embedded Systems for Biomedical Applications 190

Sena Nur Karabekiroglu, Meral Usta, Deniz Uygunoz, and Mert Akın Insel

Chapter 9 Embedded Systems in Metabolic Bariatric Surgery: From Telemonitoring to Deep Learning Applications 211

Athanasios G. Pantelis

Chapter 10 Integration of Machine Learning Techniques with Multi-Criteria Decision-Making for a Better Treatment 236

Inci Albayrak, Jale Sade, and Hale Gonce Kocken

Chapter 11 Embedded Systems in Developing Advanced Strategies in Healthcare Management 254

Selcan Karakuş, Elif Tüzün, Magdy M. Elnashar, and Sinem Özlem Enginler

Chapter 12 Human Health Status Detection from the Tongue Image Using Embedded Image Processing 272

Mohit Bhandwal, Mukesh Roy, and Pratap Pati

Index 296

Editors

Rishabha Malviya earned a Bachelor of Pharmacy degree from Uttar Pradesh Technical University and Master of Pharmacy degree (Pharmaceutics) from Gautam Buddha Technical University, Lucknow, Uttar Pradesh, India. His PhD (Pharmacy) work was in the area of Novel formulation development techniques. He has 14 years of research experience and has been an Associate Professor in the Department of Pharmacy, School of Medical and Allied Sciences, Galgotias University, India for the past 11 years. His areas of interest include formulation optimization, AI for healthcare applications, nanoformulation, targeted drug delivery, localized drug delivery, and characterization of natural polymers as pharmaceutical excipients. He has authored more than 200 research/review papers for national/international journals of repute. He has 58 patents (19 grants, 38 published, 1 filed) and publications in reputed national and international journals with a total of more than 300 cumulative impact factors. He has authored/edited/is editing 92 books and authored 165 book chapters. His name has been included in world's top 2% scientist list for the years 2020, 2021, 2022, and 2023 by Elsevier BV and Stanford University. He is Reviewer/Editor/Editorial board member of more than 50 national and international journals of repute.

Selcan Karakuş is an Associate Professor in the Department of Chemistry, at Istanbul University-Cerrahpaşa (IUC), Turkiye. She earned her Master of Science degree in physical chemistry from Istanbul University (IU) in 2006, and her PhD in physical chemistry from IU in 2011. She has been a visiting researcher at the University of Massachusetts, Department of Polymer Science and Engineering. She has research experience in drug carrier systems, nanoparticles, nanocomposites, nano-emulsion self-assembled polymeric nanostructures, and copolymer blends. She worked on a variety of projects funded by IUC and has published several research articles and book chapters.

Mukesh Roy earned his Doctor of Philosophy in Mechanical Engineering from South Dakota State University, USA, in 2021. His research concentrated on the study of the mechanics of vascular tissue to employ it as a template for engineering design and flexible biocomposites. After completing his PhD, Dr. Roy went on to complete a Postdoctoral Fellowship at the National Science Foundation's Engineering Research Center for Cellular Metamaterials (CELL-MET), Florida International University, USA in 2023. During this fellowship, Dr. Roy worked on the characterization of stem cell-laden cardiovascular patches, specifically focusing on myocardial tissue at multiple scales. Currently, Dr. Roy serves as a Clinical Researcher and Biostatistician at the Office of Clinical Research in Baptist Health South Florida-Miami, USA. Dr. Roy has research experience of 8+ years and has authored and published over 24 peer-reviewed scientific articles, conference papers, 2 book chapters, and 40+ abstracts. In addition, Dr. Roy has filed 6 patents, with one granted in the USA and 5 published in India. Dr. Roy has received 6 awards and 3 fellowships for his research, creativity, and innovations. Furthermore, Dr. Roy serves as an editorial board member and reviewer for various journals and conferences in biomaterials, computational biomechanics, biomedical devices, and public health research. Dr. Roy's research is highly interdisciplinary, and his interests include biomedical devices, clinical trials, regenerative tissues, biomaterials, and bioinspired design.

Contributors

Inci Albayrak
Department of Mathematical Engineering
Yildiz Technical University
Istanbul, Turkiye

Sündüz Alemdar
Faculty of Science, Chemistry Department
Hacettepe University
Beytepe, Ankara, Turkiye

R. Ananthakrishnan
Department of Medicine and Cardiology
INHS Asvini
Colaba, Mumbai, India

Raghav Bansal
Department of Cardiology
All India Institute of Medical Sciences
India

Nursel Pekel Bayramgil
Faculty of Science, Chemistry Department
Hacettepe University
Beytepe, Ankara, Türkiye

Mohit Bhandwal
Amity University
Tashkent
Uzbekistan

Abhinav Cardea
Dept. of Research and Innovation
Cardea Labs, Dept. of Research and Innovation
Bangalore, India

Phool Chandra
Teerthanker Mahaveer College of Pharmacy
Teerthanker Mahaveer University
Moradabad, India

Gulcicek Dere
Bahcesehir University
Turkey

Magdy M. Elnashar
Centre of Scientific Excellence-Group of Advanced Materials and Nanotechnology
National Research Centre, El-Behooth St., Dokki, Giza, Egypt
School of Medicine, Curtin University, Perth, Australia

Sinem Özlem Enginler
Faculty of Veterinary Medicine, Department of Obstetrics and Gynaecology
Istanbul University
Avcilar, Istanbul, Turkiye

Avval Gupta
Dept. of Research and Innovation
Cardea Labs
India

Mert Akın Insel
Yıldız Technical University
Turkiye

Manish Jawa
Software Consultant
India

Christian Kaunert
Dublin City University
University of South Wales
UK

Sena Nur Karabekiroglu
Faculty of Chemistry and Metallurgy, Department of Chemical Engineering
Yıldız Technical University
Istanbul, Turkiye

Gizem Karabulut
Faculty of Engineering, Department of Metallurgical and Materials Engineering,
Istanbul University - Cerrahpaşa,
Istanbul, Turkey

Selcan Karakuş
Faculty of Engineering, Department of Chemistry,
Istanbul University - Cerrahpaşa,
Avcilar, Istanbul, Turkiye

Hale Gonce Kocken
Department of Mathematical Engineering
Yildiz Technical University
Istanbul, Turkey

Arun Kumar
Global Institute of Pharmaceutical Education and Research
Kashipur, India

Rohit Kumar Kushwaha
Dept. of Research and Innovation
Cardea Labs
Bangalore, India

Rishabha Malviya
Department of Pharmacy, School of Medical and Allied Sciences
Greater Noida, Uttar Pradesh, Galgotias University
India

Nitish Naik
Department of Cardiology
All India Institute of Medical Sciences
New Delhi, India

Athanasios G. Pantelis
Surgeon, Obesity and Metabolic Disorders Department
Athens Medical Group,
Psychiko Clinic
Psychiko, Athens, Greece

Pratap Patil
Amity University
Tashkent, Uzbekistan

Mukesh Roy
Office of Clinical Research
Baptist Health South Florida
USA

Neetu Sachan
Maharana Pratap College of Pharmacy
Kanpur, Uttar Pradesh, India

Jale Sade
Department of Mathematical Engineering
Yildiz Technical University
Istanbul, Turkey

Vivek Shahi
Dept. of Research and Innovation
Cardea Labs
Bangalore, India

Shahjad
Global Institute of Pharmaceutical
Education and Research
Kashipur, India

Bhupinder Singh
Sharda University
India

Sathvik Belagodu Sridhar
RAK College of Pharmacy
RAK Medical & Health Sciences University
Ras Al Khaimah, United Arab Emirates

Elif Tüzün
Faculty of Engineering, Department of Chemistry,
Istanbul University - Cerrahpaşa,
Avcilar, Istanbul, Türkiye

Nuray Beköz Üllen
Faculty of Engineering, Department of Metallurgical and Materials Engineering,
Istanbul University - Cerrahpaşa,
Istanbul, Türkiye

Meral Usta
Faculty of Chemistry and Metallurgy, Department of Chemical Engineering
Yıldız Technical University
Istanbul, Turkiye

Deniz Uygunoz
Faculty of Chemistry and Metallurgy, Department of Chemical Engineering
Yıldız Technical University
Istanbul, Turkiye

Shristy Verma
Department of Pharmacy, School of Medical and Allied Sciences
Galgotias University
Greater Noida, Uttar Pradesh, India

Foreword

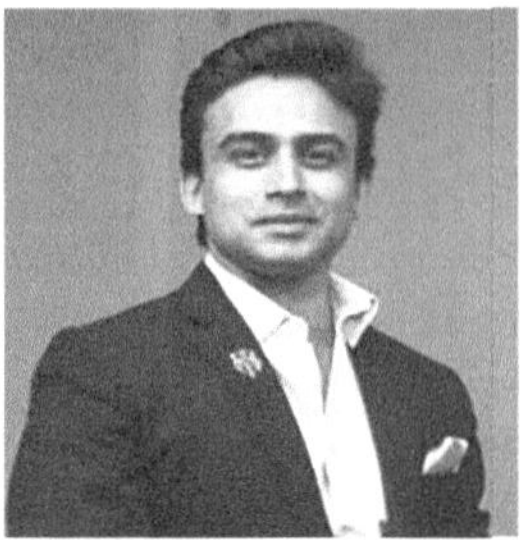

The integration of embedded systems with healthcare technology is transforming the biomedical sector by enabling real-time processing, low cost, and excellent reliability. These technologies automate medical instruments, improve diagnostic imaging, and integrate artificial intelligence. This book, "Embedded Systems for Biomedical Application: Prospective and Advances", edited by Dr. Rishabha Malviya and team provides a complete overview of these technologies, offering both theoretical foundations and practical applications that will shape the future of medicine.

The chapters explore various topics, including operational environments in healthcare settings, the pros and cons of embedded systems, automation of medical devices, and advanced imaging techniques. It also discussed the synergy between telecommunication technologies and deep learning, the role of embedded systems in clinical decision-making, and the integration of cutting-edge technologies like AI and machine learning.

One notable feature of this book is its emphasis on practical applications and case studies. For example, the integration of ATOM ECG and eSanjeevani reveals that embedded technologies might improve remote healthcare services. The study of telemonitoring and deep learning in surgery demonstrates the potential of these technologies to improve surgical outcomes and patient care.

Editors Dr. Rishabha Malviya and team as well as the contributing authors have methodically acquired their research outcomes and skills as a book that is both educational and inspiring. This book offers a thorough guide to current advancements in the subject, as well as an inspiration for future study and development.

Happy reading and best wishes.

Dr. Dhruv Galgotia
CEO, Galgotias University,
Greater Noida, India

Preface

Healthcare could be completely transformed by the quickly developing field of embedded systems integration with biological applications. This book, "Embedded Systems for Biomedical Application: Prospective and Advances", explores the integration, challenges, and advancements in the embedded system for diverse biomedical applications. It aims to bring light on the ways that cutting-edge technologies and embedded systems are reshaping healthcare management and enhancing patient outcomes.

The first chapter, titled "Introduction to Embedded Systems in Healthcare: Operational Environments in Healthcare Settings", provides an overview of the fundamental perspectives and practical contexts of embedded systems for biomedical applications. Understanding the specific requirements and barriers of healthcare settings is critical for creating effective embedded solutions. The second chapter explores the advantages and limitations of embedded systems in medical applications.

The third chapter, "Automation of Medical Devices with Embedded Systems", discusses the role of automation in improving the functionality and efficiency of medical devices, resulting in greater precision and reliability in medical processes. The fourth chapter, "Embedded Systems in Developing Imaging Devices", highlights the development and application of embedded systems in medical imaging, which has led to substantial advances in diagnostic imaging. The fifth chapter, "Deep Learning of Telecommunication Technology for the Efficient Utilisation of Embedded Systems", explores the relationship between telecommunication technologies and embedded systems, and discusses that deep learning techniques can optimize the use of embedded systems in remote healthcare applications, increasing accessibility and efficiency. Chapter six, "Role of Embedded Systems in Diagnosis and Decision Making for Better Treatment", discusses the critical role of embedded systems in the diagnostic process and clinical decision-making. Chapter seven, "Enhancing Remote Healthcare: Integration of ATOM ECG with eSanjeevani", presents a case study on the integration of specific technologies to improve remote healthcare services. Chapter eight "Artificial Intelligence in Biomedical Applications" explores the transformative role of AI with embedded systems in innovative and improved accuracy and efficiency of medical treatments. Chapter nine, "Embedded Systems in Metabolic Bariatric Surgery from Telemonitoring to Deep Learning Applications", explores the benefits of telemonitoring and deep learning in enhancing surgical outcomes and patient care.

The tenth chapter, "Integration of Machine Learning Techniques with Multi-Criteria Decision Making for a Better Treatment", discusses the integration of advanced machine learning techniques with decision-making processes in healthcare. Chapter eleventh "Embedded Systems in Developing Advanced Strategies in Healthcare Management", explores the role of embedded systems in healthcare management, improving resource management, and enhancing overall healthcare delivery. The last chapter, chapter twelve, "Health Status Detection from the Tongue

Using Embedded Image Processing", presents an innovative application of embedded systems in the image processing techniques that can be used for non-invasive health monitoring.

This book provides a comprehensive overview of the current state of the field, along with future prospects and advancements. We hope this book will inspire further research and development, ultimately contributing to the advancement of healthcare technologies.

1 Introduction to Embedded Systems in Healthcare

Operational Environments in Healthcare Settings

Bhupinder Singh, Rishabha Malviya, Christian Kaunert, and Sathvik Belagodu Sridhar

1.1 INTRODUCTION

Embedded systems which include hardware and software designed for dedicated functions are becoming increasingly important in healthcare [1]. Their ability to operate in real time, handle complex data, and ensure high reliability makes them ideal for healthcare applications [2]. This study provides an in-depth overview of the role and significance of embedded systems in healthcare settings, with a focus on their operational environment [3]. Patient care and operational effectiveness have been transformed by the introduction of embedded technology in the healthcare industry [4]. The many uses, advantages, and difficulties of embedded systems in healthcare settings are examined in this research [5]. In contemporary healthcare settings, embedded systems are essential for anything from patient monitoring to diagnostic tools [6]. This study looks at how these systems are implemented operationally and how they affect patient outcomes and healthcare delivery [7].

Embedded systems are incorporated into larger operating systems, as the name suggests. Unlike general-purpose computers, they are intended to carry out certain tasks and are a component of device systems that also involve hardware [8, 9]. Embedded systems are usually small and have low power consumption [10]. They may have microprocessors or microcontrollers as their foundation [11]. A lot of people use embedded systems on a daily basis often without even realizing it in gadgets like airplanes, digital watches, traffic lights, and MRI equipment [12]. An embedded system is a portion of a broader operating system that is designed to carry out one or two specific tasks [13, 14]. Embedded systems are widely used in the healthcare industry to store data [15]. It is critical for OEMs to use industrial-grade embedded

DOI: 10.1201/9781003508199-1

systems since healthcare applications may run in challenging environments with exposure to shocks, vibrations, and temperature changes [16]. These goods are of an industrial quality and are particularly designed to work in demanding conditions without compromising their performance [17].

1.1.1 Objectives of the Chapter

These goals need to offer a thorough synopsis of embedded systems' functions in healthcare as well as the operational contexts in which they operate. This chapter has the following objectives:

- To discuss about the ways in which embedded systems are incorporated into the current healthcare settings to guarantee smooth functioning and compatibility with various healthcare equipment and systems.
- To scrutinize the usage of embedded systems in healthcare settings for real-time monitoring of patients' vital signs, such as blood pressure, oxygen levels, and heart rate. Learn how this information is utilized for patient care and management.
- To observe the difficulties and solutions for guaranteeing the security and privacy of patient data that is gathered and sent by embedded systems in healthcare settings, taking into account adherence to laws like HIPAA.
- To scan how embedded technologies facilitate the provision of remote healthcare services, such as telemedicine and remote patient monitoring, in order to enhance patient outcomes and access to treatment.
- To study how embedded technologies affect healthcare operations, particularly how they might optimize resource allocation, cut costs, and improve operational effectiveness.

Objectives of the chapter are summarized as Figure 1.1.

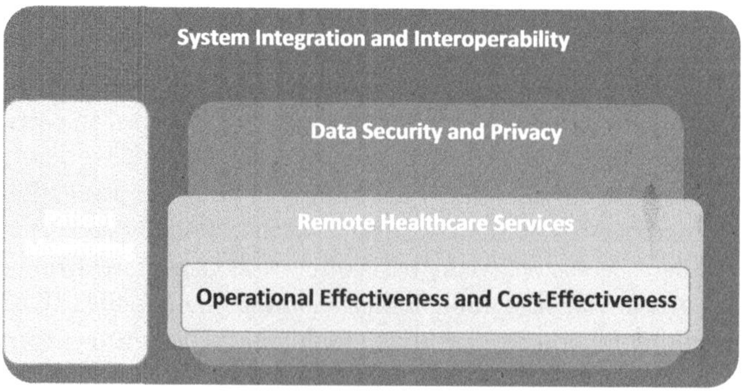

FIGURE 1.1 Objectives of the chapter.

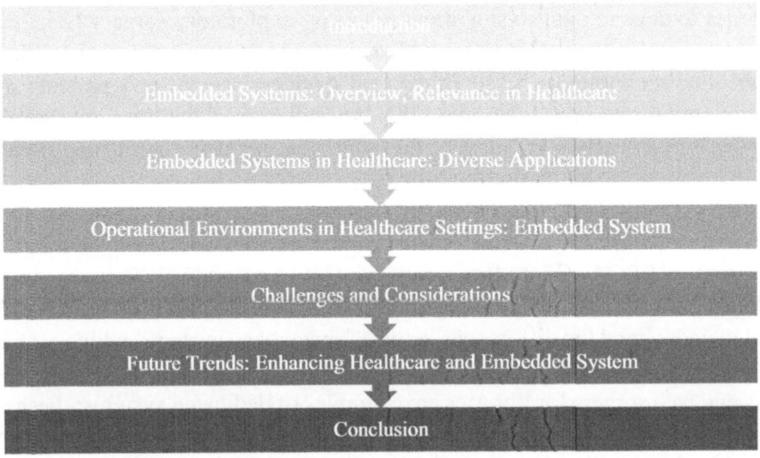

FIGURE 1.2 Flow of the chapter.

1.1.2 Structure of the Chapter

This chapter deeply dives into the diverse arena of the introduction to embedded system in healthcare: Operational Environments in Healthcare Settings (Figure 1.2). Section 1.2 explores the Embedded Systems: Overview, Relevance in Healthcare. Section 1.3 expresses the Embedded Systems in Healthcare: Diverse Applications. Section 1.4 discusses the Operational Environments in Healthcare Settings: Embedded System. Section 1.5 highlights the Challenges and Considerations. Section 1.6 specifies the Future Trends: Enhancing Healthcare and Embedded System. Finally, Section 1.7 Conclude the Chapter.

1.2 EMBEDDED SYSTEMS: OVERVIEW, RELEVANCE IN HEALTHCARE

There are several uses for embedded systems in the medical field. They are used in virtually all imaging systems, such as PET, CT, and MRI scans, as well as for monitoring vital signs and boosting sounds in electronic stethoscopes [18]. Embedded systems are also necessary for devices like glucose monitors, pacemakers, CPAP machines, and several types of biomedical sensors [19]. Through telemedicine and other remote systems, these technologies allow clinicians to diagnose diseases, treat patients, and keep an eye on their health from a distance in biomedical applications [20]. Within a larger system, an embedded system is a specialized computing system that carries out certain activities or duties [21]. Reliability, restricted user interface, real-time operation, and particular functionality are among the salient aspects [22]. These embedded systems are frequently found in complete devices along with mechanical and physical parts [23].

Both patients and physicians now feel more empowered because to the usage of embedded technology in healthcare [24]. With using embedded systems, medical professionals may monitor patients' progress throughout therapy and use imaging techniques to detect conditions without requiring exploratory surgery [25, 26]. Vital sign monitoring becomes almost immediate in the healthcare industry with the usage of embedded technologies [27]. Embedded devices have helped patients manage their ailments more easily at home [28]. For instance, diabetics can minimize the amount of finger sticks they need to do while continuously monitoring their blood sugar levels by using a glucose monitor [29].

The electronic or electromechanical systems, embedded systems are made by embedding software on microcontrollers, microprocessors, DSPs (Digital Signal Processors), or FPGAs (Field Programmable Gate Arrays) [30]. These systems typically consist of memory, input/output modules, sensors, and physical outputs. It's critical to understand the differences between specialized systems, which are selected to do a certain mission and embedded systems [31]. The larger systems like database servers and web servers for libraries are examples of dedicated systems; these are run on different computers and have distinct functions [32]. Embedded systems are programmable devices that combine development hardware and software. They are often small and have modest computing power [33]. The real-time processing capabilities and high speed of embedded systems make them the preferred choice for medical applications [34]. A microprocessor, memory for data and programs, microcontrollers or DSPs, sensors, actuators, and a variety of interfaces are all part of an embedded system, which combines hardware and software to effectively carry out particular tasks [35].

1.3 EMBEDDED SYSTEMS IN HEALTHCARE: DIVERSE APPLICATIONS

Modern medical device development now requires embedded systems as essential components. These systems are essential for improving the functionality, precision, and dependability of medical equipment used in healthcare settings [36]. They are made up of hardware and software that are specifically built to execute certain tasks within a larger system. System Embedded There are some unique elements that set programming apart from other programming systems [37]. Minimal program memory must be used by embedded software, and it must run at the system's needed speed without stuttering. It should also have a high level of readability and be simple to use [38]. Imaging devices are one of the fields in which embedded systems are used in medicine the most frequently. Imaging devices such as MRIs, CT scanners, Positron Emission Tomography scanners, and ultrasound machines are all instances of embedded systems, despite the differences in their working principles [39].

Embedded systems have a vital role in defibrillators in medicine and the devices called defibrillators are used to check a patient's heartbeat for irregularities and, if found to restart the beating at a normal rhythm [40, 41]. The personnel that react to emergency situations and the vehicles it uses, such as ambulances and helicopters, are what give emergency medical system (EMS) its most noticeable appearance [42]. However, it goes beyond merely getting you to the emergency room (ED). This system calls for the cooperation of several people and organizations in order to provide emergency medical treatment and coordinate responses [43]. Every day, an extensive

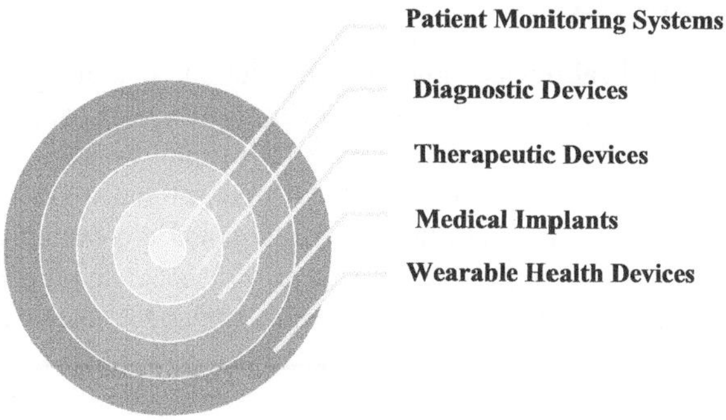

FIGURE 1.3 Diverse applications of embedded systems in healthcare.

EMS is ready to handle any kind of crisis, regardless of whether a hospital transfer is required. EMS is not isolated, even though it has a strong ecology of its own [44]. It works along with other programs and initiatives to enhance community safety and health. EMS functions at the nexus of public safety, emergency management, public health, and healthcare [45].

Figure 1.3 summarizes the various applications of embedded systems in healthcare.

1.3.1 Patient Monitoring Systems

Real-time monitoring and control of medical equipment are sometimes required to adapt to changing patient circumstances [46]. These devices' quick data collection and processing speeds are made possible by embedded systems, which allow for immediate corrections and interventions [47]. For example, embedded systems provide continuous vital sign collection in patient monitoring systems and immediately send alarms for aberrant readings, enabling healthcare practitioners to take immediate action [48]. Patient monitoring devices cannot function without embedded systems, which offer real-time data on vital indicators including blood pressure, oxygen saturation, and heart rate [49]. By facilitating immediate medical action and real-time monitoring, these tools improve patient care [50].

The medical uses for embedded systems include fetal heart monitoring machines used during pregnancy and childbirth, blood pressure monitors, glucose testing devices for systolic and diastolic pressure detection, digital flow sensors for monitoring a patient's respiratory system, and devices that let users monitor vital signs like heart rate, blood pressure, and glucose levels [51, 52]. All of these gadgets do indeed have computers; moreover, they are embedded computers [53]. Patient data may be gathered and processed by small embedded devices with the help of appropriate software [54]. These gadgets can now make control decisions that help patients receive better treatments and drugs because of the developments in size reduction and computing capacity [55]. Microcontrollers, sensors, and motor drivers are increasingly being used in compact designs. Particularly in emergency scenarios, these designs provide affordable and useful solutions [56].

1.3.2 Diagnostic Devices

Manufacturers of medical devices may design solutions that are streamlined, portable, and easy to use because of embedded systems' compact size [57]. This is especially helpful for point-of-care diagnostic instruments and wearable medical devices, where power and space constraints necessitate small, effective system designs [58]. MRI machines, CT scanners, and ultrasound equipment are examples of diagnostic equipment powered by embedded systems that provide accurate imaging and analysis. By ensuring correct diagnosis, these systems enhance patient outcomes [59].

1.3.3 Therapeutic Devices

In the increasingly linked world of healthcare, embedded systems play a critical role in enabling the integration of medical equipment with other systems, such as hospital networks and electronic health records (EHRs) [60, 61]. In the end, this connectivity improves patient care and operational efficiency in healthcare settings by enabling seamless data management, remote monitoring, and telehealth applications [62]. The embedded systems are necessary for the accurate and dependable delivery of medicine in devices like insulin pumps, pacemakers, and infusion pumps, and these technologies help patients live better lives and increase the effectiveness of treatments [63].

1.3.4 Medical Implants

Customized hardware and software are included in medical device technologies, such as embedded medical systems, to fulfill specific functional requirements [64]. Throughout the day, patients' health may be often monitored and managed, thanks to these technologies [65]. For example, sensors collect information about a patient's health, including heart rate, and send this information wirelessly to doctors for review [66]. Medical implants rely heavily on embedded technologies to provide vital functions like pacemaker heart rate management. High lifespan and dependability are needed for these implants [67].

1.3.5 Wearable Health Devices

Wireless sensors are one way to decrease wires and simplify hardware and by adding sensors like humidity and fertility check sensors, this system may be used in industrial and agricultural contexts in addition to medical ones [68, 69]. This modification increases the system's usefulness in a number of industries while enhancing its efficacy and efficiency [70]. Society depends on healthcare services, and automating these services eases the workload for humans and expedites the measurement process. Also, by increasing the system's openness, this automation promotes patient trust [71]. The healthcare system may use a lot of modifications to become more flexible, including adding more sophisticated sensors [72]. Scientists and medical researchers can access biometric data that has been kept online to evaluate its worth, spot trends, and carry out more studies [73]. Via using embedded technologies to monitor health parameters, wearables such as smartwatches and fitness trackers promote proactive health management. The usage of these gadgets for ongoing health monitoring and early illness diagnosis is growing [74].

Thus, embedded systems are essential to many medical applications, ranging from critical care equipment to imaging devices, providing effective solutions that enhance patient safety and care [75]. Applications like as camera-based social distancing monitoring systems, for instance, have brought attention to how crucial it is to maintain social distance in order to stop the spread of infectious illnesses [76]. These tools have aided in monitoring and guaranteeing compliance with social distancing standards in high-density regions as global immunization efforts advance [77].

1.4 OPERATIONAL ENVIRONMENTS IN HEALTHCARE SETTINGS: EMBEDDED SYSTEM

The development of medical equipment has made embedded systems an essential technological achievement [78, 79]. Designing and developing these devices, however, presents substantial problems due to regulatory regulations [80]. This challenge frequently results in the failure of several start-ups looking to break into the medical device industry [81]. This presents an approach for designing and developing embedded medical devices that minimizes financial investment during the technical risk stages and encourages user feedback in order to address this problem [82]. Three steps make up the suggested methodology as Medical Product Consolidation, Incremental and Iterative Prototyping, and Development Feasibility [83]. Various operational environments in healthcare settings are summarized in Figure 1.4.

Every phase is carried out adhering to relevant rules to guarantee both efficacy and safety [84, 85]. Specifically built hardware systems with an operating system and CPU that are intended to carry out a single task independently are known as embedded systems [86]. These systems use microprocessors or microcontrollers to enable the functioning of mechanical and electrical components for specific purposes. They do this by combining software and hardware. Embedded systems do not communicate with users directly [87]. With few resources, they work in real time and reactively, concentrating on a single goal. Critical tasks in their respective applications

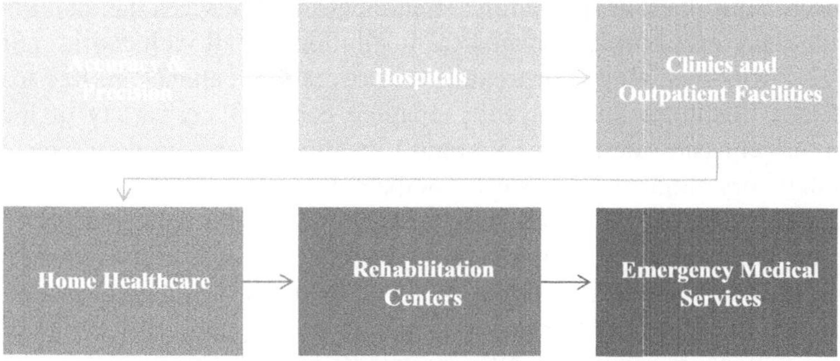

FIGURE 1.4 Operational environments in healthcare settings.

can be accomplished by them [88]. Errors in embedded systems have the ability to cause serious losses in terms of both lives and property [89]. For this reason, it is essential to make sure these systems are "reliable" and "error-tolerant" [90].

Modern medical equipment requires embedded systems in order to function properly and efficiently across a wide range of functions [91]. Embedded systems are essential to medical device operation, whether they are used for therapeutic intervention delivery, vital sign monitoring, or enabling communication between healthcare providers and equipment [92]. These systems are well-suited for incorporation into a variety of medical applications because of their small size, low power consumption, and real-time data processing capabilities [93].

1.4.1 Accuracy and Precision

Embedded systems are ideal for medical devices that require dependable and constant performance since they are designed to accomplish specific jobs with great precision and accuracy [94]. For instance, embedded systems guarantee the accurate delivery of medication or therapy in accordance with specified settings in devices like insulin pumps, pacemakers, and infusion pumps, enhancing patient safety and treatment efficacy [95].

1.4.2 Hospitals

Embedded systems are utilized in several hospital departments, such as the emergency room, intensive care unit (ICU), and operating room [96]. These systems facilitate vital life-saving treatments and provide ongoing monitoring [97]. Medical applications depend heavily on embedded systems, which frequently need industrial-grade standards because of the demanding operating environments seen in healthcare facilities [98–90]. These circumstances include fluctuating temperatures, being subjected to shock, vibration, and additional environmental strains. Industrial-grade embedded systems are made to be fully functioning even in the face of these difficulties [91].

1.4.3 Clinics and Outpatient Facilities

Healthcare consultations, procedures, treatments, and services that don't need an overnight stay at a hospital or medical institution are all included in outpatient care [92]. After receiving their treatment or operation, patients are free to depart the medical institution, unlike with inpatient care [93]. A variety of locations such as urgent care facilities, community health centers, primary care offices, and ambulatory surgical centers offer outpatient treatment [94]. When compared to inpatient services, outpatient care offers considerable cost reductions [95]. Overnight inpatient stays usually incur higher costs because of the increased need for hospital staff, medical supplies, beds, and food [96]. Outpatient care lowers the risk of infections linked to healthcare or hospital-acquired illnesses by enabling patients to recuperate after treatments and operations in the comfort of their own homes [97].

1.4.4 Home Healthcare

A hospital may be made into a robust computer system with plenty of processing power, lots of storage, and a wired or wireless local area network by installing a Hospital Information System (HIS) [98]. On the other hand, contemporary medical equipment such as an echograph operates like a computer system, with several internal components connected by an internal bus network [99]. Consequently, the hospital's local area network must be used in place of the internal bus when integrating such medical devices into the HIS [100].

1.4.5 Rehabilitation Centers

It has created two embedded systems: a networked digital camera and a pervasive echograph system. The suggested method integrates current clinical systems into the HIS significantly which increases productivity in the clinical arena as seen by the unambiguous evaluations of these systems [101, 102]. A disruptive breakthrough in healthcare might be sparked by the coupling of several embedded systems with application software customized for clinical operations, when clinical systems become modular pieces for integration into a comprehensive computer system such as the HIS [103].

1.4.6 Emergency Medical Services

EMS, or emergency medical services, is a system that reacts to situations needing highly qualified pre-hospital physicians [104]. But EMS doctors aren't simply the first medical personnel on the scene they are also frequently the first to identify a medical emergency in a community. They are becoming more and more important in community healthcare and emergency management [105].

1.5 CHALLENGES AND CONSIDERATIONS

In order to address the market need for IoT applications, it has created a variety of integrated IoT solutions and services that are speeding up the IoT ecosystem and value chain [106, 107]. Advantech provides a range of medical systems and boards that are made using cutting-edge technology to fulfill certain medical device and computing requirements [108]. Advantech is able to produce goods for a wide range of sectors since we have the most extensive ISO certifications in the IPC sector [109]. Figure 1.5 shows the various challenges associated with embedded systems for healthcare applications.

1.5.1 Security and Privacy

Embedded systems security is an all-encompassing strategy that involves design methodology, implementation, and a continuous commitment on the part of businesses to reduce the threat exposure of the devices they produce and the data they produce [110]. Embedded security is a lifecycle effort that starts far before the first

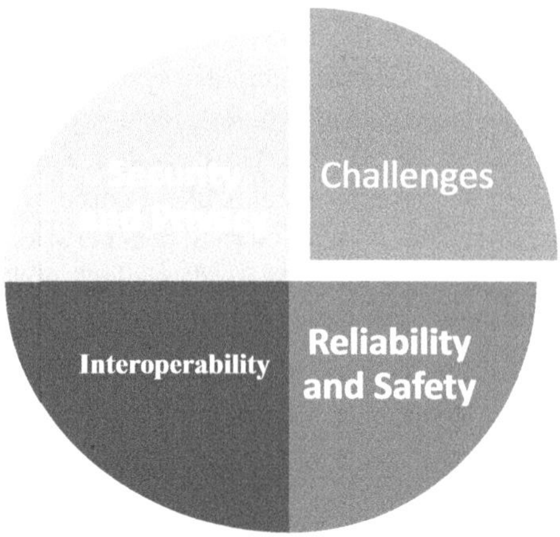

FIGURE 1.5 Challenges of embedded systems associated with healthcare applications.

line of code is generated, including defenses against device compromise, and continues all the way through to the device's decommissioning [111].

1.5.2 Reliability and Safety

With the speed at which technology is developing nowadays, embedded systems are becoming essential to modern life [112]. They span from the delicate intelligence of smart home appliances to the vital functions of the automobile and healthcare sectors [113]. Embedded systems are the hidden builders of our technology infrastructure, making sure complex systems run smoothly and without errors [114]. In the creation of embedded systems, quality assurance (QA) is crucial since accuracy and dependability are not only desirable but also necessary. It explores the role that QA plays in embedded systems and how it influences their reliable operation [115].

1.5.3 Interoperability

Specialized computing systems called embedded systems are made to carry out certain operations or duties inside bigger systems [116, 117]. Embedded systems, as opposed to general-purpose computers, are essential parts of many different sectors because of their close integration with the equipment they support [118]. They provide effective functioning without drawing much attention to them by powering industrial machinery, medical equipment, smart home gadgets, automobile systems, and more [119].

1.6 FUTURE TRENDS: ENHANCING HEALTHCARE AND EMBEDDED SYSTEM

1.6.1 Artificial Intelligence and Machine Learning

The "quadruple objective" of healthcare, which entails improving population health, improving the patient experience, improving the caregiver experience, and lowering the ever-increasing cost of treatment, presents formidable difficulties to healthcare systems throughout the globe [120]. Governments, payers, regulators, and providers are under pressure to rethink and reinvent healthcare delivery models due to aging populations, an increase in the prevalence of chronic illnesses, and rising global healthcare costs [121, 122]. Healthcare systems are also under pressure to efficiently provide high-quality treatment and improve care delivery on a massive scale by incorporating real-world data insights directly into patient care, all against the background of the global epidemic [123].

1.6.2 Internet of Medical Things (IoMT)

The proliferation of embedded systems, IoT devices, and the intelligent edge in deployments and novel use cases raises the possibility of security breaches and expands the attack surface [124]. Every connected device, regardless of its size from a simple IoT home thermostat to a sophisticated system of systems represents one or more possible ports of entry that hackers may use [125]. As there are now billions of linked devices and tens of billions more predicted, it is imperative to secure devices and safeguard the data they produce [126]. There is a great deal of expectation in the embedded market that businesses would follow and apply the most recent security and functionality standards [127]. The adopting of thorough security architecture for embedded systems used in mission-critical and safety-critical applications is crucial for the device's whole lifespan [128]. No device can be genuinely safe and keep its security throughout its operating lifespan without a security-first strategy [129].

1.6.3 Advanced Sensor Technologies

Sensor technology has advanced significantly in recent years, presenting hitherto unseen prospects in a number of important domains such as (1) early human disease diagnosis and prevention by identifying critical biomarkers; (2) health assessments by monitoring and analyzing physiological signals in healthcare and biomedical applications; and (3) effective assessment of human health-relevant environmental factors by monitoring and measuring environmental determinants [130, 131].

Figure 1.6 displays the future trends in enhancing healthcare with the utilization of embedded system.

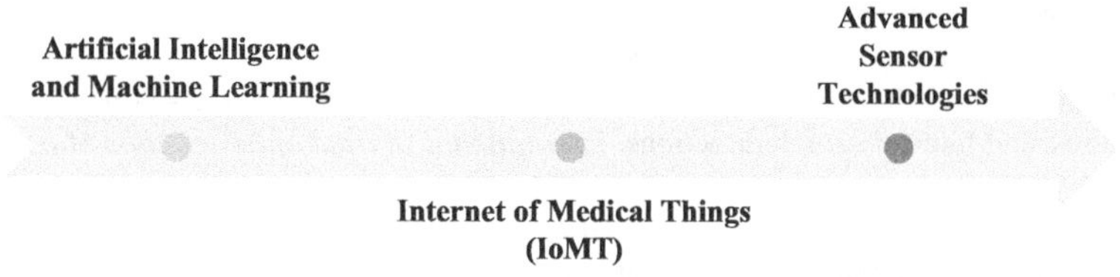

FIGURE 1.6 Future trends in enhancing healthcare with the utilization of embedded system.

1.7 CONCLUSION

The current healthcare environment would not be the same without embedded technologies, which improve patient care, operational effectiveness, and diagnostic precision. The performance and capacities of medical devices are greatly influenced by embedded systems which improve patient care, clinical effectiveness, and healthcare outcomes. Modern healthcare is expected to evolve as technology develops and embedded systems are integrated with cutting-edge technologies to enhance medical equipment' intelligence, accuracy, and connection. Although obstacles like security, dependability, and compatibility, these technologies' continued development holds great potential for improving healthcare delivery. Advanced sensors, IoT, and artificial intelligence (AI) will further transform the healthcare industry and open up new avenues for patient care and medical research.

REFERENCES

1. Singh, B., & Kaunert, C. (2024). Integration of cutting-edge technologies such as internet of things (IoT) and 5G in health monitoring systems: A comprehensive legal analysis and futuristic outcomes. *GLS Law Journal*, *6*(1), 13–20.
2. Deniz-Garcia, A., Fabelo, H., Rodriguez-Almeida, A. J., Zamora-Zamorano, G., Castro-Fernandez, M., Alberiche Ruano, M. D. P., ... & WARIFA Consortium. (2023). Quality, usability, and effectiveness of mHealth apps and the role of artificial intelligence: Current scenario and challenges. *Journal of Medical Internet Research*, *25*, e44030.
3. Singh, B. (2024). Social cognition of incarcerated women and children: Addressing exposure to infectious diseases and legal outcomes. In K. Reddy (Ed.), *Principles and Clinical Interventions in Social Cognition* (pp. 236–251). IGI Global. https://doi.org/10.4018/979-8-3693-1265-0.ch014
4. Singh, B., & Kaunert, C. (2024). Harnessing sustainable agriculture through climate-smart technologies: Artificial intelligence for climate preservation and futuristic trends. In Hemachandran Kannan, Raul Villamarin Rodriguez, Zita Zoltay Paprika, Abejide Ade-Ibijola *Exploring Ethical Dimensions of Environmental Sustainability and Use of AI* (pp. 214–239). IGI Global.
5. Istepanian, R. S., & AlAnzi, T. (2020). Mobile health (m-health): evidence-based progress or scientific retrogression. In Enrique J Gómez Aguilera, Jennifer Whetham *Biomedical information technology* (pp. 717–733). Academic Press.
6. Sharma, S. K., Al-Wanain, M. I., Alowaidi, M., & Alsaghier, H. (2022). Mobile healthcare (m-Health) based on artificial intelligence in healthcare 4.0. *Expert Systems*, 1, e13025.
7. Umapathy, V. R., Raj, R. D. S., Yadav, S., Munavarah, S. A., Anandapandian, P. A., Mary, A. V., ... & Mary, V. (2023). Perspective of artificial intelligence in disease diagnosis: A review of current and future endeavours in the medical field. *Cureus*, *15*(9), 56–59.
8. Singh, B. (2023). Tele-health monitoring lensing deep neural learning structure: Ambient patient wellness via wearable devices for real-time alerts and interventions. *Indian Journal of Health and Medical Law*, *6*(2), 12–16.
9. Sharma, R., & Kshetri, N. (2020). Digital healthcare: Historical development, applications, and future research directions. *International Journal of Information Management*, *53*, 102105.
10. Mohanta, B., Das, P., & Patnaik, S. (2019, May). Healthcare 5.0: A paradigm shift in digital healthcare system using artificial intelligence, IOT and 5G communication. In *2019 International Conference on Applied Machine Learning (ICAML)* (pp. 191–196). IEEE.

11. Aggarwal, N., Ahmed, M., Basu, S., Curtin, J. J., Evans, B. J., Matheny, M. E., … & Thadaney-Israni, S. (2020). Advancing artificial intelligence in health settings outside the hospital and clinic. *NAM Perspectives*, *2020*, 12–14.
12. Mbunge, E., Muchemwa, B., & Batani, J. (2021). Sensors and healthcare 5.0: Transformative shift in virtual care through emerging digital health technologies. *Global Health Journal*, *5*(4), 169–177.
13. Singh, B. (2024). Legal dynamics lensing metaverse crafted for videogame industry and e-sports: Phenomenological exploration catalyst complexity and future. *Journal of Intellectual Property Rights Law*, *7*(1), 8–14.
14. Dabla, P. K., Gruson, D., Gouget, B., Bernardini, S., & Homsak, E. (2021). Lessons learned from the COVID-19 pandemic: Emphasizing the emerging role and perspectives from artificial intelligence, mobile health, and digital laboratory medicine. *Ejifcc*, *32*(2), 224.
15. Galetsi, P., Katsaliaki, K., & Kumar, S. (2023). Exploring benefits and ethical challenges in the rise of mHealth (mobile healthcare) technology for the common good: An analysis of mobile applications for health specialists. *Technovation*, *121*, 102598.
16. Saif-Ur-Rahman, K. M., Islam, M. S., Alaboson, J., Ola, O., Hasan, I., Islam, N., … & Joarder, T. (2023). Artificial intelligence and digital health in improving primary health care service delivery in LMICs: A systematic review. *Journal of Evidence-Based Medicine*, *16*(3), 303–320.
17. Singh, B. (2023). Blockchain technology in renovating healthcare: Legal and future perspectives. In Keshav Kaushik, Susheela Dahiya, Ashutosh Dhar Dwivedi, Shilpi Aggarwal *Revolutionizing Healthcare Through Artificial Intelligence and Internet of Things Applications* (pp. 177–186). IGI Global.
18. Istepanian, R. S. (2022). Mobile health (m-Health) in retrospect: The known unknowns. *International Journal of Environmental Research and Public Health*, *19*(7), 3747.
19. Sulaiman, M., Håkansson, A., & Karlsen, R. (2021, November). AI-enabled proactive mHealth: A review. In *International Conference on ICT for Health, Accessibility and Wellbeing* (pp. 94–108). Springer International Publishing.
20. Singh, B. (2023). Federated learning for envision future trajectory smart transport system for climate preservation and smart green planet: Insights into global governance and SDG-9 (industry, innovation and infrastructure). *National Journal of Environmental Law*, *6*(2), 6–17.
21. Seetharam, K., Kagiyama, N., & Sengupta, P. P. (2019). Application of mobile health, telemedicine and artificial intelligence to echocardiography. *Echo Research & Practice*, *6*(2), R41–R52.
22. Manteghinejad, A., & Javanmard, S. H. (2021). Challenges and opportunities of digital health in a post-COVID19 world. *Journal of Research in Medical Sciences: The Official Journal of Isfahan University of Medical Sciences*, *26*, 77.
23. Singh, B. (2023). Unleashing alternative dispute resolution (ADR) in resolving complex legal-technical issues arising in cyberspace lensing e-commerce and intellectual property: Proliferation of e-commerce digital economy. *Revista Brasileira de Alternative Dispute Resolution-Brazilian Journal of Alternative Dispute Resolution-RBADR*, *5*(10), 81–105.
24. Senbekov, M., Saliev, T., Bukeyeva, Z., Almabayeva, A., Zhanaliyeva, M., Aitenova, N., … & Fakhradiyev, I. (2020). The recent progress and applications of digital technologies in healthcare: A review. *International Journal of Telemedicine and Applications*, *2020*, 34–48.
25. Karboub, K., Tabaa, M., Dandache, A., Dellagi, S., & Moutaouakkil, F. (2019). Toward health 4.0: Challenges and opportunities. In *International Conference on Innovation and New Trends in Information Technology* (pp. 20–21).

26. Sharma, A., & Singh, B. (2022). Measuring impact of E-commerce on small scale business: A systematic review. *Journal of Corporate Governance and International Business Law*, *5*(1), 45.
27. Gunasekeran, D. V., Tseng, R. M. W. W., Tham, Y. C., & Wong, T. Y. (2021). Applications of digital health for public health responses to COVID-19: A systematic scoping review of artificial intelligence, telehealth and related technologies. *NPJ Digital Medicine*, *4*(1), 40.
28. Kakhi, K., Alizadehsani, R., Kabir, H. D., Khosravi, A., Nahavandi, S., & Acharya, U. R. (2022). The internet of medical things and artificial intelligence: Trends, challenges, and opportunities. *Biocybernetics and Biomedical Engineering*, *42*(3), 749–771.
29. Naik, N., Hameed, B. M., Sooriyaperakasam, N., Vinayahalingam, S., Patil, V., Smriti, K., … & Somani, B. K. (2022). Transforming healthcare through a digital revolution: A review of digital healthcare technologies and solutions. *Frontiers in Digital Health*, *4*, 919985.
30. Nasr, M., Islam, M. M., Shehata, S., Karray, F., & Quintana, Y. (2021). Smart healthcare in the age of AI: Recent advances, challenges, and future prospects. *IEEE Access*, *9*, 145248–145270.
31. Singh, B. (2022). Relevance of agriculture-nutrition linkage for human healthcare: A conceptual legal framework of implication and pathways. *Justice and Law Bulletin*, *1*(1), 44–49.
32. Condry, M. W., & Quan, X. I. (2021). Digital health innovation, informatics opportunity, and challenges. *IEEE Engineering Management Review*, *49*(2), 81–88.
33. Berrouiguet, S., Barrigón, M. L., Castroman, J. L., Courtet, P., Artés-Rodríguez, A., & Baca-García, E. (2019). Combining mobile-health (mHealth) and artificial intelligence (AI) methods to avoid suicide attempts: The Smartcrises study protocol. *BMC Psychiatry*, *19*(1), 1–9.
34. Jabarulla, M. Y., & Lee, H. N. (2021, August). A blockchain and artificial intelligence-based, patient-centric healthcare system for combating the COVID-19 pandemic: Opportunities and applications. In Mohamed Yaseen Jabarulla *Healthcare* (Vol. 9, No. 8, p. 1019). MDPI.
35. Cingolani, M., Scendoni, R., Fedeli, P., & Cembrani, F. (2023). Artificial intelligence and digital medicine for integrated home care services in Italy: Opportunities and limits. *Frontiers in Public Health*, *10*, 1095001.
36. Singh, B. (2022). COVID-19 pandemic and public healthcare: Endless downward spiral or solution via rapid legal and health services implementation with patient monitoring program. *Justice and Law Bulletin*, *1*(1), 1–7.
37. Amjad, A., Kordel, P., & Fernandes, G. (2023). A review on innovation in healthcare sector (telehealth) through artificial intelligence. *Sustainability*, *15*(8), 6655.
38. Sousa, M. J., Nunes, F. G., do Nascimento, G., & Chakraborty, C. (Eds.). (2023). *Future Health Scenarios: AI and Digital Technologies in Global Healthcare Systems*. CRC Press.
39. Chakraborty, C. (Ed.). (2022). *Digital Health Transformation with Blockchain and Artificial Intelligence*. CRC Press.
40. Denecke, K., Gabarron, E., Grainger, R., Konstantinidis, S. T., Lau, A., Rivera-Romero, O., … & Merolli, M. (2019). Artificial intelligence for participatory health: Applications, impact, and future implications: Contribution of the IMIA Participatory Health and Social Media Working Group. *Yearbook of Medical Informatics*, *28*(1), 165.
41. Bhaskar, S., Bradley, S., Sakhamuri, S., Moguilner, S., Chattu, V. K., Pandya, S., … & Banach, M. (2020). Designing futuristic telemedicine using artificial intelligence and robotics in the COVID-19 era. *Frontiers in Public Health*, 1, 708.
42. Solomon, D. H., & Rudin, R. S. (2020). Digital health technologies: Opportunities and challenges in rheumatology. *Nature Reviews Rheumatology*, *16*(9), 525–535.

43. Yang, Y. C., Islam, S. U., Noor, A., Khan, S., Afsar, W., & Nazir, S. (2021). Influential usage of big data and artificial intelligence in healthcare. *Computational and Mathematical Methods in Medicine*, *2021*, 1–13.
44. Bergoeing, M., Neyem, A., Jofré, P., Hernández, C., Chacón, J., Morales, R., & Giddings, M. (2023, November). Exploring the potential of an AI-integrated cloud-based mHealth platform for enhanced type 2 diabetes mellitus management. In *International Conference on Ubiquitous Computing and Ambient Intelligence* (pp. 100–111). Springer Nature Switzerland.
45. El-Rashidy, N., El-Sappagh, S., Islam, S. R., El-Bakry, H., & Abdelrazek, S. (2021). Mobile health in remote patient monitoring for chronic diseases: Principles, trends, and challenges. *Diagnostics*, *11*(4), 607.
46. Singh, B. (2019). Profiling public healthcare: A comparative analysis based on the multidimensional healthcare management and legal approach. *Indian Journal of Health and Medical Law*, 2(2), 1–5.
47. Dinh-Le, C., Chuang, R., Chokshi, S., & Mann, D. (2019). Wearable health technology and electronic health record integration: Scoping review and future directions. *JMIR mHealth and uHealth*, *7*(9), e12861.
48. Asan, O., Choi, E., & Wang, X. (2023). Artificial Intelligence–Based Consumer Health Informatics Application: Scoping Review. *Journal of Medical Internet Research*, *25*, e47260.
49. Kadu, A., & Singh, M. (2021, October). Comparative analysis of e-health care telemedicine system based on Internet of Medical Things and artificial intelligence. In *2021 2nd International Conference on Smart Electronics and Communication (ICOSEC)* (pp. 1768–1775). IEEE.
50. Hamberger, M., Ikonomi, N., Schwab, J. D., Werle, S. D., Fürstberger, A., Kestler, A. M., ... & Kestler, H. A. (2022). Interaction empowerment in mobile health: Concepts, challenges, and perspectives. *JMIR mHealth and uHealth*, *10*(4), e32696.
51. Baker, S., & Xiang, W. (2023). Artificial intelligence of things for smarter healthcare: A survey of advancements, challenges, and opportunities. *IEEE Communications Surveys & Tutorials*, 1, 23–25.
52. Abernethy, A., Adams, L., Barrett, M., Bechtel, C., Brennan, P., Butte, A., ... & Valdes, K. (2022). The promise of digital health: Then, now, and the future. *NAM Perspectives*, *2022*, 1–24.
53. Awotunde, J. B., Folorunso, S. O., Ajagbe, S. A., Garg, J., & Ajamu, G. J. (2022). AiIoMT: IoMT-based system-enabled artificial intelligence for enhanced smart healthcare systems. *Machine Learning for Critical Internet of Medical Things: Applications and Use Cases*, 2, 229–254.
54. Uddin, M., & Syed-Abdul, S. (2021). Introduction to digital health approach and mHealth applications for participatory health. In Mohy Uddin *Digital Health* (pp. 1–6). Elsevier.
55. Shin, S. Y. (2019). Current status and future direction of digital health in Korea. *The Korean Journal of Physiology & Pharmacology*, *23*(5), 311–315.
56. Hunt, X., Tomlinson, M., Sikander, S., Skeen, S., Marlow, M., du Toit, S., & Eisner, M. (2020). Artificial intelligence, big data, and mHealth: The frontiers of the prevention of violence against children. *Frontiers in Artificial Intelligence*, *3*, 543305.
57. Perez-Pozuelo, I., Spathis, D., Clifton, E. A., & Mascolo, C. (2021). Wearables, smartphones, and artificial intelligence for digital phenotyping and health. In *Digital Health* (pp. 33–54). Elsevier.
58. Mathur, V., Purkayastha, S., & Gichoya, J. W. (2020). Artificial intelligence for global health: Learning from a decade of digital transformation in health care. *arXiv preprint arXiv:2005.12378.*

59. Chattu, V. K. (2021). A review of artificial intelligence, big data, and blockchain technology applications in medicine and global health. *Big Data and Cognitive Computing*, *5*(3), 41.
60. Bhatt, V., & Chakraborty, S. (2021, March). Real-time healthcare monitoring using smart systems: A step towards healthcare service orchestration Smart systems for futuristic healthcare. In *2021 International Conference on Artificial Intelligence and Smart Systems (ICAIS)* (pp. 772–777). IEEE.
61. Vayena, E., & Ferretti, A. (2021). Big data and artificial intelligence for global health. *Global Health: Ethical Challenges* (p. 429). WHO.
62. Li, J. P. O., Liu, H., Ting, D. S., Jeon, S., Chan, R. P., Kim, J. E., … & Ting, D. S. (2021). Digital technology, tele-medicine and artificial intelligence in ophthalmology: A global perspective. *Progress in Retinal and Eye Research*, *82*, 100900.
63. Ramesh, A., Subbaraya, C. K., & Kumar, G. R. (2023). AI based dynamic prediction model for mobile health application system. *International Journal of Advanced Computer Science and Applications*, *14*(1), 356–365.
64. Ellahham, S. (2020). Artificial intelligence: The future for diabetes care. *The American Journal of Medicine*, *133*(8), 895–900.
65. Babel, A., Taneja, R., Mondello Malvestiti, F., Monaco, A., & Donde, S. (2021). Artificial intelligence solutions to increase medication adherence in patients with non-communicable diseases. *Frontiers in Digital Health*, *3*, 669869.
66. Ramkumar, P. N., Haeberle, H. S., Bloomfield, M. R., Schaffer, J. L., Kamath, A. F., Patterson, B. M., & Krebs, V. E. (2019). Artificial intelligence and arthroplasty at a single institution: Real-world applications of machine learning to big data, value-based care, mobile health, and remote patient monitoring. *The Journal of Arthroplasty*, *34*(10), 2204–2209.
67. Brault, N., & Saxena, M. (2021). For a critical appraisal of artificial intelligence in healthcare: The problem of bias in mHealth. *Journal of Evaluation in Clinical Practice*, *27*(3), 513–519.
68. Srivastava, M., Siddiqui, A. T., & Srivastava, V. (2024). Application of artificial intelligence of medical things in remote healthcare delivery. In Priya Jeyaraj *Handbook of Security and Privacy of AI-Enabled Healthcare Systems and Internet of Medical Things* (pp. 169–190). CRC Press.
69. Wang, Q., Su, M., Zhang, M., & Li, R. (2021). Integrating digital technologies and public health to fight Covid-19 pandemic: Key technologies, applications, challenges and outlook of digital healthcare. *International Journal of Environmental Research and Public Health*, *18*(11), 6053.
70. Dahiya, S., Goyal, Y., & Sharma, C. (2022). Designing delivery of healthcare services with health management information system, artificial intelligence, big data, and innovative digital technologies. *Journal of Young Pharmacists*, *14*(4), 366–371.
71. Iqbal, J., Jaimes, D. C. C., Makineni, P., Subramani, S., Hemaida, S., Thugu, T. R., … & Hemida, S. (2023). Reimagining healthcare: Unleashing the power of artificial intelligence in medicine. *Cureus*, *15*(9), 1–14.
72. Daley, B. J., Ni'Man, M., Neves, M. R., Bobby Huda, M. S., Marsh, W., Fenton, N. E., … & McLachlan, S. (2022). mHealth apps for gestational diabetes mellitus that provide clinical decision support or artificial intelligence: A scoping review. *Diabetic Medicine*, *39*(1), e14735.
73. Manyazewal, T., Woldeamanuel, Y., Blumberg, H. M., Fekadu, A., & Marconi, V. C. (2021). The potential use of digital health technologies in the African context: A systematic review of evidence from Ethiopia. *NPJ Digital Medicine*, *4*(1), 125.
74. Kernebeck, S., Busse, T. S., Böttcher, M. D., Weitz, J., Ehlers, J., & Bork, U. (2020). Impact of mobile health and medical applications on clinical practice in gastroenterology. *World Journal of Gastroenterology*, *26*(29), 4182.

75. Burrell, D. N. (2023). Dynamic evaluation approaches to telehealth technologies and artificial intelligence (AI) telemedicine applications in healthcare and biotechnology organizations. *Merits*, *3*(4), 700–721.
76. Xie, Y., Lu, L., Gao, F., He, S. J., Zhao, H. J., Fang, Y., ... & Dong, Z. (2021). Integration of artificial intelligence, blockchain, and wearable technology for chronic disease management: A new paradigm in smart healthcare. *Current Medical Science*, *41*, 1123–1133.
77. Hackl, W. O., Neururer, S. B., Pfeifer, B., & Section Editors for the IMIA Yearbook Section on Clinical Information Systems. (2023). Transforming clinical information systems: Empowering healthcare through telemedicine, data science, and artificial intelligence applications. *Yearbook of Medical Informatics*, *32*(01), 127–137.
78. Kodama, K., Kurata, K., & Cao, J. (2022). Introduction of the concept of AI in the field of mHealth while discovering the trends in the mHealth research field. In Kota Kodama *Mobile Health (mHealth) Rethinking Innovation Management to Harmonize AI and Social Design* (pp. 3–29). Springer Nature Singapore.
79. McCool, J., Dobson, R., Whittaker, R., & Paton, C. (2022). Mobile health (mHealth) in low-and middle-income countries. *Annual Review of Public Health*, *43*, 525–539.
80. Qureshi, K. N., Din, S., Jeon, G., & Piccialli, F. (2020). An accurate and dynamic predictive model for a smart M-Health system using machine learning. *Information Sciences*, *538*, 486–502.
81. Jadi, A. (2020). Mobile health services in Saudi Arabia-challenges and opportunities. *International Journal of Advanced Computer Science and Applications*, *11*(4), 165–170.
82. Mbunge, E., & Batani, J. (2023). Application of deep learning and machine learning models to improve healthcare in sub-Saharan Africa: Emerging opportunities, trends and implications. *Telematics and Informatics Reports*, 2, 100097.
83. Pergolizzi Jr, J., LeQuang, J. A. K., Vasiliu-Feltes, I., Breve, F., & Varrassi, G. (2023). Brave new healthcare: A narrative review of digital healthcare in American medicine. *Cureus*, *15*(10), 1–14.
84. Tagde, P., Tagde, S., Bhattacharya, T., Tagde, P., Chopra, H., Akter, R., ... & Rahman, M. H. (2021). Blockchain and artificial intelligence technology in e-Health. *Environmental Science and Pollution Research*, *28*, 52810–52831.
85. Mishra, P., & Singh, G. (2023). Internet of medical things healthcare for sustainable smart cities: Current status and future prospects. *Applied Sciences*, *13*(15), 8869.
86. Blease, C., Locher, C., Leon-Carlyle, M., & Doraiswamy, M. (2020). Artificial intelligence and the future of psychiatry: Qualitative findings from a global physician survey. *Digital Health*, *6*, 1–9.
87. Monteiro, A. C. B., França, R. P., Arthur, R., & Iano, Y. (2021). An overview of medical Internet of Things, artificial intelligence, and cloud computing employed in health care from a modern panorama. In Siarry, P., Jabbar, M., Aluvalu, R., Abraham, A., Madureira, A. *The Fusion of Internet of Things, Artificial Intelligence, and Cloud Computing in Health Care* (pp. 3–23).
88. Shilpa, & Kaur, T. (2022). Digital healthcare: Current trends, challenges and future perspectives. In *Proceedings of the Future Technologies Conference (FTC) 2021, Volume 2* (pp. 645–661). Springer International Publishing.
89. Laksono, S., & Darmawan, E. S. (2021). The new leadership paradigm in digital health and its relations to hospital services. *Jurnal Ilmu Kesehatan Masyarakat*, *12*(2), 89–103.
90. Lano, K., Tehrani, S. Y., Umar, M., & Alwakeel, L. (2022). Using Artificial Intelligence for the specification of m-Health and e-Health systems. In Ehsani, S., Glauner, P., Plugmann, P., Thieringer, F.M. *The Future Circle of Healthcare: AI, 3D Printing, Longevity, Ethics, and Uncertainty Mitigation* (pp. 273–299). Springer International Publishing.

91. Kwon, H., An, S., Lee, H. Y., Cha, W. C., Kim, S., Cho, M., & Kong, H. J. (2022). Review of smart hospital services in real healthcare environments. *Healthcare Informatics Research*, *28*(1), 3–15.
92. Hinton, G., Obermeyer, Z., Emanuel, E., LeCun, Y., Bengio, Y., Hinton, G., ... & Bekhet, L. (2019). AI in health: State of the art, challenges, and future directions. *Yearbook of Medical Informatics*, *28*(1), 16–26.
93. Chew, H. S. J., & Achananuparp, P. (2022). Perceptions and needs of artificial intelligence in health care to increase adoption: Scoping review. *Journal of Medical Internet Research*, *24*(1), e32939.
94. Singh, B., & Kaunert, C. (2024). Future of digital marketing: Hyper-personalized customer dynamic experience with AI-based predictive models. In Alex Khang, Pushan Kumar Dutta, Sachin Gupta, Nishu Ayedee, Sandeep Chatterjee *Revolutionizing the AI-Digital Landscape: A Guide to Sustainable Emerging Technologies for Marketing Professionals* (p. 189).
95. Singh, B., Kaunert, C., & Vig, K. (2024). Reinventing influence of Artificial Intelligence (AI) on digital consumer lensing transforming consumer recommendation model: Exploring stimulus Artificial Intelligence on consumer shopping decisions. In T. Musiolik, R. Rodriguez, & H. Kannan (Eds.), *AI Impacts in Digital Consumer Behavior* (pp. 141–169). IGI Global. https://doi.org/10.4018/979-8-3693-1918-5.ch006
96. Dwivedi, R., Mehrotra, D., & Chandra, S. (2022). Potential of Internet of Medical Things (IoMT) applications in building a smart healthcare system: A systematic review. *Journal of Oral Biology and Craniofacial Research*, *12*(2), 302–318.
97. Vatandoost, M., & Litkouhi, S. (2019). The future of healthcare facilities: How technology and medical advances may shape hospitals of the future. *Hospital Practices and Research*, *4*(1), 1–11.
98. Bitkina, O. V., Park, J., & Kim, H. K. (2023). Application of artificial intelligence in medical technologies: A systematic review of main trends. *Digital Health*, *9*, 1–12.
99. Rodrigues, S. M., Kanduri, A., Nyamathi, A., Dutt, N., Khargonekar, P., & Rahmani, A. M. (2022). Digital health–enabled community-centered care: Scalable model to empower future community health workers using human-in-the-loop Artificial Intelligence. *JMIR Formative Research*, *6*(4), e29535.
100. Sulaiman, M., Håkansson, A., & Karlsen, R. (2022). *A framework for AI-enabled proactive mHealth with automated decision-making for a user's context.* 111–124.
101. Araiza-Garaygordobil, D., Jordán-Ríos, A., Sierra-Fernández, C., & Juárez-Orozco, L. E. (2020). On stethoscopes, patient records, artificial intelligence, and zettabytes: A glimpse into the future of digital medicine in Mexico. *Archivos de cardiología de México*, *90*(2), 177–182.
102. Kazi, A. M., Qazi, S. A., Ahsan, N., Khawaja, S., Sameen, F., Saqib, M., ... & Stergioulas, L. K. (2020). Current challenges of digital health interventions in Pakistan: Mixed methods analysis. *Journal of Medical Internet Research*, *22*(9), e21691.
103. Shajari, S., Kuruvinashetti, K., Komeili, A., & Sundararaj, U. (2023). The emergence of AI-based wearable sensors for digital health technology: A review. *Sensors*, *23*(23), 9498.
104. Gómez-González, E., & Gómez Gutiérrez, E. (2020). *Artificial Intelligence in medicine and healthcare: Applications, availability and societal impact.* Gomez Gutierrez, E., EUR 30197 EN, Publications Office of the European Union, Luxembourg. https://doi.org/10.2760/047666
105. Al Mamun, S., Kaiser, M. S., & Mahmud, M. (2021, September). An artificial intelligence based approach towards inclusive healthcare provisioning in society 5.0: A perspective on brain disorder. In Mahmud, M., Kaiser, M.S., Vassanelli, S., Dai, Q., Zhong, N. *International Conference on Brain Informatics* (pp. 157–169). Springer International Publishing.

106. Asan, O., & Choudhury, A. (2021). Research trends in artificial intelligence applications in human factors health care: Mapping review. *JMIR Human Factors*, *8*(2), e28236.
107. Limketkai, B. N., Mauldin, K., Manitius, N., Jalilian, L., & Salonen, B. R. (2021). The age of artificial intelligence: Use of digital technology in clinical nutrition. *Current Surgery Reports*, *9*(7), 20.
108. Liang, F., Yang, X., Peng, W., Zhen, S., Cao, W., Li, Q., ... & Gu, D. (2023). Applications of digital health approaches for cardiometabolic diseases prevention and management in the Western Pacific region. *The Lancet Regional Health–Western Pacific 43*, 100817.
109. Giovagnoli, M. R., & Giansanti, D. (2021, July). Artificial Intelligence in digital pathology: What is the future? Part 1: From the digital slide onwards. In Maria Rosaria *Healthcare* (Vol. 9, No. 7, p. 858). MDPI.
110. Garg, N. (2021). Technology in healthcare: Vision of smart hospitals. In Bhushan Patil, Manisha Vohra *Handbook of Research on Engineering, Business, and Healthcare Applications of Data Science and Analytics* (pp. 346–362). IGI Global.
111. Tian, S., Yang, W., Le Grange, J. M., Wang, P., Huang, W., & Ye, Z. (2019). Smart healthcare: Making medical care more intelligent. *Global Health Journal*, *3*(3), 62–65.
112. Akinola, S., & Telukdarie, A. (2023). Sustainable digital transformation in healthcare: Advancing a digital vascular health innovation solution. *Sustainability*, *15*(13), 10417.
113. Al-Shorbaji, N., & Al-Shorbaji, N. (2021). Improving healthcare access through digital health: The use of information and communication technologies. *Healthcare Access*, *10*, 1–25.
114. Alzahrani, A. S., Gay, V., Alturki, R., & AlGhamdi, M. J. (2021). Towards understanding the usability attributes of AI-enabled eHealth mobile applications. *Journal of Healthcare Engineering*, *2021*, 1–9.
115. El-Sherif, D. M., Abouzid, M., Elzarif, M. T., Ahmed, A. A., Albakri, A., & Alshehri, M. M. (2022, February). Telehealth and Artificial Intelligence insights into healthcare during the COVID-19 pandemic. In Bhushan Patil, Manisha Vohra *Healthcare* (Vol. 10, No. 2, p. 385). MDPI.
116. Niwa, M. (2022). mHealth as a component of next-generation health care. In Kota Kodama *Mobile Health (mHealth) Rethinking Innovation Management to Harmonize AI and Social Design* (pp. 189–209). Springer Nature Singapore.
117. Tadiboina, S. N. (2022). The integration of handheld and smartphone-connected technologies into the doctor-patient relationship-AI. *Journal of Positive School Psychology*, *6*(11), 2933–2940.
118. Liu, S., Huang, Y., & Shi, L. (2022). Autonomous mobile clinics: Empowering affordable anywhere, anytime healthcare access. *IEEE Engineering Management Review*, *50*(4), 147–154.
119. Maassen, O., Fritsch, S., Palm, J., Deffge, S., Kunze, J., Marx, G., ... & Bickenbach, J. (2021). Future medical artificial intelligence application requirements and expectations of physicians in German university hospitals: Web-based survey. *Journal of Medical Internet Research*, *23*(3), e26646.
120. Singh, B., & Kaunert, C. (2024). Salvaging responsible consumption and production of food in the hospitality industry: Harnessing machine learning and deep learning for zero food waste. In Amrik Singh, Pankaj Kumar Tyagi, Anshul Garg *Sustainable Disposal Methods of Food Wastes in Hospitality Operations* (pp. 176–192). IGI Global.
121. Singh, B. (2024). Evolutionary global neuroscience for cognition and brain health: Strengthening innovation in brain science. In Pranav Kumar Prabhakar *Biomedical Research Developments for Improved Healthcare* (pp. 246–272). IGI Global.
122. Singh, B., Kaunert, C., & Vig, K. (2024). Reinventing influence of Artificial Intelligence (AI) on digital consumer lensing transforming consumer recommendation model: Exploring Stimulus Artificial Intelligence on Consumer Shopping Decisions. In Thomas Heinrich Musiolik, Raul Villamarin Rodriguez, Hemachandran Kannan *AI Impacts in Digital Consumer Behavior* (pp. 141–169). IGI Global.

123. Singh, B., & Kaunert, C. (2024). Revealing green finance mobilization: Harnessing FinTech and blockchain innovations to surmount barriers and foster new investment avenues. In Syed Hasan Jafar, Raul Villamarin Rodriguez, Hemachandran Kannan, Shakeb Akhtar, Philipp Plugmann *Harnessing Blockchain-Digital Twin Fusion for Sustainable Investments* (pp. 265–286). IGI Global.
124. Al-Marridi, A., Mohamed, A., & Erbad, A. (2020). AI-based techniques on edge devices to optimize energy efficiency in m-health applications. In Abeer Ziad Al-Marridi *Energy Efficiency of Medical Devices and Healthcare Applications* (pp. 1–23). Academic Press.
125. Pap, I. A., & Oniga, S. (2022). A review of converging technologies in eHealth pertaining to Artificial Intelligence. *International Journal of Environmental Research and Public Health, 19*(18), 11413.
126. Patra, R., Bhattacharya, M., & Mukherjee, S. (2021). IoT-based computational frameworks in disease prediction and healthcare management: Strategies, challenges, and potential. *IoT in Healthcare and Ambient Assisted Living*, 1, 17–41.
127. Singh, K., Singh, P., & Angurala, M. (2023). Future directions in healthcare research. In Aryan Chaudhary Sardar M. N. Islam, *Computational Health Informatics for Biomedical Applications* (pp. 287–313). Apple Academic Press.
128. Vervoort, D., Tam, D. Y., & Wijeysundera, H. C. (2022). Health technology assessment for cardiovascular digital health technologies and artificial intelligence: Why is it different? *Canadian Journal of Cardiology, 38*(2), 259–266.
129. Busnatu, Ș. S., Niculescu, A. G., Bolocan, A., Andronic, O., Pantea Stoian, A. M., Scafa-Udriște, A., ... & Jinga, V. (2022). A review of digital health and biotelemetry: Modern approaches towards personalized medicine and remote health assessment. *Journal of Personalized Medicine, 12*(10), 1656.
130. Sun, G., & Zhou, Y. H. (2023). AI in healthcare: Navigating opportunities and challenges in digital communication. *Frontiers in Digital Health, 5*, 1291132.
131. Singh, B. (2024). Evolutionary global neuroscience for cognition and brain health: Strengthening innovation in brain science. In P. Prabhakar (Ed.), *Biomedical Research Developments for Improved Healthcare* (pp. 246–272). IGI Global. https://doi.org/10.4018/979-8-3693-1922-2.ch012

2 Embedded Systems in the Medical Field

Pros and Cons

Gizem Karabulut Şevk, Elif Tüzün, and Nuray Beköz Üllen

2.1 INTRODUCTION

Embedded systems represent a crucial aspect of modern technological landscapes, permeating various facets of our daily lives. These specialized computing systems designed to perform specific tasks or functions are embedded deeply within larger systems and devices [1]. The overarching goal of embedded systems is to execute predefined tasks efficiently, often with real-time constraints, making them indispensable in numerous applications [2]. This task can be many different things, such as providing control of a device, automating a process, collecting and processing data, or optimizing a device's features. They are characterized by their real-time operation, reliability, low power consumption, and often, a compact form factor [3]. Unlike general-purpose computers, embedded systems are purpose-built for specific applications, optimizing performance for the targeted tasks. Parts of embedded systems may vary depending on the needs of a particular application or task. These core components are usually a combination of processors, sensors, and application software. Microcontrollers/Microprocessors, which are the heart of embedded systems, are responsible for executing instructions and managing tasks [4]. Embedded systems are used in many areas such as automotive systems, home appliances, and industrial control systems. These systems are designed to suit the needs of specific applications and generally focus on long-term, reliable operation requirements. Embedded systems are prevalent in smartphones, smart televisions, digital cameras, and home automation systems, enhancing user experience and functionality [5]. In Figure 2.1, the usage areas of embedded systems are presented schematically. In-car entertainment, engine control units, and safety systems heavily rely on embedded systems. Embedded systems control machinery and processes in manufacturing, enhancing efficiency and precision. Networking equipment, routers, and switches incorporate embedded systems for seamless communication [6]. Due to the recent increasing technology and requirements, their use in the medical field is becoming increasingly widespread. In recent times, there has been a growing fascination with embedded computing systems within the realm of medical and biomedical applications. The swift progress in communication technologies, processors, and sensors/actuators,

DOI: 10.1201/9781003508199-2

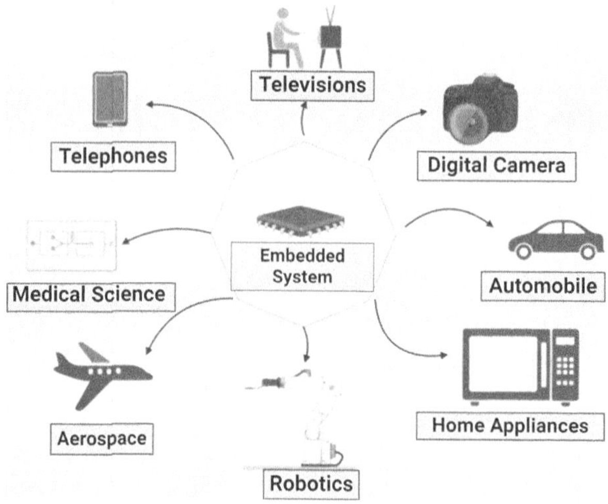

FIGURE 2.1 Usage areas of embedded systems.

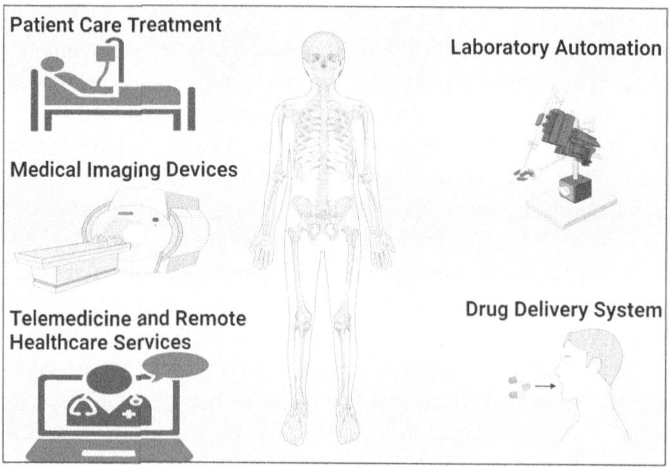

FIGURE 2.2 Applications of embedded systems in healthcare.

coupled with the advent of artificial intelligence, Internet of Things (IoT), artificial intelligence, and machine learning has empowered biomedical applications [6]. These advancements have facilitated activities such as disease diagnosis, telemedicine, and the characterization of biological materials [7–9].

Today, embedded systems have now become indispensable in modern healthcare, completely transforming the methods through which medical practitioners observe, diagnose, and provide care to patients [9, 10]. In Figure 2.2, the usage areas of embedded systems in the medical field are presented schematically. This integration brings forth a myriad of advantages, yet it is not without its share of challenges. On the positive side, embedded systems excel in enhancing patient monitoring. Real-time data acquisition allows healthcare providers to access vital information instantaneously, leading to more informed decision-making. Continuous health tracking ensures a comprehensive overview of a patient's well-being, enabling early detection of anomalies and timely intervention. In diagnostics and treatment, embedded systems contribute to unprecedented precision in medical imaging. This accuracy leads to more precise diagnoses and the capacity to customize treatment plans according to the individual requirements of each patient. This individualized method signifies a notable progression in the provision of healthcare services. The increased efficiency in healthcare delivery is another notable advantage. Streamlined workflows and a reduction in human errors improve overall patient care and optimize resource utilization. Remote patient management, facilitated by telemedicine applications and remote monitoring, expands access to healthcare services, particularly in remote or underserved areas [8]. However, these advancements come with a set of challenges. Security concerns loom large, as the sensitive nature of medical data makes healthcare systems a prime target for cyber threats. Safeguarding patient information and ensuring the integrity of embedded systems is a paramount challenge that demands continuous innovation in cybersecurity. Cost implications present another hurdle. The initial implementation of embedded systems in healthcare settings can be capital-intensive, and ongoing expenses for maintenance and upgrades must be carefully considered. Striking a balance between technological innovation and fiscal responsibility is an ongoing concern for healthcare institutions. Integration challenges also surface as healthcare systems evolve. Compatibility issues with existing infrastructure and the broader problem of interoperability between different systems may hinder the seamless integration of embedded technologies. Ensuring a harmonious coexistence with legacy systems is crucial for a smooth transition. Ethical considerations add another layer of complexity. Patient consent, autonomy, and the responsible use of data are paramount in an era where embedded systems play a pivotal role in healthcare decision-making. Striking a balance between leveraging technology for improved patient outcomes and respecting individual rights is an ongoing challenge.

In essence, embedded systems are the silent workhorses behind the seamless functioning of countless devices, contributing to the efficiency, reliability, and innovation in various industries. As technology progresses further, the influence and significance of embedded systems are set to expand, influencing the trajectory of intelligent and interconnected systems in the future. In conclusion, embedded systems in the medical field usher in a new era of possibilities, providing unprecedented insights and efficiencies. The advantages of enhanced patient monitoring, improved diagnostics, and increased efficiency in healthcare delivery are clear. However, addressing the challenges of security, cost, integration, and ethics is crucial to realizing the full potential of embedded systems while ensuring the highest standards of patient care and data integrity. This chapter aims to provide a comprehensive exploration of the embedded systems' role in the medical field, analyzing both the positive and negative aspects. By delving into case studies and future trends, the chapter will contribute valuable insights for researchers, healthcare professionals, and policymakers seeking to navigate the evolving landscape of healthcare technology.

2.2 PROS OF EMBEDDED SYSTEMS IN THE MEDICAL FIELD

Embedded systems have brought forth numerous advantages in the medical field, revolutionizing patient care and healthcare delivery. One significant pro lies in the enhanced patient monitoring capabilities enabled by these systems. Real-time data acquisition provides healthcare professionals with instantaneous access to critical information, fostering more informed decision-making. The precision offered by embedded systems in medical imaging contributes to highly accurate diagnoses, allowing for tailored and effective treatment plans for individual patients. Moreover, the increased efficiency in healthcare delivery is evident through streamlined workflows, a reduction in human errors, and optimized resource utilization. Remote patient management, facilitated by telemedicine applications, extends healthcare services to remote or underserved areas. The continuous health tracking provided by embedded systems ensures early anomaly detection, enabling proactive interventions and personalized care. Overall, embedded systems play a pivotal role in advancing patient-centric healthcare, offering benefits that range from improved diagnostics to optimized resource allocation [6, 9].

2.2.1 Patient Monitoring

Embedded systems have significantly enhanced patient monitoring in healthcare, providing real-time data acquisition and improving the overall quality of care. Embedded systems facilitate uninterrupted and instantaneous monitoring of critical indicators such as heart rate, blood pressure, oxygen saturation, and other vital signs [7, 11]. This immediate data acquisition empowers healthcare professionals with real-time information regarding a patient's physiological condition, enabling prompt and informed decision-making. With embedded systems, healthcare providers can continuously track a patient's health status over extended periods. This continuous monitoring ensures a comprehensive overview of the patient's well-being and allows for the early detection of any anomalies or deviations from normal parameters. Real-time data provided by embedded systems grants healthcare professionals immediate access to critical patient information. Rapid access to this information is essential for making well-informed and timely decisions regarding patient care, particularly in critical and emergency scenarios. Embedded systems enable healthcare providers to remotely monitor patients, extending healthcare oversight beyond conventional healthcare environments. This is especially advantageous for individuals with chronic illnesses or residing in remote or underserved regions, enabling healthcare providers to intervene promptly when needed [12]. The data collected by embedded systems can be analyzed in real-time or through retrospective analysis. This analytical capability aids in the early detection of trends, abnormalities, or potential health risks, empowering healthcare providers to take preventive measures [13]. Embedded systems can be configured to produce customized alerts and notifications according to predetermined thresholds. This feature ensures that healthcare professionals are promptly notified of any deviations from normal parameters, enabling swift responses to changes in a patient's condition [14]. Embedded systems are often integrated into wearable devices, allowing patients to monitor their health in real time outside of healthcare facilities. This promotes patient engagement and empowers individuals to take an active role in their own healthcare management. Automation through embedded systems reduces the likelihood of errors in data collection and recording, ensuring that the information available to healthcare professionals is accurate and reliable [14]. In summary, embedded systems have revolutionized patient monitoring by providing immediate access to real-time data, enabling continuous health tracking, and facilitating proactive interventions. These advancements contribute to improved patient outcomes, enhanced quality of care, and a more patient-centric approach to healthcare.

2.2.2 Diagnosis and Treatment

Embedded systems offer a range of advantages in the field of diagnosis and treatment, contributing to more accurate diagnostics, personalized treatment plans, and overall improvements in healthcare [7]. Embedded are pivotal in advancing the capabilities of high-precision medical imaging devices. This precision leads to more accurate diagnoses by providing detailed and clear images, aiding healthcare professionals in identifying and understanding various medical conditions [15]. The data gathered and analyzed by embedded systems empower healthcare providers to tailor treatment plans according to the specific needs of each patient. This individualized strategy guarantees that interventions are more targeted, efficient, and aligned with the specific characteristics of each patient's condition. Embedded systems offer real-time decision support to healthcare professionals throughout the diagnosis and treatment process. This includes analyzing patient data, suggesting potential treatment options, and aiding in the decision-making process for timely and informed interventions. Embedded systems automate various diagnostic processes, reducing the time and effort required for analysis. This automation enhances the efficiency of diagnostics, allowing for quicker turnaround times and facilitating a more rapid response to patients' healthcare needs. In laboratory settings, embedded systems integrate with diagnostic equipment to automate and streamline testing processes. This not only increases the speed of obtaining results but also ensures accuracy and consistency in diagnostic procedures. Embedded systems enable remote diagnostics through telemedicine applications, extending diagnostic capabilities beyond traditional healthcare settings [8]. This is especially advantageous for patients in remote areas, enabling access to specialized expertise without requiring physical presence. For patients with chronic conditions, embedded systems allow continuous monitoring of key parameters. This continuous data collection supports ongoing assessment and adjustment of treatment plans, promoting better management of chronic diseases. Embedded systems enable advanced data analysis, facilitating the development of predictive models for disease progression. This capability allows healthcare providers to anticipate potential complications and adjust treatment strategies preemptively. Embedded systems are integrated into drug delivery systems, ensuring precise dosage and timing of medications. This level of control enhances the efficacy of treatment regimens while minimizing the risk of adverse effects. In surgical applications, embedded systems enhance precision through robotic-assisted surgeries and other technologies. This optimization leads to less invasive procedures, reduced recovery times, and improved overall surgical outcomes. In summary, embedded systems significantly contribute to the advancement of diagnosis and treatment in healthcare by improving precision, personalization, and efficiency. These technologies empower healthcare professionals with the tools and insights needed to provide more effective and tailored care to patients.

2.2.3 Increased Efficiency of Healthcare

Increased efficiency in healthcare delivery is achieved through embedded systems in several ways, streamlining processes, reducing errors, and optimizing resource utilization. Embedded systems automate routine tasks and administrative processes, reducing manual workload for healthcare professionals. This automation streamlines workflows, allowing medical staff to focus more on patient care and critical decision-making. Automation and decision support features in embedded systems minimize the potential for human errors. By automating data entry, medication administration, and other tasks, these systems enhance accuracy, reducing the risk of mistakes in healthcare delivery. Embedded systems assist in the efficient allocation of resources such as medical equipment, personnel, and facilities. Real-time data analysis helps healthcare administrators make informed decisions about resource distribution, ensuring that resources are utilized where they are most needed. Telemedicine applications, facilitated by embedded systems, allow for remote patient monitoring and consultations. This diminishes the necessity for face-to-face appointments, conserving time for both patients and healthcare providers, all the while upholding the quality of care. Embedded systems enable rapid access to patient data by storing and processing information instantaneously. This quick access ensures that healthcare professionals have the most up-to-date information when making decisions about patient care. Embedded systems automate and expedite diagnostic processes, reducing the time required for tests and analyses. This efficiency is particularly crucial for timely diagnosis and treatment planning. Embedded systems facilitate seamless communication between different departments within a healthcare facility. This ensures that critical information is shared promptly, enhancing coordination and collaboration among healthcare professionals. Through real-time monitoring and data analysis, embedded systems contribute to the efficient management of patient flow within hospitals. This includes optimizing appointment scheduling, reducing waiting times, and ensuring timely patient discharges. Embedded systems seamlessly integrate with electronic health records, providing a centralized platform for comprehensive patient information. This integration improves the continuity of care, as healthcare providers can access complete patient histories and treatment plans. In summary, embedded systems play a vital role in increasing efficiency in healthcare delivery by automating tasks, reducing errors, optimizing resource allocation, and improving overall communication and coordination within healthcare facilities. These technologies contribute to a more streamlined and effective healthcare system, ultimately benefiting both healthcare professionals and patients.

2.2.4 Remote Patient Management

Remote patient management with embedded systems offers a range of advantages, transforming healthcare delivery by enhancing patient care, improving accessibility, and optimizing resource utilization. Remote patient management with embedded systems involves using technology to monitor and manage patients' health remotely. Embedded systems suitable for remote patient management should be selected [16]. These systems should include sensors, communication modules, and data processing capabilities to securely monitor and transmit relevant health data [17]. Embedded systems facilitate the continuous and real-time monitoring of patients' vital signs and health metrics. This constant surveillance allows for early detection of anomalies or changes in health conditions. Healthcare providers can receive immediate alerts and notifications through embedded systems, enabling them to intervene promptly in case of critical health events or deviations from normal parameters. This results in timely and potentially life-saving interventions. Remote patient management is especially advantageous for individuals dealing with chronic conditions. Embedded systems facilitate the ongoing monitoring of chronic diseases, allowing healthcare professionals to make proactive adjustments to treatment plans and reduce the risk of complications. By monitoring patients remotely, unnecessary hospital visits and readmissions can be minimized. This leads to cost savings for both healthcare providers and patients, particularly for those with chronic illnesses requiring continuous care. Patients actively engage in their healthcare by routinely monitoring their health metrics through embedded systems. This heightened engagement nurtures a sense of accountability for one's health, resulting in improved adherence to treatment plans and lifestyle recommendations. Remote patient management extends healthcare services beyond traditional settings, especially in remote or underserved areas. This improves accessibility, ensuring that patients can receive quality healthcare without the need for frequent travel to healthcare facilities. The data collected by embedded systems enables healthcare providers to customize treatment plans according to the specific needs of each patient. This individualized approach enhances the effectiveness of interventions and promotes better patient outcomes. Continuous monitoring and data analysis empower healthcare professionals to detect potential health risks at an early stage. This facilitates preventive care strategies and reduces the likelihood of complications, hospitalizations, or emergency situations. In summary, remote patient management with embedded systems revolutionizes healthcare by providing continuous monitoring, prompt interventions, and individualized care. These advantages contribute to better patient outcomes, improved healthcare accessibility, and increased efficiency in the delivery of healthcare services.

2.3 CONS OF EMBEDDED SYSTEMS IN THE MEDICAL FIELD

The integration of embedded systems in the medical field, while transformative, is face to face some challenges. One prominent concern revolves around the security of patient data, as the sensitive nature of medical information makes healthcare systems susceptible to cyber threats. The substantial costs associated with the initial implementation, maintenance, and updates of embedded systems pose financial challenges for healthcare institutions [7]. Integration hurdles arise due to the diverse existing infrastructure, leading to compatibility issues and potential disruptions. Ethical considerations, such as patient privacy and data consent, demand careful navigation. Additionally, the lack of standardized protocols may hinder interoperability and result in data silos. The dependency on technology raises the risk of disruptions in healthcare delivery during system failures. Handling the large volumes of patient data generated by embedded systems can be daunting, potentially resulting in information overload for healthcare professionals. Addressing these cons requires a comprehensive approach that encompasses cybersecurity, financial planning, ethical guidelines, and the development of standardized practices in the integration of embedded systems into medical practices [6, 9, 15].

2.3.1 Security Concerns

The integration of embedded systems in the medical field introduces security concerns primarily related to the protection of sensitive patient data [18]. The healthcare sector is an attractive target for cybercriminals due to the valuable and sensitive information stored in medical records [8]. Embedded systems, which often involve interconnected devices and networks, become vulnerable to various cyber threats such as ransomware, data breaches, and unauthorized access. The compromised security of embedded systems poses a direct threat to patient privacy. Medical records contain highly personal information, and unauthorized access or data breaches can lead to identity theft, fraud, or other malicious activities that infringe upon patient confidentiality. Ensuring the integrity of medical data is crucial for accurate diagnoses and treatment plans. If embedded systems are not adequately protected, there is a risk of data manipulation or tampering, leading to incorrect patient information and potentially harmful consequences. The sector is governed by rigorous regulatory frameworks, such as the Health Insurance Portability and Accountability Act (HIPAA) in the United States [19]. Security breaches may result in non-compliance, leading to legal consequences and fines for healthcare institutions. Embedded systems often involve the interconnection of medical devices and equipment. If security measures are not robust, a vulnerability in one embedded system or device could be exploited to gain unauthorized access to the entire network, putting patient data and safety at risk. Healthcare professionals may not always be well-versed in cybersecurity practices. Lack of awareness and training can lead to inadvertent security lapses, such as weak passwords, improper device configurations, or failure to update software promptly, leaving embedded systems susceptible to attacks. Many healthcare facilities still use legacy systems that may lack the advanced security features found in newer technologies. Integrating modern embedded systems with legacy infrastructure poses challenges in maintaining a uniform and robust security posture across the entire healthcare network. Embedded systems often rely on a complex supply chain, involving multiple vendors and components. Each element introduces a potential point of vulnerability. If not carefully managed, the supply chain itself can become a source of security threats, including the introduction of compromised components. Encryption is a critical aspect of securing patient data during transmission and storage. Inadequate or outdated encryption practices within embedded systems may expose patient information to interception and unauthorized access. Addressing these security concerns requires a holistic approach involving the implementation of robust cybersecurity measures, continuous monitoring, regular training for healthcare professionals, and adherence to regulatory standards. It's essential for healthcare institutions to prioritize cybersecurity as an integral part of their overall strategy when adopting embedded systems.

2.3.2 Cost Implications

The integration of embedded systems in the medical field presents challenges related to cost implications, impacting both initial implementation and ongoing maintenance [6]. The initial implementation of embedded systems in healthcare settings can be capital-intensive. Acquiring the necessary hardware, software, and infrastructure, along with the costs of system integration and deployment, can place a significant financial burden on healthcare institutions. Beyond the initial setup, embedded systems require continuous maintenance, updates, and technical support. These ongoing expenses can include software updates, security patches, and hardware maintenance. Healthcare providers must allocate resources to ensure the reliability and optimal performance of embedded systems over time. Healthcare facilities often have existing legacy systems and diverse technologies. Integrating new embedded systems with this pre-existing infrastructure can be complex and costly. Compatibility issues may arise, necessitating additional investments to ensure seamless integration. Healthcare professionals and staff members may need training to effectively use and manage embedded systems. Training programs, workshops, and educational materials incur additional costs, and the time required for staff members to become proficient in using new technologies may temporarily impact productivity. To address security concerns associated with embedded systems, healthcare institutions must invest in robust cybersecurity measures. This includes the implementation of encryption, firewalls, intrusion detection systems, and ongoing monitoring, adding to the overall cost of system integration. Healthcare organizations must comply with strict regulatory standards, and adherence to these standards may require additional investments. Ensuring that embedded systems meet regulatory requirements, such as those outlined by HIPAA or other healthcare data protection laws, can involve significant financial commitments. As technology evolves, healthcare institutions may need to upgrade or scale their embedded systems to keep pace with industry advancements. The costs associated with upgrading software, hardware, and expanding system capabilities to meet growing demands can strain financial resources. Demonstrating a clear and tangible return on investment can be challenging, especially in the short term. While embedded systems offer long-term benefits, healthcare institutions may face difficulty justifying the upfront costs to stakeholders without a clear and measurable return on investment.

Economic factors and budget constraints within the healthcare sector can limit the available funds for adopting embedded systems. Competing priorities, such as patient care, facility upgrades, and staff salaries, may divert resources from investing in advanced technologies. Addressing the cost implications of integrating embedded systems in the medical field requires careful financial planning, transparent communication about the expected benefits, and a long-term strategy that considers both initial expenses and ongoing operational costs. Healthcare organizations must weigh the potential advantages against the financial investments required to ensure a sustainable and efficient integration of embedded systems. Embedded systems necessitate regular updates to address security vulnerabilities, enhance functionality, and remain compatible with evolving technologies. Coordinating these updates with existing systems while ensuring minimal downtime can be challenging. Overcoming integration challenges necessitates a comprehensive approach involving careful planning, collaboration between vendors and healthcare providers, adherence to interoperability standards, and a commitment to ongoing system optimization. Addressing these challenges is vital to realizing the full potential of embedded systems in the medical field and ensuring a smooth and efficient healthcare delivery process.

2.3.3 Ethical Considerations

Ethical considerations in the integration of embedded systems in the medical field involve navigating complex issues related to patient autonomy, privacy, consent, and responsible use of data. The collection, storage, and sharing of patient data through embedded systems raise significant concerns about privacy. Protecting patient confidentiality is paramount, and healthcare institutions must enforce stringent security measures to prevent unauthorized access or breaches that might compromise sensitive medical data. Ethical considerations dictate that patients have the right to be fully informed about the use of embedded systems in their healthcare. Securing informed consent is essential, guaranteeing that patients comprehend the methods of data collection, processing, and utilization. Transparent communication about the potential risks and benefits is essential for maintaining trust. Clear ethical guidelines must address the ownership and stewardship of patient data. It should be explicit whether the data belongs to the patients, healthcare providers, or the embedded system providers. Transparency in data ownership ensures accountability and responsible use. Protecting patient data from cyber threats is an ethical imperative. Embedding systems should adhere to high standards of data security and incorporate robust cybersecurity measures to safeguard against unauthorized access, breaches, and potential harm to patients. The use of embedded systems should respect patient dignity and ensure that individuals are not reduced to mere data points. Ethical considerations involve maintaining a human-centric approach to healthcare and recognizing the unique needs, values, and experiences of each patient. Addressing these ethical considerations necessitates a joint endeavor involving healthcare professionals, technology developers, policymakers, and patients. Establishing clear ethical guidelines, incorporating patient input, and fostering an ongoing dialogue about the responsible use of embedded systems are essential for ensuring that technological advancements align with ethical principles in the medical field.

2.3.4 Dependency on Technology

Dependency on technology in the integration of embedded systems in the medical field refers to the reliance of healthcare providers on these systems for essential functions and decision-making processes. Healthcare professionals depend on the accuracy and reliability of data collected and processed by embedded systems for making clinical decisions. Any inaccuracies or errors in the data can lead to incorrect diagnoses, treatment plans, and patient outcomes. Embedded systems play a crucial role in various aspects of healthcare delivery, including patient monitoring, diagnostics, and treatment. Healthcare providers rely on the functionality and performance of these systems to deliver timely and effective care to patients. However, healthcare professionals may become heavily reliant on these systems for routine tasks, potentially impacting their ability to perform tasks manually or adapt to system failures. Dependency on technology introduces the risk of system failures or malfunctions, which can disrupt healthcare operations and compromise patient care. Healthcare providers must have contingency plans in place to mitigate the impact of system failures and ensure continuity of care. Healthcare professionals need adequate training and competency in using embedded systems effectively. Dependence on technology requires ongoing training and skill development to ensure healthcare providers can effectively navigate and troubleshoot these systems. Healthcare organizations need to adapt to rapid technological developments and innovations in embedded systems. Dependence on specific technologies may require healthcare providers to constantly update their skills and infrastructure to remain competitive and provide high-quality care. Healthcare organizations invest significant resources in the integration and maintenance of embedded systems. Dependence on technology requires ongoing financial commitments to upgrades, maintenance, and cybersecurity measures that must be carefully managed to ensure sustainability and return on investment. Overall, while dependency on technology offers numerous benefits in the medical field, healthcare providers must be mindful of the potential risks and challenges associated with reliance on embedded systems. Balancing technological advancements with human-centric care and adopting a proactive approach to addressing system vulnerabilities is essential for ensuring safe, effective, and ethical healthcare delivery.

2.3.5 Regulatory Compliance

Regulatory compliance in the integration of embedded systems in the medical field refers to adhering to the laws, regulations, and standards set forth by regulatory bodies governing healthcare and technology. Regulatory bodies such as the HIPAA set strict guidelines for the protection of patient health information. Embedded systems must adhere to these laws to guarantee the confidentiality, integrity, and accessibility of healthcare data. Embedded systems that qualify as medical devices are subject to regulations governing their design, manufacturing, labeling, and performance. Organizations such as the Food and Drug Administration (FDA) mandate that medical devices undergo thorough testing and certification procedures to ensure their safety and efficacy. Regulatory efforts aim to promote interoperability between healthcare systems and devices, allowing seamless exchange of data and information. Compliance with interoperability standards, such as those developed by organizations like Digital Imaging and Communications in Medicine (DICOM) and Health Level Seven International (HL7), ensures that embedded systems can communicate effectively with other healthcare technologies. Regulatory bodies increasingly focus on cybersecurity standards for healthcare systems, including embedded systems.

Adhering to cybersecurity regulations entails implementing measures to safeguard against unauthorized access, data breaches, and cyber threats that may jeopardize patient safety and privacy. Regulatory compliance extends to ethical considerations surrounding the use of embedded systems in healthcare. Adherence to ethical guidelines involves respecting patient autonomy, ensuring informed consent, and promoting transparency in data-handling practices. Regulatory compliance often requires healthcare organizations to implement quality management systems (QMS) to oversee the development, deployment, and maintenance of embedded systems. QMS frameworks, such as ISO 13485, provide guidelines for ensuring product quality and regulatory compliance throughout the product lifecycle. Compliance with regulatory standards necessitates thorough documentation of design, development, testing, and deployment processes related to embedded systems. Healthcare organizations must maintain comprehensive records and report any adverse events or non-compliance incidents as required by regulatory authorities. Non-compliance with regulatory requirements can result in legal repercussions, fines, reputational damage, and barriers to market access for embedded systems in the medical field. Therefore, ensuring regulatory compliance is essential for healthcare organizations and technology developers involved in the integration of embedded systems in healthcare settings.

2.4 CASE STUDIES

There are numerous case studies showcasing the successful integration of embedded systems in various aspects of the medical field. These case studies illustrate the diverse applications and benefits of integrating embedded systems in the medical field, ranging from improved patient monitoring and personalized treatment to enhanced healthcare accessibility and efficiency. By showcasing real-world examples of successful implementations, these case studies provide valuable insights and best practices for healthcare organizations, technology developers, and policymakers seeking to leverage embedded systems to transform healthcare delivery. Table 2.1 shows a summary of the application areas of embedded systems in the medical field.

TABLE 2.1
General Usage Points of the Embedded System in Medical Field

Application	Reference
Blood Pressure Monitor	Mahmood [20]
Oximetry	Devarshi et al. [21]
Sleep Monitor	Liu and Yang [22]
Telehealth	Dabiri et al. [23]
Medical Image Analysis	Niepceron et al. [24] and Li et al. [25]
Blood Sugar Monitor	Al-Odat et al. [26]
Electrocardiogram [ECG] Monitor	Kim et al. [27] and Mhamdi et al. [28]
Wearable Systems	Hu [29] and Diab and Rodriguez-Villegas [30]
Information Systems	Kuroda et al. [31]

2.4.1 Remote Patient Monitoring Systems

These systems are advanced healthcare solutions that enable the continuous tracking of patients' health metrics outside traditional clinical settings. Utilizing a combination of wearable devices, mobile apps, and telehealth platforms, these systems collect vital signs such as heart rate, blood pressure, and glucose levels, transmitting this data in real-time to healthcare providers. This technology enhances patient care by allowing for early detection of potential health issues, timely medical interventions, and personalized treatment plans, all while improving convenience for patients and reducing the burden on healthcare facilities. These systems are particularly beneficial for managing chronic diseases, post-operative care, and elderly patients, ultimately leading to better health outcomes and more efficient use of healthcare resources.

Chen [11] introduced a user-friendly web-based interface for observing real-time pulse signals and heart rate, facilitating remote treatment at the client end. Additionally, the system ensures accurate measurement and transmission of pulse signals to the human physiological database, making it suitable for daily home health care. The system, developed using embedded system technology, has been successfully implemented, enabling the creation of compact, lightweight, and affordable portable heart rate monitoring systems.

Chiuchisan and Geman [13] conducted a study on monitoring a morbidly obese patient using a system that collects health parameters from sensors and transfers the data to a device. The study involved processing data by collecting health parameters such as blood pressure and heart rate. Additionally, the patient was monitored throughout the night for signs of sleep apnea. Remote patient monitoring and follow-up were successfully carried out with the system used in the study, allowing patients at severe risk to remain under constant monitoring.

2.4.2 Implantable Medical Devices

These are case studies focusing on implantable medical devices (IMDs), such as pacemakers, insulin pumps, and neurostimulators, which incorporate embedded systems to deliver therapeutic interventions. These devices continuously monitor physiological parameters, deliver medication or electrical stimulation, and provide data for long-term disease management, enhancing patients' quality of life and treatment efficacy.

The most important development in medical devices is the placement of these devices into the body through surgical operations. With the combination of many technologies, interest in this field has increased recently. As a result of developing chips in very small sizes and integrating them into the body, compatible devices that consume minimum power for medical applications have been obtained [32]. In recent years, significant advances have been made in the field of health by surgically implanting a device or object for health problems in certain parts of the body [33].

One of the most important contributions in the fields of health and engineering is to make implantable devices useful and compatible with the human body. These devices need to be reduced in size for compatibility and to eliminate difficulties during and after implantation. For this reason, integrated chips must be produced for implantable devices. These IMDs are used in the diagnosis and treatment of many diseases. The use of these IMDs in pain management, heart diseases, Parkinson's and epilepsy, gastrointestinal and bladder control, many autoimmune diseases and psychological disorders makes it possible to treat them at low cost [34, 35]. However, as a result of advances in the field of nanotechnology and submicron-scale applications, more compatible implanted devices have been developed. For the patients we mentioned, IMDs such as brain and pacemakers, which need to be implanted through surgical intervention, are gaining great importance in finding cures for diseases of the age such as Parkinson's and heart diseases, which make patients' lives difficult. The smaller the size of these IMDs, the more advantages they will have, as the smaller they are, the easier they will be to adapt to the body and to remain for a long time. The desired features of the produced IMDs include long life, reliability in terms of biocompatibility, and low power consumption. In line with the developments in engineering and medicine, implanted devices are increasingly in demand in miniature form. As a result, thanks to the latest technological developments of these devices, the diagnosis and treatment processes of physicians have become easier and the quality of life of the patient has increased [33]. Improvements have been made through many studies to ensure that IMDs produced in smaller sizes have better performance and efficiency for treatment and diagnosis processes [36, 37]. Different methodologies have been developed for the produced chip and studies have been carried out to develop the applications of the implanted product. Power consumption control after IMDs is produced is also very important. For this reason, power consumption should be reduced, and the duration of the battery used should be increased and the frequency of replacement should be minimum. The highest cost of the state-of-the-art IMDs is due to surgical implantation. For this reason, it is aimed to develop more cost-effective and reliable products for IMDs in the future [32].

2.4.3 Smart Wearable Health Devices

These are case studies highlighting smart wearable health devices, such as fitness trackers, smartwatches, and health monitoring patches, which integrate embedded sensors and connectivity features to monitor users' activity levels, sleep patterns, and vital signs. These devices empower individuals to take control of their health, track their wellness goals, and provide valuable data for preventive healthcare strategies.

Wearable health systems (WHS), which emerged as a result of the coming together of many disciplines in the field of health, are a subject that needs to be developed so that the patient's controls can be carried out in the patient's own living space. Otherwise, there will be a loss of time for simple procedures in hospitals. WHS is an interesting subject in order to make the patient use his time and make his life easier. In smart technology, WHS are systems that can come into contact with the human body, detect any change in the body, transmit this data to us as processed, and signal us with instant voice systems. Multidisciplinary studies are an important issue for WHS. As a result, WHS must constantly update itself in line with the ever-increasing demand. As a result of interdisciplinary studies of nano and micro technologies in chemistry, materials, biomedical, computer, and industry fields, new approaches have been developed to facilitate the lives of WHS people. Although the work and time loss in the healthcare field may not be noticeable, it is important for the patient. In order to prevent this and diagnose the disease early, biochemical tests, follow-up, and post-treatment stages can be done more personally and easily thanks to WHS. In the field of healthcare, service management and its coordinated progress are gaining importance in terms of the service to be provided to the patient. Since the individual patient has a stronger role in the disease process, new ways are being sought for the application of wearable technology. People have to face these socioeconomic challenges, especially considering the care expectations of the elderly population, the increase in diseases and, their costs to the health sector [38]. It is very difficult for an unhealthy individual to manage his own illness and reach healthcare teams. Personal Health Systems (PHS), a new concept that has emerged recently, has emerged to meet this need and to contribute to the patient and healthcare teams and make their work easier on both sides. Increasing the quality of care given to individuals, increasing the efficiency of the technology used, and reducing the costs while doing these are among the duties of PHS. Wearable biomedical materials produce solutions in the healthcare industry to give us instant information about our body. Increasing the technological (ICT) application areas in the field of information and communication and improving the quality through wrist-integrated wearable devices are among the positive services that WHS provides to users. In the future, WHS will be an interesting subject as a special subsidiary of PHS with an innovative approach in the field of health with multidisciplinary solutions in the fields of ICT, biotechnology, and nanotechnology focused on the wishes of the user [39].

If we want to briefly list the aims of WHS in the health sector [40]:

- To provide healthcare services to all patients and prospective patients using inexpensive treatment methods.
- Being able to monitor long-term health and not reduce the patient's quality of life and continue their social life without interrupting them.
- Producing wearable materials to improve the quality of care for patients.
- Making a correct diagnosis during the disease period and ensuring the reliability of the treatment process.

To ensure that the person's risks are reduced in personalized health applications (such as drug allergy) with the right approach and without error.

2.4.4 Medical Imaging Systems

These are case studies showcasing advanced medical imaging systems, such as magnetic resonance image machines, computed tomography scanners, and ultrasound devices, which utilize embedded systems to acquire, process, and visualize high-resolution medical images [2]. These systems enable healthcare providers to accurately diagnose and monitor various medical conditions, guide surgical procedures, and plan personalized treatment strategies.

Obeidat and Alqudah [41] present the creation of a groundbreaking embedded system using Raspberry Pi, which transforms the monitoring of ECG signals in clinical settings. This device provides a quicker and more effective method for ECG monitoring, requiring only three leads that can be effortlessly connected to the human body. Once connected and powered on, the ECG signal is instantly displayed on the screen, enabling swift monitoring. To ensure signal accuracy, factors affecting it are considered, implementing necessary filter stages, designing a well-structured PCB layout, and incorporating a protective covering for shielding components from external noise. Extensive testing employing both simulated and real human ECG signals demonstrates the device's success in measuring ECG signals across a range of heart rates accurately. The obtained ECG results can be easily shown on a graphical LCD screen and accessed via a Virtual Network Computing (VNC) viewer on a smartphone or PC. Data can be securely stored on the cloud via a mobile application, aiding doctors in future diagnostics. The device integrates Raspberry Pi's power, enabling wireless and wired interfaces for real-time detection and response to heart abnormalities. The system comprises analog and digital components for signal conditioning, amplification, noise filtering, and analog-to-digital conversion, ensuring compatibility with Raspberry Pi. The device aims to be portable, cost-effective, and user-friendly, catering to the growing need for affordable medical diagnostic solutions. In conclusion, this Raspberry Pi-based embedded system offers significant advancements in ECG monitoring, providing a faster, more efficient, and comprehensive solution for healthcare professionals. Future plans involve employing the device for heart arrhythmia classification using a hybrid model and deploying it in hospitals and clinical applications with institutional Review Board (IRB) approval.

2.4.5 Health Information Systems

These are case studies focusing on health information systems, electronic health records (EHRs), and medical data analytics platforms, which incorporate embedded systems to manage, analyze, and exchange vast amounts of patient data securely. These systems support clinical decision-making, population health management, and healthcare resource optimization, leading to more efficient and coordinated care delivery.

Wang et al. [42] evaluated the coding technology of the international classification of diseases and the implementation of the embedded electronic medical record (EMR) system through clinical diagnosis selection and medical record information management with artificial intelligence algorithm in their study. The study analyzed the causes of major diagnostic selection errors in the fields of obstetrics and gynecology, endocrinology, oncology, orthopedics, and neurosurgery, before and after training, as well as disease coding errors in the fields of obstetrics and gynecology, endocrinology, cardiovascular medicine, burns, orthopedics, and ophthalmology. The study shows that the implemented system does not yet fully understand various diseases and their special classifications, and at the same time, medical personnel cannot clearly fill in medical records of diseases. It has been stated that small sample numbers are insufficient and more efficient results are obtained with increasing sample numbers. In the next stage, the study conclusion is presented that scientists should expand the scope of sample collection in order to provide certain support for future research on main diagnostic selection and disease coding.

Ricci et al. [43] presented an embedded system for the digital processing of ultrasound (US) signals in real time in their study. The system is stated to be capable of transmitting arbitrary waveforms, demodulating echoes to multiple channels simultaneously, and processing the received data through programmable algorithms. With these features, it has been reported to be used in various applications such as embolism detection, characterization of contrast agents, arterial mechanical studies, and hemodynamic evaluations. The implementation of the system on a single electronic board makes it an ideal tool for any ultrasound research activity that requires flexible transmission and reception strategies.

Mahmood et al. [44] proposed a four-layer hierarchical design for analyzing lung sounds and extracting various features in their study. They noted the difficulty even for individuals with relevant training to interpret these results, prompting the examination of sound analysis by a programmed system. According to their findings, the system achieved high average accuracy rates, such as 100% for COPD, 99.83% for Healthy, 99.62% for URTI, 99.88% for Bronchiectasis, and 99.87% for Pneumonia diseases. This underscores the potential benefits of utilizing embedded systems in the diagnosis phase, highlighting the need for further research in this area.

2.5 FUTURE TRENDS AND DEVELOPMENTS

Future embedded systems are expected to become even smaller and more lightweight, leading to the development of wearable medical devices. These devices can be seamlessly integrated into clothing or accessories, allowing for monitoring and control of vital parameters without interfering with the user's daily activities. The Internet of Medical Things (IoMT) describes an interconnected network of medical devices and applications that collect and transmit health data. Future trends in embedded systems involve leveraging IoMT technologies to enable real-time monitoring, remote patient management, and personalized healthcare interventions. Embedded systems in the medical field are increasingly incorporating artificial intelligence algorithms to analyze patient data and derive actionable insights. These technologies enable predictive analytics, disease detection, and personalized treatment recommendations based on individual patient characteristics. Edge computing, which involves processing data closer to its source rather than relying on centralized servers, is emerging as a key trend in embedded systems. Future embedded medical devices may leverage edge computing capabilities to perform real-time data analysis and decision-making, while also integrating with cloud-based platforms for storage and collaboration. As the healthcare ecosystem becomes more interconnected, interoperability and standards compliance are critical considerations for future embedded systems. Efforts to establish common data exchange formats, communication protocols, and interoperability standards will facilitate the seamless integration of embedded devices with existing healthcare infrastructure. The growing demand for telemedicine and remote patient monitoring is driving the development of embedded systems that support virtual consultations, remote diagnostics, and telehealth services. Future trends in this area involve enhancing the capabilities of embedded devices to enable more comprehensive and personalized remote healthcare delivery. Blockchain technology holds promise for enhancing data security and integrity in embedded medical systems. By creating a tamper-proof ledger that is resistant to complex systems that are not connected to the central system, blockchain can help ensure the privacy, authenticity, and traceability of health data generated by embedded devices. Future embedded systems will focus on improving human-machine interaction to enhance user experience and usability. Technologies such as natural language processing, gesture recognition, and haptic feedback will enable more intuitive and user-friendly interfaces for medical devices. Embedded systems will play a crucial role in the advancement of personalized medicine and precision healthcare. By integrating genomic data, biomarkers, and other personalized health information, future embedded devices will enable tailored treatment strategies and interventions based on individual patient needs and characteristics. With the increasing adoption of embedded systems in medical applications, regulatory compliance and ethical considerations will remain paramount. Future trends involve addressing regulatory challenges, ensuring data privacy and security, and upholding ethical standards in the development and deployment of embedded medical devices. Overall, the future of embedded systems in the medical field is characterized by innovation, integration, and the pursuit of improved patient outcomes through advanced technologies and methodologies. By embracing these trends, healthcare providers, technology developers, and policymakers can work together to harness the full potential of embedded systems for the benefit of patients and healthcare systems worldwide.

2.6 CONCLUSIONS

This chapter focuses on the use of embedded systems in the medical field and tries to clarify the subject by discussing the pros and cons of embedded systems. Embedded systems used in the medical field with advancing technology play an important role in monitoring the patient and managing the treatment process. In addition, it has positively affected the occupational safety and efficiency of medical personnel. If embedded systems are designed well, efficient and effective reconstruction resources that provide a balance between power and memory consumption can be efficiently utilized. In addition to the use of embedded systems in many commercial applications, their applications in medicine and biomedical fields are becoming increasingly widespread. It is very important to develop tools to increase the safety of healthcare workers, especially in the case of the emergence of epidemics and infectious diseases such as the pandemic process. Embedded system design will make them more preferred due to the release of better versions, increase in software libraries, and lowering the cost of embedded systems in healthcare services and their portability. Moreover, introducing artificial intelligence applications into systems integrated with embedded systems will enable them to serve more purposes. Other expectations in the biomedical field; include monitoring of vital health parameters, wearable devices in the healthcare sector, sensors that increase portability, in vivo measurement systems, teleradiology, telerehabilitation, bio-signal collection and processing, virtual reality systems, 3D education and training.

The benefits of applying embedded technology to medical diagnosis and treatment are clear. Performing the treatment, which can be done manually by doctors, with machines, and in an unlimited period allows the correct diagnosis to be achieved by constantly monitoring the health parameters. With embedded technology, shipping costs for sending medical records are reduced. Medical reports can be viewed instantly with embedded software support; this means that the doctor–patient consultation will take place in a very short time. All these benefits show how important embedded systems are for both patients and healthcare personnel. Since the medical field will always be looking for new treatments and diagnoses, the future of embedded system technology is very bright in this field. The role of embedded systems in the development of future biomedical devices is indisputably important. This process sees embedded systems as a way to integrate signal processing, computer programming, and electronic concepts during the application phase of medical devices. By using these, time and cost will be saved. That perform or monitor the process remotely over mobile networks. Its main purpose is to provide medical services to places with low socio-economic levels.

Most embedded systems have a complex design with the use of multiple people in concurrent processes. The details of the process are a critical process that determines the requirements of the system. Embedded systems used in the medical field have both pros and cons. These can be considered as limited support, hardware dependency, limited resources, difficulties in programming, limited application area, and difficulties in complying with standardization. The main difficulty of embedded systems is the limited size of the embedded medical device and the materials used. The problem encountered in this process can be resolved by optimizing the software and hardware. This optimization increases energy efficiency and extends battery life. Another negative aspect relates to medical device security and privacy security. With the inclusion of artificial intelligence in embedded systems, it is seen that applications in the field of medicine are developing toward intelligence, miniaturization, and personalization. Embedded systems that improve with technological developments in increasing the quality and efficiency of healthcare services aim to meet the expectations of patients and healthcare personnel. Embedded systems in the field of medicine can be used in various fields such as medical data collection and data processing, medical monitoring and diagnosis systems, and medical treatment and rehabilitation systems. Embedded systems used in medical equipment greatly increase its accuracy and efficiency by making the equipment easy to use. Medical electronic devices are used extensively to monitor the patient's values and to collect data about the patient's sleep pattern and drug use period. These systems require the use of various devices such as electrical stimulators, prostheses, and rehabilitation robots. Embedded systems are necessary to control the functions of these devices and make the operations more precise and efficient. Robot-assisted therapy is possible with the embedded system.

Following technological developments, it is thought that embedded systems will make significant progress in the fields of artificial intelligence, miniaturization, and personalization. Sustainable practices also determine the future of embedded systems used in the medical field. Energy-saving designs, optimization of power usage, and environmentally friendly technology solutions are critical issues to be solved.

REFERENCES

1. White E. *Making Embedded Systems*. O'Reilly Media; 2012.
2. Dere G. Data Acquisition – Recent Advances and Applications in Biomedical Engineering. In: Płaczek B, editor. *Data Acquisition – Recent Advances and Applications in Biomedical Engineering* [Internet]. IntechOpen; 2021 [cited 2024 Apr 3]. Available from: undefined/chapters/75395

3. Caffarena G, Raya R, Urendes E, Otero A, Mennard D. Teaching Embedded Systems in Biomedical Engineering degrees: A case study. *2021 IEEE Mysore Sub Sect Int Conf MysuruCon 2021*. 2021; 58–64.
4. Marques Soudré M, Hultmann Ayala HV, Melo AC, Llanos CH. A novel GPU-based approach for embedded NARMAX/FROLS system identification. *Mech Syst Signal Process*. 2024 Apr;211:111261.
5. Toulson R, Wilmshurst T. Embedded systems, microcontrollers, and ARM. *Fast Eff Embed Syst Des*. 2017 Jan;3–18. https://doi.org/10.1016/B978-0-08-100880-5.00001-3
6. Nandini KP, Seshikala G. Role of embedded computing systems in biomedical applications-opportunities and challenges. *2021 IEEE Int Conf Distrib Comput VLSI, Electr Circuits Robot Discov 2021 – Proc*. 2021;332–5.
7. Awotunde JB, Chakraborty C, AbdulRaheem M, Jimoh RG, Oladipo ID, Bhoi AK. Internet of medical things for enhanced smart healthcare systems. In: Chinmay Chakraborty, Subhendu Kumar Pani, Mohd Abdul Ahad, and Qin Xin *Implementation of Smart Healthcare Systems using AI, IoT, and Blockchain*. Academic Press; 2023. pp. 1–28.
8. Murillo-Escobar D, Cruz-Hernández C, López-Gutiérrez RM, Murillo-Escobar MA. Chaotic encryption of real-time ECG signal in embedded system for secure telemedicine. *Integration*. 2023 Mar 1;89:261–70.
9. Zhao H. Applications of embedded systems in medicine: Challenges and future trends. Highlights Sci Eng Technol [Internet]. 2023 Jul 27 [cited 2024 Apr 3];62:31–5. Available from: https://drpress.org/ojs/index.php/HSET/article/view/10416
10. Joshi V. The role of embedded systems in revolutionizing healthcare: A comprehensive analysis. 2023. https://medium.com/@vedjoshi03/the-role-of-embedded-systems-in-revolutionizing-healthcare-a-comprehensive-analysis-df1713323c5a
11. Chen CM. Web-based remote human pulse monitoring system with intelligent data analysis for home health care. *Expert Syst Appl*. 2011 Mar 1;38 [3]:2011–9.
12. Remote patient monitoring – FasterCapital [Internet]. [cited 2024 Apr 3]. Available from: https://fastercapital.com/keyword/remote-patient-monitoring.html
13. Chiuchisan I, Geman O. Trends in embedded systems for e-Health and biomedical applications. *Proc 2016 Int Conf Expo Electr Power Eng EPE 2016*. 2016 Dec 9;304–8.
14. Williamson K. Health on the horizon: The power of remote patient monitoring [Internet]. [cited 2024 Apr 3]. Available from: https://www.asianhhm.com/articles/health-on-the-horizon-the-power-of-remote-patient-monitoring
15. Panneerselvam P. Application of embedded system for a genetic disease, sickle cell anemia. *2014 Int Conf Adv Electr Eng* [Internet]. 2014 Jan [cited 2024 Apr 3];1–4. Available from: https://ieeexplore.ieee.org/document/6838446/
16. Cheikhrouhou O, Mershad K, Jamil F, Mahmud R, Koubaa A, Moosavi SR. A lightweight blockchain and fog-enabled secure remote patient monitoring system. *Internet of Things*. 2023 Jul;22:100691.
17. Ghasemzadeh H, Ostadabbas S, Guenterberg E, Pantelopoulos A. Wireless medical-embedded systems: A review of signal-processing techniques for classification. *IEEE Sens J*. 2013;13 [2]:423–37.
18. Koopman P. Embedded system security. *Computer [Long Beach Calif]*. 2004 Jul;37 [7]:95–7.
19. Research T. MRI contrast media agents market – Global industry size, share, trends, opportunity, and forecast, 2018–2028 segmented by products [superparamagnetic agents, paramagnetic agents], by type [clinical, preclinical], by application [gastrointestinal, intraven] [Internet]. 2023 [cited 2024 Apr 3]. p. 1–171. Available from: https://www.marketresearch.com/TechSci-Research-v3895/MRI-Contrast-Media-Agents-Global-35295318/

20. Mahmood SN, Ercelecbi E. Development of blood pressure monitor by using capacitive pressure sensor and microcontroller. *Int Iraqi Conf Eng Technol its Appl IICETA 2018.* 2018 Sep 7;96–100.
21. Das DM, Gupta A, Srivastava A, Vidwans A, Ahmad M, Shelke A, et al. A pulse oximeter system, OxiSense, with embedded signal processing using an ultra-low power ASIC designed for testability. *Microelectronics J.* 2018 Feb 1;72:1–10.
22. Liu J, Yang Y. Implement and design on the embedded sleep monitoring system based on fuzzy control. *2010 Int Conf Comput Des Appl ICCDA 2010.* 2010;1.
23. Dabiri F, Massey T, Noshadi H, Hagopian H, Lin CK, Tan R, et al. A telehealth architecture for networked embedded systems: A case study in In Vivo health monitoring. *IEEE Trans Inf Technol Biomed.* 2009;13 [3]:351–9.
24. Niepceron B, Nait-Sidi-Moh A, Grassia F. Moving medical image analysis to GPU embedded systems: Application to brain tumor segmentation. *Appl Artif Intell* [Internet]. 2020 Oct 14 [cited 2024 Apr 30];866–79. Available from: https://www.tandfonline.com/doi/abs/10.1080/08839514.2020.1787678
25. Li C, Balla-Arabé S, Yang F. Embedded multi-spectral image processing for real-time medical application. *J Syst Archit.* 2016 Mar 1;64:26–36.
26. Al-Odat ZA, Srinivasan SK, Al-Qtiemat EM, Shuja S. A reliable IoT-based embedded health care system for diabetic patients. 2019 Aug 16 [cited 2024 Apr 30]; Available from: https://arxiv.org/abs/1908.06086v1
27. Kim J, Kim E, Kyung Y, Ko H. A study on ECG monitoring embedded systems. *Int Conf ICT Converg. 2022.* 2022 October:1671–3.
28. Mhamdi L, Dammak O, Cottin F, Dhaou I Ben. Artificial Intelligence for cardiac diseases diagnosis and prediction using ECG images on embedded systems. Biomed. 2022;10:2013 [Internet]. Available from: https://www.mdpi.com/2227-9059/10/8/2013/htm
29. Hu J. Development of wearable health monitoring devices based on embedded technology. *2024 Int Conf Integr Circuits Commun Syst* [Internet]. 2024 Feb 23 [cited 2024 Apr 30];1–5. Available from: https://ieeexplore.ieee.org/document/10498459/
30. Diab MS, Rodriguez-Villegas E. Embedded machine learning using microcontrollers in wearable and ambulatory systems for health and care applications: A review. *IEEE Access.* 2022;10:98450–74.
31. Kuroda T, Sasaki H, Suenaga T, Masuda Y, Yasumuro Y, Hori K, et al. Embedded ubiquitous services on hospital information systems. *IEEE Trans Inf Technol Biomed.* 2012;16 [6]:1216–23.
32. Kakkar V. An ultra low power system architecture for implantable medical devices. *IEEE Access.* 2019 Jan 26;7:111160–7.
33. Khan W, Muntimadugu E, Jaffe M, Domb AJ. Implantable medical devices. 2014 [cited 2024 Apr 29];33–59. Available from: https://link.springer.com/chapter/10.1007/978-1-4614-9434-8_2
34. Ahmed S, Kakkar V. An electret-based angular electrostatic energy harvester for battery-less cardiac and neural implants. *IEEE Access.* 2017 Aug 12;5:19631–43.
35. Santa W, Jensen R, Miesel K, Carlson D, Avestruz A, Molnar G, et al. Radios for the brain? A practical micropower sensing and algorithm architecture for neurostimulators. *Proc – IEEE Int Symp Circuits Syst* [Internet]. 2008 [cited 2024 Apr 30];348–51. Available from: https://experts.umn.edu/en/publications/radios-for-the-brain-a-practical-micropower-sensing-and-algorithm
36. Wang A, Chandrakasan A. A 180mV FFT processor using subthreshold circuit techniques. *Dig Tech Pap – IEEE Int Solid-State Circuits Conf.* 2004;47, 292–529.
37. Zhai B, Hanson S, Blaauw D, Sylvester D. A variation-tolerant sub-200 mV 6-T subthreshold SRAM. *IEEE J Solid-State Circuits.* 2008 Oct;43 [10]:2338–48.

38. Doughty K, Cameron K, Garner P. Three generations of telecare of the elderly. *J Telemed Telecare*. 1996 Jun 1;2 [2]:71–80.
39. Wilkinson M. Medical market for microsystems. *MST News*. 2002; 12[1]:37–8.
40. Lymberis A, Gatzoulis L. Wearable health systems: From smart technologies to real applications. *Annu Int Conf IEEE Eng Med Biol – Proc*. 2006;6789–92.
41. Obeidat YM, Alqudah AM. An embedded system based on Raspberry Pi for effective electrocardiogram monitoring. *Appl Sci*. 2023 Jul;13 [14]:8273.
42. Wang C, Yao C, Chen P, Shi J, Gu Z, Zhou Z. Artificial Intelligence algorithm with ICD coding technology guided by embedded electronic medical record system in medical record information management. *Microprocess Microsyst* [Internet]. 2023 Oct 13 [cited 2024 Apr 3];104962. Available from: https://linkinghub.elsevier.com/retrieve/pii/S0141933123002065
43. Ricci S, Dallai A, Boni E, Bassi L, Guidi F, Cellai A, et al. Embedded System for Real-Time Digital Processing of Medical Ultrasound Doppler Signals. *EURASIP J Adv Signal Process 2008 20081* [Internet]. 2008 Apr 30 [cited 2024 Apr 3];2008 [1]:1–7. Available from: https://asp-eurasipjournals.springeropen.com/articles/10.1155/2008/418235
44. Mahmood AF, Alkababji AM, Daood A. Resilient embedded system for classification respiratory diseases in a real time. *Biomed Signal Process Control*. 2024 Apr 1;90:105876.

3 Automation of Medical Devices with Embedded Systems

Phool Chandra, Shahjad, Neetu Sachan, and Arun Kumar

3.1 INTRODUCTION

Embedded systems have become an integral part of modern medical devices, enabling precise control, monitoring, and advanced functionality. These specialized computer systems are designed to perform specific tasks within the medical device, ensuring reliable and efficient operation. The integration of embedded systems has revolutionized the healthcare industry, providing advanced diagnostic and therapeutic capabilities, improving patient care, and enhancing overall treatment outcomes. Embedded systems in medical devices typically consist of a microprocessor or microcontroller, memory, input/output (I/O) interfaces, and specialized software or firmware. They are designed to be compact, energy-efficient, and capable of executing specific functions with high reliability and performance. These systems are often required to operate in real time, ensuring timely response and accurate execution of critical tasks. The applications of embedded systems in medical devices are vast and diverse, ranging from simple devices like thermometers and blood pressure monitors to complex life-support systems, surgical robots, and advanced imaging equipment. In patient monitoring devices, such as electrocardiographs (ECGs), pulse oximeters, and respiratory monitors, embedded systems collect and process physiological data from sensors, enabling real-time monitoring and alerting healthcare professionals to any abnormalities. Therapeutic devices like insulin pumps, pacemakers, and defibrillators rely on embedded systems for precise control and delivery of medications or electrical stimuli, ensuring accurate dosing and timely interventions. Advanced imaging modalities, including computed tomography (CT) scanners, magnetic resonance imaging (MRI) machines, and ultrasound systems, leverage embedded systems for data acquisition, image reconstruction, and user interface control. Robotic-assisted surgery is another area where embedded systems play a crucial role, enabling precise control of robotic arms, real-time visual feedback, and integration with surgical planning software. Additionally, implantable medical devices, such as cochlear implants, deep brain stimulators, and implantable cardioverter-defibrillators (ICDs), rely on embedded systems for precise control and monitoring, ensuring the safe and effective operation of these life-saving devices (1–6).

DOI: 10.1201/9781003508199-3

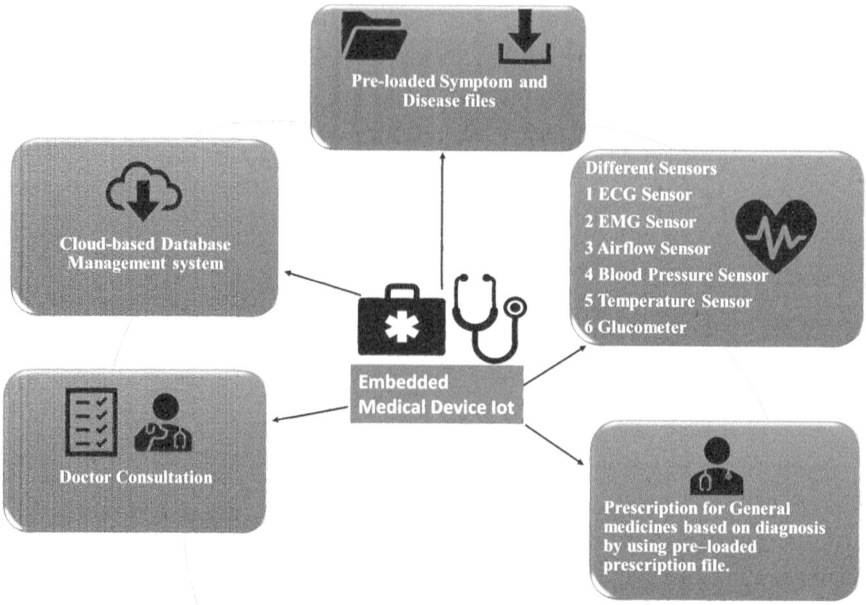

FIGURE 3.1 Embedded medical devices.

Embedded systems are computer systems designed to perform specific dedicated functions within larger systems or devices (Figure 3.1). These systems are ubiquitous and found in a wide range of applications, from consumer electronics and industrial automation to automotive and medical devices. Embedded systems are characterized by their compact size, low power consumption, real-time performance, and reliable operation. At the heart of an embedded system is a microprocessor or microcontroller, which executes the system's software or firmware. These systems often have limited memory and processing resources compared to general-purpose computers, requiring optimization for efficient performance and resource utilization. Embedded systems typically integrate various peripherals, such as sensors, actuators, communication interfaces, and user interfaces, to interact with the external environment and perform their intended functions. Embedded systems can be classified based on their performance, complexity, and application domains. Some examples include: Microcontroller-based Systems: These systems are based on low-power microcontrollers and are used in simple applications like home appliances, toys, and basic control systems. Real-time Embedded Systems: These systems are designed to respond to events within specific time constraints, ensuring deterministic behavior. Examples include industrial control systems, robotics, and automotive control systems. Networked Embedded Systems: These systems incorporate communication capabilities, enabling them to exchange data and interact with other devices or systems over various networks, such as the Internet of Things (IoT) devices. Safety-critical Embedded Systems: These systems demand high levels of reliability and fault tolerance, as their failure could result in catastrophic consequences. Examples include medical devices, aerospace systems, and nuclear power plant control systems (7–9).

The evolution of medical device technology has been driven by the integration of embedded systems, enabling advanced capabilities, improved patient care, and enhanced treatment outcomes. Embedded systems have become indispensable components in modern medical devices, facilitating precise control, real-time monitoring, and seamless integration with various sensors, actuators, and user interfaces. The adoption of embedded systems in medical devices has been fueled by several factors, including technological advancements, increasing healthcare demands, and the need for improved patient safety and efficacy. These specialized computer systems have revolutionized the healthcare industry by providing advanced diagnostic and therapeutic capabilities, enabling remote monitoring, and enhancing overall treatment efficiency. One of the key roles of embedded systems in medical devices is real-time data acquisition and processing. These systems collect and analyze physiological data from various sensors, such as electrocardiograms (ECGs), pulse oximeters, and respiratory monitors, enabling real-time monitoring and alerting healthcare professionals to any abnormalities. This real-time monitoring capability is crucial in critical care settings, allowing for timely interventions and potentially life-saving decisions. Embedded systems also play a vital role in therapeutic devices, such as insulin pumps, pacemakers, and defibrillators. These systems precisely control the delivery of medications or electrical stimuli, ensuring accurate dosing and timely interventions. Furthermore, embedded systems are essential components in implantable medical devices, like cochlear implants, deep brain stimulators, and ICDs, enabling precise control and monitoring of these life-saving devices. Advanced imaging modalities, including CT scanners, MRI machines, and ultrasound systems, heavily rely on embedded systems for data acquisition, image reconstruction, and user interface control. Additionally, robotic-assisted surgery leverages embedded systems for precise control of robotic arms, real-time visual feedback, and integration with surgical planning software (10–12).

3.2 SIGNIFICANCE OF AUTOMATION IN HEALTHCARE

The healthcare industry has witnessed a profound transformation driven by the integration of automation and embedded systems in medical devices. Automation has become a significant driving force, enabling enhanced patient care, improved efficiency, and better treatment outcomes. Embedded systems, as specialized computer systems designed to perform dedicated functions within medical devices, play a crucial role in facilitating automation and revolutionizing healthcare delivery (Table 3.1) (13, 14).

3.2.1 Real-time Monitoring and Decision Support

Embedded systems in medical devices enable real-time monitoring and decision support by continuously collecting and analyzing physiological data from various sensors, such as electrocardiograms (ECGs), pulse oximeters, and respiratory monitors. This data is processed using advanced algorithms and artificial intelligence (AI) techniques, allowing for the detection of patterns and anomalies that may indicate potential health risks or deteriorating conditions. For example, in intensive care units (ICUs), embedded systems integrated into patient monitoring devices can analyze

TABLE 3.1
Applications of Automation in Healthcare

S. No.	Applications	Description	Ref.
1.	Compile the patient's medical history accurately	• Accurately gathering a patient's medical history is one of a physician's most important responsibilities. Because the patient is not a specialist and is unaware of the data, this is frequently challenging. With the use of machine learning (ML), medical professionals can precisely gather patient history and healthcare management data to determine the most pertinent questions to pose to patients depending on a number of variables. • It provides a forecast of the most likely circumstances in addition to helping to gather crucial data.	(15)
2.	Boost the quality of the experience of receiving medical care	• The main objective of platforms with machine learning assistance is to enhance the quality of healthcare services for the largest possible group of individuals. • Maximizing profit is the ultimate goal of systems that have previously been implemented in traditional businesses. Strong machine learning technologies hospital operations management needs to set itself apart from conventional systems by fusing compassion with a desire to turn a profit. • The pharmaceutical industry is using machine learning (ML) techniques more and more to tackle the incredibly difficult task of finding effective new drugs.	(16)
3.	Enhance the process of treatment	• By increasing patient involvement, machine learning (ML) can enhance the therapy process and, thus, Adoption of health outcomes can greatly enhance almost every procedure in the healthcare industry. • When hundreds of handwritten document scans are mixed with fragmented, duplicated, or missing data, it might result in a lack of understanding and inaccurate conclusions. For ML algorithms to effectively use the data, it must therefore first be cleaned and presented correctly.	(17, 18)
4.	Robotic surgery and more image-guided medical procedures	• ML tools are very valuable since they improve the surgeon's display by providing data such as where the cancer is during robotic surgery and other image-guided treatments. • ML platforms and technologies are very helpful to radiologists. Many healthcare organizations are currently digitizing exabytes of medical data. To support robotics treatments, robust and flexible AI-enabled solutions are needed to link to many patient databases and analyze a complex range of data types. • The systems that have been built ought to have the capacity to fully reveal hidden patterns. In order to allow physicians and other healthcare professionals to work on their output with complete confidence and transparency and to support the better implementation of robotic and image-guided processes, they should also be able to convert and depict their findings into human-readable forms.	(19)

5.	Find a health issue	• By analyzing vast amounts of patient data, doctors can use machine learning (ML) to identify health issues before they develop into diseases. This is one of the main uses of ML in healthcare. Clinical facilities can use machine learning (ML) in healthcare to evaluate heart health, identify other problems, and predict strokes based on pre-existing medical disorders. • Since ML algorithms provide real-time data and analysis, medical professionals and specialists can diagnose potential much earlier. Healthcare workers may automate a lot of administrative tasks with machine learning (ML) to improve patient care. Early on in the study of medications, this technology can be useful. Research and development technologies like next-generation sequencing and precision medicine already have a significant influence on it. These technologies are used to find alternate therapeutic pathways for complex ailments.	(20)
6.	Clinical trials	• ML has many uses in the healthcare industry, including research and clinical trials. It helps researchers by predicting which patients would be the best candidates for clinical trials, which lowers the chance of error. It looks at a variety of data points, including medical history, therapies, and health, and determines who can participate in clinical trials. Businesses can provide real-time data about study participants in the healthcare industry. It's an efficient way to make decisions and adjust testing procedures when new predictions emerge. ML improves patient health by responding to common questions via apps. Artificial intelligence bots can identify patterns in patients' requests and forward them to the relevant doctor.	(21)
7.	Radiology	• ML has shown to be quite helpful in radiology. Numerous discrete variables can be found in medical image analysis that are always ready to go. In this case, ML-based algorithms are useful. ML algorithms are able to diagnose and identify the variables of interest more accurately because they are trained on a broad variety of data samples. • Machine learning (ML) is used in medical image analysis to classify objects, such as lesions, into multiple categories, including normal, aberrant, lesion or non-lesion, benign, malignant, and so on. • ML enables devices and machines to complete their tasks. One of the things machine learning (ML) has brought to the healthcare industry is robotic surgery. • A lot of experts think the application has promise. It is beneficial for robotic surgery, surgeon skill assessment, and workflow patterns.	(22)
8.	Creation of innovative medical techniques	• ML is currently on its way to being an essential part of healthcare systems, helping with everything from the creation of new medical treatments to the administration of patient data and records. • The emergence of machine learning software makes it possible to foresee a time when medical practitioners would use analytics and data to streamline processes and complete tasks. Globally, epidemic monitoring and prediction is currently being done using ML and AI-based technologies. • These days, scientists have access to a vast amount of information gathered from websites, social media posts made in real time, and satellite data. Data collection and prediction for a wide range of topics, including severe chronic infectious diseases and malaria outbreaks, are facilitated by artificial neural networks.	(23)

(Continued)

TABLE 3.1 (CONTINUED)
Applications of Automation in Healthcare

S. No.	Applications	Description	Ref.
9.	Boost the precision of the diagnosis	• It is anticipated that machine learning (ML) would increase diagnostic accuracy and reduce over-testing as the algorithm learns to send patients exclusively for high-value tests. • Machine learning algorithms based on medical imaging recognition will be a big help to radiologists and anatomic pathologists in their work. With the use of ML models on streaming data, many of the jobs currently carried out by anesthesiologists and critical care staff are probably going to be automated. • As machine learning (ML) technology develops, new ecosystems and solutions—like augmented reality and the Internet of Things—are penetrating the life sciences and healthcare sectors. • Because machine learning (ML) uses sophisticated algorithms, white-box testing is more important than functional testing. • As ML becomes more popular, a number of businesses are attempting to establish themselves in the healthcare industry.	(24, 25)
10.	Treats blood cancer with assistance	• Blood cancer and other diseases are now treated by ML. With their well-known cancer knowledge, all patients can choose the optimal course of action. Even while data entry is now easier to access thanks to technology, some tasks still take a long time. Keeping current health records requires a lot of work and attention every day. • By keeping track of medical records, ML has joined the market to save time, money, and effort. Many machine learning techniques are being employed globally to track and predict epidemics. This has access to the enormous volumes of data gathered from social networking sites, websites, satellites, and other sources. With the use of artificial neural networks, humans can communicate with information and predict anything from small illnesses to serious, long-term infectious diseases.	(26, 27)

multiple data streams simultaneously, including heart rate, blood pressure, oxygen saturation levels, and respiratory rates. By leveraging machine learning algorithms, these systems can identify early warning signs of sepsis, a life-threatening condition caused by the body's response to infection. Early detection and intervention can significantly improve patient outcomes and reduce mortality rates associated with sepsis. Similarly, embedded systems in wearable devices can monitor patients' activity levels, sleep patterns, and vital signs, providing valuable insights into their overall health and well-being. This continuous monitoring can aid in the early detection of chronic conditions, such as heart disease or diabetes, allowing for timely interventions and improved disease management (28–30).

3.2.2 Automated Therapeutic Interventions

The integration of embedded systems in therapeutic devices has enabled precise control and automated delivery of medications or therapeutic interventions, significantly improving patient safety and treatment efficacy. Insulin pumps, for instance, leverage embedded systems to monitor blood glucose levels in real time and automatically deliver the appropriate insulin dosage based on sophisticated algorithms and patient-specific parameters. This closed-loop system, often referred to as an artificial pancreas, can maintain optimal blood glucose levels, reducing the risk of complications associated with diabetes, such as hypoglycemia and hyperglycemia. Implantable medical devices, like pacemakers and defibrillators, rely on embedded systems for precise control and monitoring of heart function. These systems can detect abnormal heart rhythms and automatically deliver electrical impulses to restore normal heart function, potentially preventing life-threatening arrhythmias and cardiac arrests. Advanced algorithms and machine learning techniques can be employed to personalize the therapy based on individual patient characteristics and response to treatment. Furthermore, embedded systems in drug delivery systems can automate the administration of medications, ensuring accurate dosing and adherence to treatment regimens. This is particularly beneficial for patients with chronic conditions or those requiring complex medication schedules, reducing the risk of medication errors and improving treatment outcomes (31, 32).

3.2.3 Robotic-Assisted Surgery and Precision Medicine

The integration of embedded systems in robotic-assisted surgical systems has revolutionized the field of precision medicine, enabling surgeons to perform complex procedures with enhanced precision, dexterity, and control. Embedded systems play a crucial role in controlling the robotic arms, providing real-time visual feedback, and integrating with surgical planning software. These systems allow for minimally invasive procedures, reducing patient trauma, blood loss, and recovery times. Additionally, robotic-assisted surgery can enhance surgical precision, enabling more accurate tumor resections or delicate procedures, such as those performed in neurosurgery or cardiovascular surgery. Advanced imaging modalities, like CT scanners and MRI machines, heavily rely on embedded systems for data acquisition, image reconstruction, and visualization. These systems enable precise diagnosis and treatment planning, contributing to the development of personalized treatment plans tailored to individual patient needs. Moreover, embedded systems can integrate with surgical navigation systems, providing real-time guidance and visualization during procedures. This integration enhances surgical accuracy and reduces the risk of complications, leading to improved patient outcomes (33–36).

3.2.4 Remote Patient Monitoring and Telehealth

The COVID-19 pandemic has accelerated the adoption of telehealth and remote patient monitoring, further highlighting the significance of embedded systems in medical devices. Wearable devices and mobile health (mHealth) applications, powered by embedded systems, enable continuous monitoring of patients' vital signs, activity levels, and adherence to treatment plans, even in remote settings. These embedded systems can securely transmit data to healthcare providers, enabling real-time monitoring and timely interventions without the need for in-person visits. For instance, patients with chronic conditions, such as heart failure or chronic obstructive pulmonary disease (COPD), can be monitored remotely, allowing healthcare providers to track their condition and adjust treatment plans as needed. Remote patient monitoring can also be valuable in post-operative care, enabling healthcare providers to monitor patients' recovery and detect potential complications early, reducing the need for hospital readmissions. Furthermore, telehealth solutions powered by embedded systems can facilitate virtual consultations, enabling patients to access healthcare services from the comfort of their homes, particularly in remote or underserved areas. This not only improves access to healthcare but also reduces the risk of exposure to infectious diseases and minimizes the burden on healthcare facilities (37, 38).

3.2.5 Cybersecurity and Privacy Considerations

As the integration of embedded systems in medical devices continues to grow, addressing cybersecurity and privacy concerns becomes paramount. Embedded systems can be vulnerable to cyber threats, such as hacking, malware, and unauthorized access, which can compromise patient data and potentially disrupt critical medical devices. Researchers are actively developing secure boot mechanisms, data encryption techniques, access control mechanisms, and vulnerability detection methods to enhance the cybersecurity of embedded systems in medical devices. Additionally, privacy-preserving techniques, such as differential privacy and secure multi-party computation, are being explored to ensure the protection of sensitive patient data while enabling collaborative data analysis and research. Regulatory bodies and industry standards play a crucial role in establishing guidelines and best practices for cybersecurity and privacy in medical devices, ensuring the safe and secure deployment of these embedded systems (39, 40).

3.2.6 Interoperability and Integration

The seamless integration of medical devices with healthcare information systems and other devices is crucial for enabling effective automation and data exchange. Embedded systems must be designed to support standardized communication protocols, data formats, and interoperability frameworks to facilitate the exchange of data and ensure compatibility between different devices and systems. Researchers are exploring plug-and-play interoperability solutions, enabling medical devices to

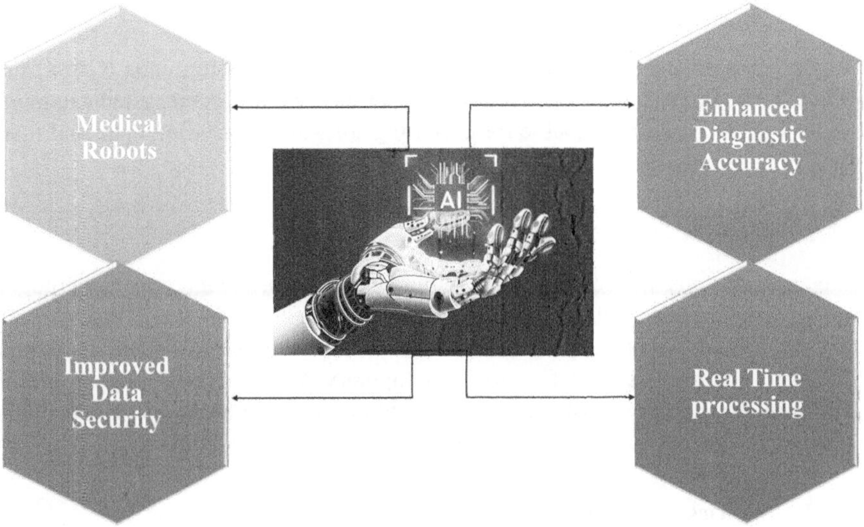
Medical Robots
Enhanced Diagnostic Accuracy
AI
Improved Data Security
Real Time processing

FIGURE 3.2 Embedded AI applications in the healthcare industry.

automatically discover and connect with other devices or systems, streamlining the integration process, and reducing the risk of errors. Furthermore, the development of standard-based patient data exchange models and interoperability frameworks can facilitate the efficient exchange of patient data across different healthcare providers and systems, enabling coordinated care and improved treatment outcomes. Overall, the significance of automation in healthcare, driven by embedded systems in medical devices, cannot be overstated. From real-time monitoring and decision support to automated therapeutic interventions, robotic-assisted surgery, remote patient monitoring, and telehealth, these systems have the potential to revolutionize healthcare delivery, improve patient outcomes, and enhance access to quality care (Figure 3.2) (41, 42).

Embedded systems are at the heart of modern medical devices, enabling precise control, monitoring, and advanced functionality. These specialized computer systems are designed to perform specific tasks within the medical device, ensuring reliable and efficient operation. The integration of embedded systems has revolutionized the healthcare industry by providing advanced diagnostic and therapeutic capabilities, improving patient care, and enhancing overall treatment outcomes (43).

The key components and technologies that enable embedded systems in medical devices are as given in the following section.

3.3 HARDWARE COMPONENTS OF EMBEDDED SYSTEMS

Embedded systems in medical devices rely on various hardware components to perform their functions effectively and reliably. These components work together to enable precise control, monitoring, data processing, and communication capabilities. The hardware components commonly found in embedded systems for medical devices include (44).

3.3.1 Microprocessors and Microcontrollers

Microprocessors and microcontrollers are the central processing units (CPUs) that execute instructions and control the overall operation of embedded systems in medical devices. They are responsible for executing software, processing data, and managing peripherals (45).

3.3.2 Memory Technologies

Embedded systems in medical devices require various types of memory technologies to store program code, data, and configuration settings. Flash Memory: Non-volatile memory used for storing program code and firmware. RAM (Random Access Memory): Volatile memory for storing temporary data and executing programs. EEPROM (Electrically Erasable Programmable Read-Only Memory): Non-volatile memory for storing configuration settings and calibration data (46).

3.3.3 Sensors and Actuators

Embedded systems in medical devices often interact with various sensors and actuators to monitor physiological parameters, deliver therapies, or control device functions. Sensors: Electrocardiogram (ECG), pulse oximeters, blood pressure monitors, temperature sensors, and imaging sensors. Actuators: Insulin pumps, pacemakers, robotic surgical tools, and drug delivery systems (47).

3.3.4 Communication Interfaces

Embedded systems in medical devices often require communication interfaces to exchange data with other devices, healthcare information systems, or remote monitoring platforms. Wired Interfaces: USB, Ethernet, serial ports (UART, SPI, I2C). Wireless Interfaces: Bluetooth, Wi-Fi, Zigbee, and cellular networks (3G, 4G, 5G). Power Management and Energy Efficiency.

Power management and energy efficiency are crucial considerations for medical devices, particularly implantable and wearable devices with limited battery life (48).

3.3.5 Security Hardware

Ensuring the security and privacy of patient data and device operations is a critical requirement for medical devices. Embedded systems may incorporate dedicated hardware security components, such as: Secure Enclaves: Isolated hardware environments for secure execution and data protection. Cryptographic Accelerators: Hardware modules for efficient encryption and decryption operations. Trusted Platform Modules (TPM): Hardware-based security solutions for secure boot, key storage, and platform integrity verification (49).

3.3.6 Input/Output (I/O) Interfaces

Embedded systems in medical devices often require various input/output (I/O) interfaces to interact with users, display information, or control external devices. User Input Interfaces: Buttons, switches, touchscreens, and voice recognition modules.

Display Interfaces: LCD screens, LED displays, and graphical user interfaces (GUI). Device Control Interfaces: General-purpose input/output (GPIO) pins, analog-to-digital converters (ADCs), and digital-to-analog converters (DACs) (50).

3.3.7 Real-Time Clocks (RTC)

Real-time clocks (RTCs) are essential components in embedded systems for medical devices, providing accurate timekeeping and scheduling capabilities for time-critical tasks and event logging (51).

3.3.8 Printed Circuit Boards (PCBs)

Printed circuit boards (PCBs) serve as the foundation for integrating and interconnecting the various hardware components of embedded systems in medical devices. They provide physical support, power distribution, and signal routing (52).

3.4 SOFTWARE FOR MEDICAL DEVICE AUTOMATION

Software plays a vital role in enabling automation in medical devices, allowing for precise control, monitoring, and decision support. As embedded systems in medical devices become more sophisticated, the software components have evolved to provide advanced functionality, interoperability, and compliance with regulatory standards. The following sections delve into various aspects of software for medical device automation, supported by recent research papers and studies (53).

3.4.1 Real-Time Operating Systems (RTOS)

Real-time operating systems (RTOS) are essential for medical devices that require deterministic behavior and predictable response times. These operating systems are designed to handle time-critical tasks, multitasking, and resource management efficiently, ensuring that critical operations are executed within specified time constraints. This comprehensive survey paper examines the role of RTOS in medical embedded systems. It provides an overview of RTOS concepts, architectures, and scheduling algorithms, and discusses their applications in various medical devices, such as patient monitoring systems, surgical robots, and implantable devices (54).

3.4.2 Device Drivers and Firmware

Device drivers and firmware are low-level software components that interact directly with the hardware components of medical devices. They provide an abstraction layer, enabling higher-level software to communicate with sensors, actuators, and other peripherals. This chapter provides a comprehensive overview of ARM-based microcontrollers and their applications in biomedical systems. It covers firmware development, device driver implementation, and interfacing techniques for various biomedical sensors and actuators, such as ECG sensors, pulse oximeters, and insulin pumps (55).

3.4.3 Data Acquisition and Processing

Medical devices often require software for data acquisition and processing, including algorithms for signal processing, data filtering, and feature extraction. These software components enable accurate interpretation of physiological data and facilitate decision-making processes. This research paper proposes an AI-based embedded system for healthcare cyber-physical systems. It discusses the integration of machine learning algorithms and data processing techniques for accurate physiological signal analysis, anomaly detection, and decision support, while ensuring data protection and privacy (56).

3.4.4 Control Systems and Automation

Control systems and automation software are essential for medical devices that deliver therapies or perform automated tasks. These software components implement control algorithms, decision logic, and safety mechanisms to ensure precise and reliable operation. This research paper focuses on embedded actuators and control systems for smart medical devices. It discusses various control strategies, such as proportional-integral-derivative (PID) control, model predictive control, and adaptive control, for precise and reliable actuation in applications like robotic surgery, prosthetics, and drug delivery systems (57).

3.4.5 Communication and Networking

Software for communication and networking is crucial for medical devices that need to exchange data with other systems or remote monitoring platforms. This includes protocols, middleware, and interfaces for wired and wireless communication. This paper discusses the role of wireless body area networks (WBANs) in enabling integrated remote healthcare IoT applications. It covers various communication protocols, such as Bluetooth, ZigBee, and Wi-Fi, and their suitability for different medical device applications, considering factors like data rate, power consumption, and reliability (58).

3.4.6 Security and Cybersecurity

Ensuring the security and privacy of patient data and device operations is a critical requirement for medical device software. This includes secure boot mechanisms, data encryption, access control, and vulnerability detection and mitigation techniques. This review paper provides a comprehensive overview of the current challenges and solutions in medical device cybersecurity. It discusses various security threats, such as unauthorized access, malware attacks, and data breaches, and presents techniques for secure boot, data encryption, access control, and vulnerability management in medical devices (59).

3.5 SENSOR TECHNOLOGIES AND DATA ACQUISITION

In the field of medical devices, sensor technologies and data acquisition play a crucial role in enabling accurate monitoring, diagnosis, and treatment. These technologies are essential for collecting and processing physiological data, providing healthcare professionals with valuable insights and facilitating informed decision-making. The integration of advanced sensor technologies and data acquisition systems has revolutionized various medical applications, from patient monitoring and diagnostics to therapeutic interventions and surgical procedures (60).

3.5.1 Wearable and Implantable Sensors

Wearable and implantable sensors have gained significant attention in recent years, enabling continuous monitoring of vital signs and physiological parameters in real time. These sensors can be integrated into medical devices or worn as standalone devices, allowing for remote patient monitoring and personalized healthcare. This research paper provides a comprehensive review of wearable sensors and their applications in remote monitoring of physiological signals in healthcare. It covers various types of wearable sensors, such as electrocardiogram (ECG), electromyogram (EMG), electroencephalogram (EEG), and photoplethysmogram (PPG) sensors, and discusses signal processing techniques for accurate data acquisition and analysis (61).

3.5.2 Biomedical Imaging Sensors

Biomedical imaging sensors play a vital role in medical diagnostics and treatment planning. These sensors are employed in various imaging modalities, such as CT, MRI, and ultrasound, providing detailed visualizations of internal structures and facilitating accurate diagnosis and monitoring of various medical conditions. This research paper reviews the recent advances in biomedical imaging sensors and signal processing techniques for healthcare applications. It covers various imaging modalities, including CT, MRI, and ultrasound, and discusses the latest developments in sensor technologies, image reconstruction algorithms, and signal processing methods for improved image quality and clinical utility (62).

3.5.3 Biosignal Acquisition and Processing

Biosignal acquisition and processing are essential components in medical devices for monitoring and analyzing physiological signals, such as electrocardiograms (ECG), electromyograms (EMG), and electroencephalograms (EEG). These systems involve specialized sensors, signal conditioning circuits, and advanced signal processing algorithms to extract meaningful information from the acquired data. This research paper, in addition to covering wearable sensors, also discusses various signal-processing techniques for accurate biosignal acquisition and analysis. It covers topics such as noise reduction, feature extraction, and classification algorithms for ECG, EMG, and EEG signals (63).

3.5.4 Sensor Fusion and Multi-sensor Integration

Sensor fusion and multi-sensor integration are emerging trends in medical devices, combining data from multiple sensors to obtain a more comprehensive understanding of physiological processes and improve diagnostic accuracy. These techniques leverage advanced data fusion algorithms and machine learning approaches to enhance the reliability and robustness of the acquired data. This research paper, in addition to presenting the LCP-based multi-sensor platform, discusses the challenges and opportunities in multi-sensor integration for continuous health monitoring. The authors explore sensor fusion techniques and data fusion algorithms for integrating data from multiple sensors, such as ECG, bioimpedance, and temperature sensors (64).

3.5.5 Data Acquisition Systems and Interfaces

Data acquisition systems and interfaces play a crucial role in medical devices by providing the necessary infrastructure for collecting, transmitting, and processing sensor data. These systems often involve various communication protocols, data formats, and interfaces to ensure seamless integration with other components and systems. This research paper discusses the role of wireless body area networks (WBANs) in enabling integrated remote healthcare IoT applications. It covers various communication protocols and data acquisition interfaces, such as Bluetooth, ZigBee, and Wi-Fi, for transmitting and processing sensor data in medical devices and healthcare systems. This survey paper explores the concept of plug-and-play interoperability for medical devices, which enables seamless integration and data exchange among different devices and systems. It discusses various communication protocols, data formats, and interoperability standards, such as HL7, DICOM, and IHE, that facilitate data acquisition and integration in healthcare environments. The integration of advanced sensor technologies and data acquisition systems in medical devices has revolutionized the healthcare industry, enabling more accurate monitoring, diagnosis, and treatment. However, challenges such as sensor reliability, data security, and interoperability remain, and ongoing research efforts aim to address these issues and further enhance the capabilities of medical devices (65, 66).

3.6 DESIGN AND DEVELOPMENT OF AUTOMATED MEDICAL DEVICES

Automated medical devices have become increasingly important in modern healthcare, offering improved efficiency, accuracy, and patient safety. These devices leverage cutting-edge technologies, such as robotics, AI, and machine learning, to automate various medical procedures and processes. From robotic-assisted surgeries to intelligent diagnostic systems, automated medical devices are revolutionizing the way healthcare is delivered (67).

3.6.1 Robotic-Assisted Surgery

Robotic-assisted surgery has emerged as a game-changer in the field of minimally invasive procedures. These systems provide surgeons with enhanced dexterity, precision, and visualization capabilities, enabling them to perform complex operations with greater accuracy and control. One notable example is the da Vinci Surgical System, which has been widely adopted for procedures such as prostatectomies, hysterectomies, and cardiac surgeries (68). Researchers are continuously working on improving the capabilities of robotic surgical systems. For instance, a study by scientists explored the use of AI and machine learning algorithms to enhance the autonomous control of surgical robots, enabling them to adapt to dynamic environments and make real-time adjustments during procedures (69). Additionally, efforts are underway to develop smaller and more versatile robotic systems that can access hard-to-reach areas of the body, expanding the range of procedures that can benefit from robotic assistance (70).

3.6.2 Intelligent Diagnostic Systems

Advancements in AI and machine learning have paved the way for the development of intelligent diagnostic systems that can assist healthcare professionals in making accurate and timely diagnoses. These systems leverage vast amounts of medical data, including patient records, imaging studies, and laboratory results, to identify patterns and provide diagnostic recommendations. One notable example is the use of deep learning algorithms for image analysis in radiology. Researchers have developed AI-powered systems that can analyze medical images, such as X-rays, CT scans, and MRI scans, to detect abnormalities and assist radiologists in making more accurate diagnoses (71).

3.6.3 Automated Drug Delivery Systems

Automated drug delivery systems have become increasingly important in ensuring patient safety and adherence to medication regimens. These systems leverage advanced technologies to precisely control the dosage and timing of drug administration, reducing the risk of medication errors and potentially improving treatment outcomes. One example is the development of closed-loop insulin delivery systems for the management of diabetes. These systems combine continuous glucose monitoring (CGM) devices with insulin pumps, using algorithms to automatically adjust insulin delivery based on real-time glucose levels (72). This approach not only improves glycemic control but also reduces the burden on patients and caregivers, leading to better quality of life. Researchers are also exploring the use of automated drug delivery systems in other areas, such as pain management and chemotherapy administration (73).

3.7 CONCEPTUALIZATION AND PROTOTYPING

Conceptualization is the initial stage in the development of automated medical devices, where ideas are generated, evaluated, and refined. This phase lays the groundwork for subsequent stages by defining the problem, exploring potential solutions, and establishing design requirements. Effective conceptualization involves a multidisciplinary approach, drawing upon expertise from various fields, including medicine, engineering, computer science, and human factors. Needs Assessment and Problem Definition: The first step in conceptualization is to identify and define the specific healthcare problem or need that the automated medical device aims to address. This process involves gathering input from various stakeholders, including healthcare professionals, patients, and domain experts, to gain a comprehensive understanding of the problem (74). Ideation and Concept Generation: Once the problem is well-defined, the next step is to generate various conceptual solutions through ideation sessions. These sessions leverage techniques such as brainstorming, mind mapping, and design thinking methodologies to encourage creative thinking and foster innovation (75). Concept Evaluation and Selection: After generating multiple conceptual solutions, a rigorous evaluation process is undertaken to assess their feasibility, potential impact, and alignment with design requirements. This evaluation often involves techniques such as Pugh matrix analysis, analytical hierarchy process (AHP), or multi-criteria decision analysis (MCDA) (76). Preliminary Design and Refinement: The selected concept undergoes further refinement and development, resulting in a preliminary design that incorporates technical specifications, functional requirements, and user considerations. This stage may involve the creation of low-fidelity prototypes or computer-aided design (CAD) models to facilitate communication and gather feedback from stakeholders (77).

3.7.1 Prototyping: Bringing Concepts to Life

Prototyping is an iterative process that follows conceptualization, enabling developers to transform abstract ideas into tangible representations of the proposed automated medical device. Prototypes serve as a means to validate design concepts, identify potential issues, and gather feedback from users and stakeholders, ultimately improving the final product (78).

3.7.2 Rapid Prototyping Techniques

3D Printing: This technology has revolutionized prototyping by enabling the rapid and cost-effective production of physical models and components. 3D printing allows for the creation of intricate and customized designs, facilitating iterative refinement and testing. Virtual and Augmented Reality (VR/AR): VR and AR technologies provide immersive environments for prototyping and simulating the use of automated medical devices. These techniques enable designers and stakeholders to visualize and interact with virtual prototypes, facilitating evaluation and iteration (79).

3.7.3 Functional Prototyping

Breadboard Prototyping: This approach involves creating functional prototypes using off-the-shelf components and breadboards, allowing developers to test and refine the electronic and software aspects of the automated medical device (80). Rapid Control Prototyping: This technique focuses on developing and testing control systems and algorithms for automated medical devices. It leverages hardware-in-the-loop (HIL) simulations and rapid control prototyping platforms to evaluate performance and refine control strategies (81).

3.7.4 User Testing and Feedback

Usability Studies: Prototypes serve as valuable tools for conducting usability studies, enabling developers to gather feedback from potential users, including healthcare professionals and patients. These studies help identify usability issues, assess user experiences, and inform design improvements (82).

Clinical Simulations: In the context of medical devices, clinical simulations using prototypes are crucial for evaluating the device's performance and safety in controlled environments. These simulations involve role-playing scenarios with healthcare professionals and standardized patients to assess the device's functionality and potential risks (83).

3.7.5 Iterative Refinement

Design Iterations: Based on the feedback and insights gathered through prototyping and user testing, the design undergoes iterative refinement. This cyclical process allows developers to make necessary modifications, address identified issues, and incrementally improve the automated medical device's design (Figure 3.3) (84). Risk Mitigation: Prototyping plays a vital role in risk mitigation by enabling the identification and resolution of potential hazards and failure modes early in the development process. This proactive approach helps minimize risks and ensures a safer final product (85).

3.7.6 Robotic Exoskeleton for Stroke Rehabilitation

Conceptualization: The initial concept for this robotic exoskeleton emerged from the need to provide more effective and personalized rehabilitation for stroke patients. A multidisciplinary team, including neurologists, physical therapists, and robotics engineers, collaborated to define the design requirements, such as range of motion, adjustability, and integration with virtual reality environments (86). Prototyping: Early prototypes of the exoskeleton were developed using 3D printing and rapid prototyping techniques, allowing for iterative refinement of the design based on feedback from clinicians and patients. Virtual reality simulations were also used to test and optimize the integration of the exoskeleton with immersive therapy environments (87).

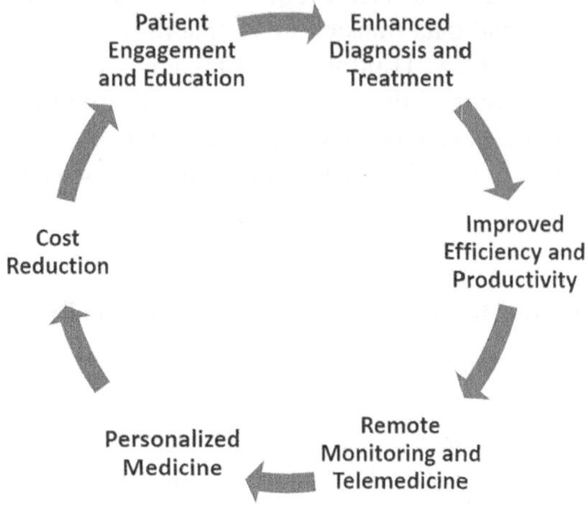

FIGURE 3.3 Benefits of AI and robotics in healthcare.

3.7.7 Automated Medication Dispensing System for Hospitals

Conceptualization: The concept for this automated medication dispensing system arose from the need to improve medication safety, efficiency, and inventory management in hospitals. A team of healthcare professionals, pharmacists, and software engineers defined the system requirements, such as barcode scanning, user authentication, and real-time inventory tracking (88). Prototyping: Functional prototypes were developed using breadboard prototyping and rapid control prototyping techniques, allowing for the testing and refinement of the system's hardware and software components. User testing with nurses and pharmacists was conducted to evaluate the system's usability, workflow integration, and potential for reducing medication errors (89).

3.7.8 AI-Powered Diagnostic System for Radiology

Conceptualization: The concept for this AI-powered diagnostic system emerged from the need to enhance the accuracy and efficiency of radiological image analysis. A team of radiologists, data scientists, and computer vision experts collaborated to define the system's requirements, such as the ability to detect and classify various abnormalities, integrate with existing medical imaging systems, and provide interpretable results. Prototyping: Initial prototypes were developed using machine learning algorithms and publicly available medical image datasets for training and validation. These prototypes were iteratively refined based on feedback from radiologists and performance evaluations. Virtual simulations were also used to test the integration of the AI system with existing radiology workflows and user interfaces (90, 91).

3.7.9 Wearable Sensor for Continuous Vital Sign Monitoring

Conceptualization: The concept for this wearable sensor emerged from the need for continuous and non-invasive monitoring of vital signs in various healthcare settings. A team comprising biomedical engineers, physiologists, and user experience designers defined the sensor's requirements, such as form factor, sensor accuracy, battery life, and data transmission capabilities. Prototyping: Rapid prototyping techniques, such as 3D printing and breadboard prototyping, were used to develop early prototypes of the wearable sensor. These prototypes were tested in simulated environments and on volunteers to evaluate the sensor's performance, comfort, and usability. Iterative refinements were made based on feedback and data analysis (92).

3.8 DESIGN CONSIDERATIONS FOR RELIABILITY AND SAFETY

The field of medical technology has witnessed a remarkable surge in the development of automated medical devices, revolutionizing the way healthcare is delivered. These devices play a crucial role in diagnosis, treatment, and monitoring, offering enhanced precision, efficiency, and patient care. However, ensuring their reliability and safety is of paramount importance, as any malfunction or error could have severe consequences for patients' well-being (93).

3.8.1 Risk Analysis and Management

Effective risk analysis and management are foundational to the design and development of reliable and safe automated medical devices. A comprehensive risk assessment should be conducted to identify potential hazards, evaluate their likelihood and severity, and implement appropriate risk control measures. This process involves systematic techniques such as Failure Mode and Effects Analysis (FMEA) and Fault Tree Analysis (FTA) to identify potential failure modes, their causes, and their effects on the device's performance and patient safety (94).

3.8.2 Human Factors Engineering

The integration of human factors engineering principles is crucial in the design of automated medical devices. These principles aim to optimize the interaction between the device, its users (healthcare professionals and patients), and the intended use environment. Considerations such as usability, intuitive user interfaces, ergonomics, and effective training and documentation can significantly reduce the risk of human errors, which are a major contributing factor to adverse events (95).

3.8.3 Redundancy and Fault Tolerance

Incorporating redundancy and fault tolerance mechanisms into the design of automated medical devices can enhance their reliability and safety. Redundancy involves the inclusion of backup components or systems that can take over in case of failure, ensuring continuous operation and minimizing the risk of complete system failure. Fault tolerance involves the ability of the device to detect and recover from faults, enabling it to continue functioning, albeit with reduced capabilities, until the fault is rectified or the device is replaced (96).

3.8.4 Software Validation and Verification

The software components of automated medical devices play a critical role in their functionality and performance. Rigorous software validation and verification processes are essential to ensure the software meets the specified requirements, functions as intended, and is free from defects or vulnerabilities. This includes comprehensive testing, code reviews, and the use of formal methods and model-checking techniques to verify the correctness and robustness of the software (97).

3.8.5 Cybersecurity and Data Privacy

With the increasing connectivity and integration of automated medical devices into healthcare networks, cybersecurity, and data privacy have become paramount concerns. Effective security measures must be implemented to protect these devices from unauthorized access, data breaches, and potential cyber-attacks. This includes robust authentication and encryption mechanisms, secure communication protocols, regular software updates and patching, and adherence to data privacy regulations such as HIPAA (Health Insurance Portability and Accountability Act) and GDPR (General Data Protection Regulation) (98).

3.8.6 Maintenance and Lifecycle Management

Proper maintenance and lifecycle management strategies are crucial for ensuring the reliable and safe operation of automated medical devices throughout their intended lifespan. This involves regular inspections, calibrations, and preventive maintenance to detect and address potential issues before they escalate. Additionally, effective obsolescence management and timely upgrades or replacements are necessary to keep up with technological advancements and evolving safety and regulatory requirements (99).

3.8.7 Regulatory Compliance and Quality Assurance

Automated medical devices are subject to stringent regulatory requirements and quality assurance standards to ensure their safety and efficacy. Adherence to regulatory guidelines, such as those set by the U.S. Food and Drug Administration (FDA) and international standards like IEC 60601 (Medical Electrical Equipment Safety), is crucial throughout the device's lifecycle. Implementing robust quality assurance processes, including design reviews, documentation, and post-market surveillance, can help maintain compliance and facilitate continuous improvement (100).

3.8.8 User Training and Education

Effective user training and education are essential for ensuring the safe and proper use of automated medical devices. Healthcare professionals and patients should receive comprehensive training on the device's operation, safety features, and troubleshooting procedures. Clear and concise user manuals, instructional videos, and ongoing training programs can help mitigate the risk of user errors and promote responsible device usage (101).

3.8.9 Post-market Surveillance and Incident Reporting

Continuous post-market surveillance and incident reporting systems are critical for monitoring the performance and safety of automated medical devices in real-world settings. Collecting and analyzing data on device failures, adverse events, and user feedback can help identify potential issues and inform necessary improvements or corrective actions. Establishing robust incident reporting mechanisms and fostering a culture of transparency and collaboration among manufacturers, regulatory bodies, and healthcare providers can contribute to enhanced device safety and patient well-being (102).

3.8.10 Ethical Considerations and Patient Safety

The design and development of automated medical devices should be guided by ethical principles and a steadfast commitment to patient safety. Considerations such as autonomy, beneficence, non-maleficence, and justice must be carefully weighed to ensure that the devices respect patient autonomy, maximize benefits, minimize risks and harm, and promote equitable access to healthcare. Additionally, safeguards should be implemented to prevent unintended harm, preserve patient privacy, and maintain human oversight and control over critical decision-making processes (103).

3.9 USER INTERFACE AND EXPERIENCE

In the rapidly evolving landscape of healthcare technology, automated medical devices have become indispensable tools for diagnosis, treatment, and monitoring. However, the efficacy and safety of these devices hinges not only on their technical capabilities but also on their user interface (UI) and user experience (UX) design. A well-designed UI and UX can significantly enhance the usability, efficiency, and safety of automated medical devices, ultimately leading to better patient outcomes (104).

3.9.1 Human Factors Engineering and Usability

Human factors engineering and usability are foundational principles that should guide the UI and UX design of automated medical devices. These principles aim to optimize the interaction between the device and its users, ensuring intuitive operation, minimizing the risk of user errors, and promoting efficient workflows. Conducting user research, task analyses, and usability testing can help identify potential usability issues and inform design iterations to enhance the overall user experience (105).

3.9.2 User-Centered Design Approach

Adopting a user-centered design approach is crucial for creating effective UI and UX solutions in automated medical devices. This approach involves actively engaging end-users (healthcare professionals, patients, or caregivers) throughout the design process, gathering their insights, and incorporating their feedback to ensure the final product meets their needs and expectations Collaborative design sessions, prototyping, and iterative testing can facilitate a deeper understanding of user requirements and preferences (106).

3.9.3 Intuitive Navigation and Information Architecture

The navigation and information architecture of automated medical devices should be intuitive and organized in a logical manner. Clear and consistent labeling, well-structured menus, and hierarchical organization of information can enhance the discoverability of features and reduce cognitive load for users. Incorporating familiar design patterns and adhering to industry standards can further improve the learnability and usability of the device's interface (107).

3.9.4 Visual Design and Accessibility

Effective visual design principles are essential for creating accessible and user-friendly interfaces in automated medical devices. This includes considerations such as legible typography, high-contrast color schemes, appropriate use of icons and symbols, and adherence to accessibility guidelines (e.g., WCAG) to accommodate users with disabilities Additionally, incorporating adjustable display settings and multimodal feedback (e.g., auditory and haptic cues) can enhance the overall user experience (107).

3.9.5 Error Prevention and Recovery

UI and UX design plays a crucial role in preventing and mitigating user errors in automated medical devices. Incorporating error-prevention mechanisms, such as input validation, confirmations for critical actions, and clear error messages, can help users avoid mistakes Additionally, providing guidance and recovery mechanisms, such as undo/redo functions and context-sensitive help, can enable users to correct errors and regain control of the device (108).

3.9.6 Workflow Integration and Context Awareness

Automated medical devices often operate within complex healthcare environments and workflows. Designing UI and UX solutions that seamlessly integrate with existing workflows and provide context-aware functionality can significantly enhance efficiency and reduce cognitive load for users. This may involve features such as customizable interfaces, adaptive displays based on user roles or clinical contexts, and interoperability with other healthcare systems and devices (109).

3.9.7 Training and User Support

Comprehensive training and user support are essential components of effective UI and UX design for automated medical devices. Providing clear and accessible user manuals, interactive tutorials, and ongoing training programs can help users develop proficiency with the device's interface and features. Additionally, offering responsive technical support and regular software updates can ensure users receive timely assistance and access to the latest improvements and bug fixes (110).

3.9.8 Continuous Improvement and Feedback Loops

UI and UX design for automated medical devices should be an iterative and ongoing process, driven by continuous improvement and feedback loops. Collecting and analyzing user feedback, usage data, and incident reports can help identify areas for enhancement and inform future design iterations. Establishing robust post-market surveillance mechanisms and fostering open communication channels with end-users can facilitate a culture of continuous learning and improvement (111).

3.9.9 Regulatory Compliance and Standards

The UI and UX design of automated medical devices must comply with relevant regulatory requirements and industry standards. Adherence to guidelines and standards, such as those set by the U.S. Food and Drug Administration (FDA), International Electrotechnical Commission (IEC), and International Organization for Standardization (ISO), is crucial to ensure the safety, effectiveness, and usability of these devices. Close collaboration with regulatory bodies and active participation in the development of relevant standards can help drive best practices in UI and UX design (112).

3.9.10 Ethical Considerations and User Empowerment

UI and UX design for automated medical devices should be guided by ethical principles that prioritize user autonomy, transparency, and empowerment. Providing clear and accessible information about the device's capabilities, limitations, and potential risks can enable users to make informed decisions and maintain appropriate levels of trust and control. Additionally, incorporating user preference settings, customization options, and shared decision-making features can foster a sense of ownership and engagement among users (113).

3.10 UNDERSTANDING REGULATORY FRAMEWORKS

Automated medical devices are subject to stringent regulatory requirements and industry standards to ensure their safety, effectiveness, and quality. Compliance with these regulations and standards is crucial throughout the entire product lifecycle, from design and development to manufacturing, marketing, and post-market surveillance. Failure to adhere to regulatory guidelines and industry norms can have severe consequences, including product recalls, legal liabilities, and compromised patient safety (114).

The rapid advancement of automated medical devices has revolutionized the healthcare industry, offering unprecedented opportunities for improved patient care, streamlined processes, and enhanced efficiency. However, the integration of these cutting-edge technologies into clinical settings necessitates robust regulatory frameworks to ensure their safety, efficacy, and reliability. Regulatory bodies around the world have established comprehensive guidelines and standards to govern the development, manufacturing, and deployment of automated medical devices, safeguarding public health and promoting trust in these innovative solutions (115).

3.10.1 Risk-Based Classification and Premarket Approval

Regulatory frameworks typically employ a risk-based classification system for medical devices, with higher-risk devices subjected to more stringent premarket approval processes. Automated medical devices, particularly those involved in critical functions such as diagnosis, treatment, or life support, are often classified as high-risk devices and require extensive clinical data, testing, and documentation to obtain regulatory approval This rigorous evaluation aims to ensure that the benefits of the device outweigh potential risks and that adequate measures have been taken to mitigate safety concerns (116).

3.10.2 Software and Cybersecurity Regulations

The software components of automated medical devices are subject to specific regulatory requirements and industry standards. Regulatory bodies like the U.S. Food and Drug Administration (FDA) and international organizations like the International Medical Device Regulators Forum (IMDRF) have issued guidance documents and standards for software validation, risk management, and cybersecurity. These guidelines aim to ensure the safety, security, and reliability of software-controlled medical devices, addressing potential vulnerabilities and minimizing the risk of cyber threats (117).

3.10.3 Quality Management Systems (QMS)

Implementing and adhering to Quality Management Systems (QMS) is a fundamental requirement for medical device manufacturers. Regulatory frameworks, such as the FDA's Quality System Regulation (QSR) and the ISO 13485 standard, provide guidelines and best practices for ensuring the quality and consistency of medical devices throughout their lifecycle QMS encompasses processes for design control, risk management, supplier management, production and process control, and post-market surveillance, ensuring adherence to regulatory requirements and industry best practices (118).

3.10.4 Human Factors Engineering and Usability

Usability and human factors engineering play a crucial role in the design and development of automated medical devices. Regulatory bodies and industry standards, such as the FDA's guidance on human factors and usability engineering and the IEC 62366-1 standard, provide frameworks and best practices for incorporating user-centered design principles, conducting usability testing, and mitigating the risk of use-related errors. These guidelines aim to promote intuitive and safe interactions between users and automated medical devices, reducing the potential for human errors and improving patient outcomes (119).

3.10.5 Labeling and Instructional Materials

Proper labeling and instructional materials are essential for the safe and effective use of automated medical devices. Regulatory frameworks mandate specific requirements for labeling, including clear and concise instructions for use, warnings, precautions, and contraindications. Standards like IEC 82079-1 provide guidelines for the design and development of instructional materials, ensuring they are clear, comprehensible, and user-friendly, minimizing the risk of misuse or misinterpretation (120).

3.10.6 Post-Market Surveillance and Reporting

Regulatory compliance extends beyond the premarket approval stage and encompasses post-market surveillance and reporting requirements. Manufacturers are obligated to monitor and report adverse events, product complaints, and device malfunctions to regulatory authorities. Robust post-market surveillance systems, such as those outlined in the FDA's Quality System Regulation and ISO 13485, are crucial for identifying and addressing safety issues, implementing corrective and preventive actions, and ensuring the continued safe and effective use of automated medical devices (121).

3.10.7 International Harmonization and Mutual Recognition

With the globalization of medical device markets, efforts have been made to harmonize regulatory requirements and establish mutual recognition agreements between different regions and countries. Organizations like the International Medical Device Regulators Forum (IMDRF) and the Global Harmonization Task Force (GHTF) work toward promoting regulatory convergence and reducing regulatory burdens while maintaining high standards of safety and quality. This harmonization facilitates the efficient introduction of automated medical devices into multiple markets while ensuring consistent levels of regulatory oversight (122).

3.10.8 Emerging Technologies and Regulatory Challenges

The rapid pace of technological advancements in automated medical devices presents unique regulatory challenges. Novel technologies, such as AI, machine learning, and advanced robotics, may not fit neatly into existing regulatory frameworks, necessitating adaptations and updates to ensure appropriate oversight and risk mitigation. Regulatory bodies and industry stakeholders collaborate to develop guidance and standards that address these emerging technologies' unique characteristics and potential risks (123).

3.10.9 Continuous Improvement and Regulatory Updates

Regulatory frameworks for automated medical devices are not static; they require continuous improvement and adaptation to evolving regulations, technological advancements, and industry best practices. Manufacturers must stay abreast of regulatory updates, guidance document revisions, and emerging standards to ensure their automated medical devices remain compliant throughout their lifecycle. Fostering a culture of continuous learning and improvement, as well as active participation in industry forums and regulatory discussions, is essential for maintaining regulatory compliance and promoting patient safety (124).

3.10.10 Ethical Considerations and Patient Safety

Regulatory frameworks for automated medical devices are underpinned by ethical principles that prioritize patient safety, autonomy, and well-being. Considerations such as transparency, accountability, and informed consent are paramount when introducing automated medical devices into clinical settings. Regulatory bodies and manufacturers must collaborate to ensure that these devices respect patient autonomy, minimize risks and potential harm, and promote equitable access to healthcare while maximizing the benefits of these innovative technologies (125).

3.11 COMPLIANCE WITH GLOBAL STANDARDS

The rapid advancement of automated medical devices has revolutionized the healthcare industry, offering unprecedented opportunities for improved patient care, streamlined processes, and enhanced efficiency. However, the integration of these cutting-edge technologies into clinical settings necessitates robust regulatory frameworks and adherence to global standards to ensure their safety, efficacy, and reliability. Regulatory bodies and international organizations have established comprehensive guidelines and standards to govern the development, manufacturing, and deployment of automated medical devices, safeguarding public health and promoting trust in these innovative solutions (126).

3.11.1 International Organization for Standardization (ISO)

The International Organization for Standardization (ISO) plays a pivotal role in developing and disseminating global standards for medical devices, including automated systems. The ISO 13485 standard, which specifies requirements for quality management systems in the medical device industry, is widely adopted by manufacturers worldwide. Additionally, standards such as ISO 14971 for risk management and ISO 62304 for medical device software lifecycle processes provide guidelines for ensuring the safety and quality of automated medical devices (127).

3.11.2 International Electrotechnical Commission (IEC)

The International Electrotechnical Commission (IEC) is a leading global organization responsible for developing international standards and conformity assessment systems in the field of electrotechnology. The IEC 60601 series of standards, specifically IEC 60601-1 for general safety and essential performance requirements, is widely recognized and adopted for automated medical devices. Other relevant IEC standards include IEC 62304 for medical device software lifecycle processes and IEC 62366-1 for usability engineering (128).

3.11.3 Usability and Human Factors Engineering

Usability and human factors engineering play a crucial role in the design and development of automated medical devices. The IEC 62366-1 standard and the FDA's guidance on human factors and usability engineering provide frameworks and best practices for incorporating user-centered design principles, conducting usability testing, and mitigating the risk of use-related errors. These guidelines aim to promote intuitive and safe interactions between users and automated medical devices, reducing the potential for human errors and improving patient outcomes (129).

3.11.4 Software and Cybersecurity Standards

The software components of automated medical devices are subject to specific regulatory requirements and industry standards. Standards such as IEC 62304 for medical device software lifecycle processes and ISO/IEC 27001 for information security management systems address software validation, risk management, and cybersecurity. These guidelines ensure the safety, security, and reliability of software-controlled medical devices, addressing potential vulnerabilities and minimizing the risk of cyber threats (130).

3.11.5 Risk Management and Safety Standards

Effective risk management is essential for ensuring the safety and reliability of automated medical devices. Standards such as ISO 14971 and IEC 60601-1 provide guidance on risk management processes, including risk analysis, evaluation, control, and post-production monitoring. These standards help manufacturers identify and mitigate potential hazards, ensuring that the benefits of the device outweigh potential risks (131).

3.11.6 Labeling and Instructional Materials

Proper labeling and instructional materials are critical for the safe and effective use of automated medical devices. Standards like IEC 82079-1 provide guidelines for the design and development of instructional materials, ensuring they are clear, comprehensible, and user-friendly, minimizing the risk of misuse or misinterpretation. Adherence to these standards promotes transparency and enables users to make informed decisions when operating automated medical devices (132).

3.11.7 International Medical Device Regulators Forum (IMDRF)

The International Medical Device Regulators Forum (IMDRF) is a voluntary group of medical device regulators from around the world that aims to promote international regulatory alignment and convergence. The IMDRF develops harmonized guidelines and standards for medical device regulation, facilitating global regulatory cooperation and reducing regulatory burdens while maintaining high standards of safety and quality. This harmonization effort is particularly beneficial for automated medical device manufacturers operating in multiple markets (133).

3.11.8 Emerging Technologies and Standard Development

The rapid pace of technological advancements in automated medical devices presents challenges for existing global standards. Novel technologies, such as AI, machine learning, and advanced robotics, may require the development of new standards or the adaptation of existing ones to address their unique characteristics and potential risks. International organizations and industry stakeholders collaborate to ensure that standards remain relevant and address the evolving needs of the medical device industry (134).

3.11.9 Continuous Improvement and Standard Updates

Compliance with global standards for automated medical devices is an ongoing process that requires continuous improvement and adaptation to evolving regulations, technological advancements, and industry best practices. Manufacturers must stay abreast of standard updates, guidance document revisions, and emerging best practices to ensure their automated medical devices remain compliant throughout their lifecycle. Fostering a culture of continuous learning and improvement, as well as active participation in industry forums and standard development processes, is essential for maintaining compliance and promoting patient safety (135).

3.11.10 Ethical Considerations and Patient Safety

Global standards for automated medical devices are underpinned by ethical principles that prioritize patient safety, autonomy, and well-being. Considerations such as transparency, accountability, and informed consent are paramount when introducing automated medical devices into clinical settings. Manufacturers and regulatory bodies must collaborate to ensure that these devices respect patient autonomy, minimize risks and potential harm, and promote equitable access to healthcare while maximizing the benefits of these innovative technologies (136).

3.12 ETHICS AND PATIENT SAFETY

The rapid integration of automated medical devices into healthcare systems has the potential to revolutionize patient care, enhance diagnostic accuracy, and streamline treatment processes. However, the deployment of these cutting-edge technologies raises significant ethical concerns and patient safety considerations that must be carefully addressed. As these devices become increasingly sophisticated and autonomous, it is imperative to ensure that they align with ethical principles and prioritize patient well-being (137).

3.12.1 Ethical Principles and Frameworks

Automated medical devices should be developed and deployed within the context of well-established ethical principles and frameworks. These include respect for patient autonomy, beneficence (promoting well-being), non-maleficence (minimizing harm), and justice (ensuring fair and equitable access). Additionally, ethical considerations such as transparency, accountability, and informed consent must be integrated into the design, development, and implementation processes of these devices (138).

3.12.2 Algorithmic Bias and Fairness

The algorithms and decision-making processes employed by automated medical devices must be rigorously evaluated for potential biases that could lead to unfair or discriminatory outcomes. Biases can arise from various sources, including the training data used to develop machine learning models, inherited biases from the developers, or societal biases reflected in the data. Addressing algorithmic bias and promoting fairness in automated medical devices is crucial to ensure equitable and non-discriminatory healthcare delivery (139).

3.12.3 Privacy and Data Protection

Automated medical devices often collect, process, and transmit sensitive patient data, raising significant privacy and data protection concerns. Robust measures must be implemented to safeguard patient privacy, ensure data security, and comply with relevant regulations such as the Health Insurance Portability and Accountability Act (HIPAA) and the General Data Protection Regulation (GDPR). This includes secure data storage, transmission protocols, access controls, and transparent data handling practices (140).

3.12.4 Cybersecurity and Resilience

The increasing connectivity and reliance on automated medical devices heighten the risk of cyber threats, such as hacking, malware attacks, and data breaches. Robust cybersecurity measures, including encryption, authentication protocols, and real-time monitoring, are essential to protect these devices from unauthorized access and ensure their resilience against potential attacks. Failure to address cybersecurity vulnerabilities can compromise patient safety and potentially lead to catastrophic consequences (141).

3.12.5 Human Oversight and Control

While automated medical devices offer significant advantages in terms of efficiency and accuracy, maintaining appropriate human oversight and control is crucial to ensure patient safety and ethical decision-making. Healthcare professionals should retain the ability to override automated systems when necessary, and clear protocols should be established for human intervention in critical situations. Additionally, ensuring transparency in the decision-making processes of these devices can foster trust and facilitate effective collaboration between humans and automated systems (142).

3.12.6 Liability and Accountability

The introduction of automated medical devices raises complex questions regarding liability and accountability in the event of errors, malfunctions, or adverse patient outcomes. Establishing clear guidelines and legal frameworks for assigning responsibility and ensuring appropriate compensation for harm is essential. This may involve revisiting existing liability laws and regulations to account for the unique challenges posed by automated medical technologies (143).

3.12.7 Informed Consent and Patient Education

Patients have a right to be fully informed about the use of automated medical devices in their care and the potential risks and benefits associated with these technologies. Obtaining informed consent and providing comprehensive patient education are ethical imperatives. Healthcare providers must ensure that patients understand the capabilities and limitations of automated devices, as well as their role in the decision-making process, empowering them to make informed choices about their care (144).

3.12.8 Equitable Access and Socioeconomic Considerations

The deployment of automated medical devices raises concerns about equitable access to healthcare and potential socioeconomic disparities. Efforts must be made to ensure that these technologies are accessible and affordable to all segments of the population, regardless of socioeconomic status, geographic location, or other factors. Failing to address these disparities could exacerbate existing healthcare inequalities and undermine the ethical principle of justice (145).

3.12.9 Continuous Monitoring and Improvement

The ethical and patient safety considerations surrounding automated medical devices are not static; they require continuous monitoring and improvement as these technologies evolve and new challenges emerge. Establishing robust post-market surveillance systems, analyzing real-world performance data, and fostering open dialogues among stakeholders (manufacturers, healthcare providers, regulators, and patients) are crucial for identifying and addressing emerging ethical and safety concerns (146).

3.12.10 Interdisciplinary Collaboration and Public Discourse

Addressing the ethical and patient safety challenges posed by automated medical devices necessitates interdisciplinary collaboration and public discourse. Bringing together expertise from various fields, including biomedical engineering, healthcare, ethics, law, and public policy, can foster a holistic understanding of the implications and facilitate the development of comprehensive guidelines and best practices. Additionally, engaging the public and fostering open discussions can raise awareness, build trust, and shape the responsible development and deployment of these technologies (147).

3.13 APPLICATIONS IN HEALTHCARE

The healthcare industry has seen a rapid evolution of automated medical devices in recent years, driven by advancements in AI, robotics, and sensor technologies. These automated systems are designed to improve patient care, enhance diagnostic accuracy, and streamline therapeutic procedures.

3.13.1 Diagnostic Devices

Automated medical imaging analysis systems have gained significant traction in recent years. These systems leverage deep learning algorithms and computer vision techniques to analyze medical images such as X-rays, CT scans, MRI scans, and ultrasound images. By detecting and classifying abnormalities, these systems assist radiologists in making more accurate and efficient diagnoses. A study published in Radiology demonstrated the effectiveness of an AI-powered system in detecting breast cancer from mammograms, achieving an area under the receiver operating characteristic curve (AUC) of 0.92, comparable to experienced radiologists (148).

Automated pathology analysis systems utilize AI and machine learning algorithms to analyze digital pathology slides, enabling faster and more consistent diagnoses. These systems can identify and classify various tissue abnormalities, such as cancerous cells, and provide quantitative measurements to aid pathologists in their decision-making process. A research paper published in Nature Machine Intelligence described an AI-based system that achieved human-level performance in detecting and grading prostate cancer from biopsy samples, with an AUC of 0.98 (149).

Wearable diagnostic devices, such as smartwatches and fitness trackers, are equipped with sensors that can continuously monitor vital signs and physiological parameters. These devices can detect abnormalities, such as irregular heart rates or sleep disturbances, and alert healthcare providers or the wearer for further evaluation. A study published in JAMA Network Open evaluated the accuracy of a wearable ECG monitor in detecting atrial fibrillation, reporting a sensitivity of 92% and a specificity of 88% compared to clinical ECG readings (150).

3.13.2 Therapeutic Devices-Robotic Surgery Systems

Robotic surgery systems have revolutionized minimally invasive surgical procedures. These systems consist of robotic arms controlled by a surgeon through a console, providing enhanced precision, dexterity, and visualization during complex operations. Robotic surgery is commonly used in various specialties, including urology, gynecology, and cardiothoracic surgery. A systematic review published in The Lancet analyzed the outcomes of robotic-assisted radical prostatectomy compared to open surgery, concluding that robotic surgery resulted in lower blood loss, shorter hospital stays, and faster recovery times (151).

3.13.3 Automated Drug Delivery Systems

Automated drug delivery systems are designed to ensure accurate and timely administration of medications to patients. These systems integrate smart infusion pumps, electronic health records, and automated medication dispensing cabinets to reduce medication errors and improve patient safety. A study published in the Journal of Patient Safety reported a significant reduction in medication administration errors after implementing an automated drug delivery system, with a 67% decrease in potential adverse drug events (152).

3.13.4 Automated Rehabilitation Devices

Automated rehabilitation devices are designed to assist patients in regaining mobility and function after injuries or neurological conditions. These devices include robotic exoskeletons, powered orthoses, and virtual reality systems that provide task-specific training and real-time feedback to patients during their rehabilitation process.

A randomized controlled trial published in The New England Journal of Medicine evaluated the effectiveness of a robotic exoskeleton in improving walking ability in individuals with spinal cord injuries, demonstrating significant improvements in walking speed and endurance compared to conventional therapy (153).

3.13.5 Automated Ventilators

Automated ventilators are essential devices in ICUs and respiratory therapy. These devices provide mechanical ventilation to patients with respiratory failure or during surgical procedures. Advanced automated ventilators incorporate AI and machine learning algorithms to optimize ventilation settings based on the patient's physiological parameters and response to therapy. A study published in Critical Care Medicine compared the performance of an AI-powered automated ventilator to manually adjusted ventilation in patients with acute respiratory distress syndrome (ARDS). The AI-powered ventilator achieved better oxygenation and ventilation outcomes while reducing the risk of ventilator-induced lung injury (154).

3.13.6 Wearable Health Technologies

Wearable health technologies have seen rapid advancement and adoption in recent years, revolutionizing the way we monitor and manage various medical conditions. These devices, integrated seamlessly into our daily lives, are transforming the healthcare landscape by enabling continuous, real-time data collection and analysis, leading to improved patient outcomes and more personalized care. One of the most prominent applications of wearable health technologies is in the field of automated medical devices. These devices leverage the power of wearable sensors, machine learning algorithms, and advanced data analytics to provide real-time monitoring, diagnosis, and even treatment recommendations, effectively bridging the gap between patients and healthcare professionals (155).

3.13.6.1 Continuous Glucose Monitoring (CGM) Devices

Diabetes management has been significantly enhanced by the advent of CGM devices. These wearable sensors continuously measure glucose levels in the interstitial fluid, providing patients with real-time data and alerts for highs and lows. CGM devices have been shown to improve glycemic control, reduce the risk of hypoglycemic events, and increase overall quality of life for individuals with diabetes. Additionally, researchers are exploring the integration of CGM data with automated insulin delivery systems, known as closed-loop systems or artificial pancreas devices. These systems use advanced algorithms to automatically adjust insulin delivery based on real-time glucose levels, minimizing the need for manual intervention (156).

3.13.6.2 Cardiac Monitoring Wearables

Cardiovascular diseases are a leading cause of mortality worldwide, and early detection and monitoring are crucial for effective management. Wearable cardiac monitoring devices, such as electrocardiogram (ECG) patches and smartwatches, have become increasingly popular in recent years. These devices can continuously monitor heart rate, rhythm, and other vital signs, alerting patients and healthcare providers to potential abnormalities or cardiac events. Advanced algorithms can detect atrial fibrillation, a common arrhythmia associated with an increased risk of stroke, enabling timely intervention and treatment. Furthermore, wearable cardiac monitors are being integrated with AI systems to improve the accuracy of diagnosis and risk stratification. These systems can analyze vast amounts of data from multiple sources, including wearable devices, electronic health records, and patient demographics, to provide personalized risk assessments and treatment recommendations (157).

3.13.6.3 Neurological Monitoring Wearables

Wearable technologies have also made significant strides in the field of neurological monitoring and rehabilitation. Devices such as electroencephalogram (EEG) headsets and motion sensors can track brain activity, sleep patterns, and motor function, providing valuable insights into neurological disorders like epilepsy, Parkinson's disease, and stroke. For instance, wearable EEG devices can detect and alert patients and caregivers of impending seizures, enabling timely intervention and potentially reducing the risk of injury. Additionally, these devices can be integrated with automated seizure detection and treatment systems, delivering targeted therapies or alerting emergency services when necessary. In the realm of rehabilitation, wearable motion sensors and virtual reality (VR) systems are being used to track and guide patients through personalized exercise programs, enhancing recovery and improving functional outcomes (158).

3.13.6.4 Respiratory Monitoring Wearables

Respiratory disorders, such as asthma, COPD, and sleep apnea, can significantly impact a patient's quality of life and pose serious health risks. Wearable respiratory monitoring devices, like respiratory rate sensors and spirometers, can provide continuous monitoring of lung function, enabling early detection of exacerbations and timely intervention. These devices can be paired with AI-powered systems that analyze respiratory patterns, environmental factors, and patient-reported symptoms to provide personalized treatment recommendations and alerts for potential adverse events. Furthermore, wearable respiratory monitors are being integrated with automated drug delivery systems, such as smart inhalers, which can release medication based on real-time data and predetermined algorithms, ensuring optimal treatment and reducing the risk of complications (159).

3.13.7 Remote Monitoring and Telemedicine

The integration of remote monitoring and telemedicine technologies with automated medical devices has revolutionized healthcare delivery, enabling continuous patient monitoring and real-time interventions, regardless of geographical barriers. This fusion of cutting-edge technologies has the potential to improve patient outcomes, reduce healthcare costs, and enhance access to quality care, particularly in remote or underserved areas (160).

3.13.7.1 Remote Patient Monitoring (RPM)

Remote patient monitoring (RPM) systems leverage wearable sensors, mobile devices, and wireless communication technologies to collect and transmit patient data from their homes or remote locations to healthcare providers. These systems enable continuous monitoring of various physiological parameters, such as heart rate, blood pressure, glucose levels, and respiratory function, allowing for early detection of potential health issues and timely interventions. One notable application of RPM is in the management of chronic conditions like heart failure, diabetes, and COPD. Wearable sensors and automated devices can continuously track vital signs, medication adherence, and disease-specific markers, transmitting this data to healthcare providers for analysis and decision-making. For instance, in heart failure management, RPM systems equipped with weight scales, blood pressure monitors, and electrocardiogram (ECG) sensors can detect early signs of decompensation, such as weight gain or arrhythmias, allowing for prompt adjustment of treatment plans and potentially reducing hospitalization rates. Similarly, in diabetes management, CGM devices can be integrated with RPM systems, providing real-time glucose data and alerts to patients and healthcare providers. This allows for timely adjustments to insulin dosages, dietary recommendations, and lifestyle modifications, improving glycemic control and preventing complications. RPM systems are also being used in post-operative care and rehabilitation settings, enabling healthcare providers to monitor patients' recovery progress, medication adherence, and functional status remotely. This not only reduces the need for in-person follow-up visits but also ensures timely intervention in case of complications or setbacks (161, 162).

3.13.7.2 Telemedicine and Virtual Consultations

Telemedicine, the delivery of healthcare services through telecommunication technologies, has gained significant traction in recent years, particularly in the wake of the COVID-19 pandemic. Telemedicine platforms enable virtual consultations, remote diagnosis, and treatment recommendations, bridging the gap between patients and healthcare providers, especially in areas with limited access to specialized care. One application of telemedicine in automated medical devices is in the field of remote monitoring and diagnosis. Patients can transmit data from wearable devices or implanted medical devices, such as pacemakers or insulin pumps, to healthcare providers for real-time analysis and adjustment of treatment plans. For instance, in cardiac care, patients with ICDs or pacemakers can securely transmit device data, including heart rhythms and device performance, to their healthcare providers through telemedicine platforms. This allows for remote monitoring and adjustment of device settings, reducing the need for in-person visits and enabling timely interventions in case of emergencies. Telemedicine platforms are also being integrated with AI and machine learning algorithms to enhance diagnostic capabilities and treatment recommendations. These AI-powered systems can analyze patient data, including medical images, lab results, and device data, to provide clinical decision support and personalized treatment plans. Furthermore, telemedicine is being employed in mental health care, enabling virtual therapy sessions, remote monitoring of patient well-being, and automated interventions. Wearable sensors and mobile applications can track patient mood, sleep patterns, and behavioral data, which can be analyzed by AI algorithms to detect early signs of mental health issues and provide personalized support or interventions (163).

3.14 CHALLENGES

3.14.1 Ensuring Safety and Reliability

One of the biggest challenges is ensuring the safety and reliability of automated medical devices, as any failure or inaccuracy could have severe consequences for patient health. Key issues include: Rigorous testing and validation to identify potential risks and failure modes Dealing with uncertain inputs, noise, and artifact data that could confuse AI systems Verifying the robustness and generalizability of machine learning models across diverse patient populations Maintaining cybersecurity and preventing malicious attacks on networked medical devices (164).

3.14.2 Interpretability and Trust

For clinicians to trust and adopt automated medical devices, the decision-making process needs to be interpretable and explainable. Challenges include: Developing transparent AI models that show the reasoning behind predictions/decisions, providing clear confidence estimates to indicate when human oversight is needed, aligning AI system behavior with clinician mental models and expectations (165).

3.14.3 Data Quality and Availability

Many automated medical devices rely on large, high-quality datasets for training AI models. Obstacles include: Data silos and lack of interoperability between medical systems/institutions, privacy concerns around sharing patient data and the need for data de-identification, class imbalances, noise, and artifacts in medical data that require cleaning/preprocessing (166).

3.14.4 Human–AI Interaction

Automated devices still require human oversight and integration into clinical workflows. Issues involve: Designing intuitive interfaces that reduce cognitive load on clinicians; clearly defining human roles versus automated roles to avoid disengagement or over-reliance; providing effective decision support that enhances rather than disrupts clinician workflows; and ethical and social implications. The increasing use of "black box" AI systems in healthcare raises ethical concerns such as potential bias and discrimination in datasets and algorithms; need for oversight, accountability, and legal frameworks around AI failures; and ensuring patient privacy, data rights, and transparency about AI usage (167).

3.14.5 Improved AI Techniques

Advances in AI and machine learning could help overcome many current challenges: use of causality to make AI models more robust and interpretable; federated learning to enable collaborative AI training without sharing raw data; self-supervised and multimodal learning to leverage diverse unlabeled data sources; and online/continual learning to allow AI systems to adapt to new data over time (168).

3.14.6 Human-Centered Design

More focus on integrating automated devices into real-world clinical environments, including: human factors testing and clinician involvement throughout design process; adaptive interfaces that personalize information for each user; and augmented intelligence that combines AI capabilities with human expertise (169).

3.14.7 Regulatory Standards and Validation

There is a need for clear regulatory frameworks and standards for validating automated medical devices: developing consensus benchmarks and evaluation protocols across diverse settings; real-world performance monitoring and post-deployment surveillance; and defining responsible practices around data usage, ethics, and patient rights (170).

3.14.8 Data Ecosystems and Infrastructure

Improving data quality/access is key for powering AI systems: common data standards and interoperability between platforms; secure data sharing mechanisms and federated learning frameworks; and next-generation data annotation tools and synthetic data generators (171).

3.14.9 Multidisciplinary Collaboration

Effective healthcare AI requires bridging diverse domains: close coordination between clinicians, data scientists, engineers, and ethicists; combined medical and technical education/training programs; and public–private partnerships between hospitals, universities, and industry (172).

3.15 OVERCOMING TECHNICAL AND ETHICAL CHALLENGES

3.15.1 Ensuring Safety and Robustness

A key priority is ensuring automated medical devices operate safely and reliably across diverse clinical environments: rigorous testing and validation procedures to identify potential risks and failure modes; adversarial training and robustness verification to make models resilient to noisy or adversarial inputs; uncertainty quantification to indicate when human oversight is needed; online monitoring and anomaly detection to catch errors during deployment; and improving Model Performance. Boosting the accuracy and generalization of AI models is crucial for high-stakes medical tasks: self-supervised and multimodal learning to leverage all available data sources; domain adaptation techniques to transfer knowledge from data-rich to data-poor settings; and causal reasoning and disentangled representations to build more robust hybrid neuro-symbolic approaches combining deep learning with structured knowledge (173, 174).

3.15.2 Model Interpretability and Explainability

For clinicians to trust AI systems, the decision process needs to be interpretable: developing inherently transparent models like decision trees/rules; post-hoc explainers like SHAP, LIME, and concept activation vectors; and example-based explanations highlighting similar cases to justify predictions interactive interfaces for exploring and querying model behavior (175).

3.15.3 Federated Learning and Privacy

Protecting patient data privacy while enabling collaborative model training: federated learning frameworks to train models on decentralized data; homomorphic encryption and secure multi-party computing approaches; differential privacy mechanisms for sharing privatized data; and synthetic data generation techniques preserving statistical properties Human-AI Interaction (176).

3.16 CASE STUDIES (SUCCESS STORIES OF AUTOMATED MEDICAL DEVICES)

3.16.1 Automated Diabetic Retinopathy Screening

Diabetic retinopathy is a leading cause of blindness, but requires expert analysis of retinal images to detect. An automated AI system developed by researchers at Google and Verily showed performance on par with expert ophthalmologists in identifying diabetic retinopathy and macular edema from retinal fundus images. When deployed at clinics in Thailand and India, the system was able to provide affordable, accessible screening to over 240,000 patients in underserved rural areas with limited access to specialists. This allowed for early detection and treatment to prevent vision loss (177).

3.16.2 AI-Guided Robotic Surgical Assistance

Researchers at Johns Hopkins developed an AI system integrated with a surgical robot to assist with situational awareness and guidance during procedures. Using real-time video feeds and preoperative imaging data, the AI could identify key anatomical structures, track surgical instruments, and provide data overlays and safety boundaries to the surgeon. In clinical studies across over 300 robotic procedures, this system helped reduce surgical duration, error rates, and surgeon fatigue and stress levels compared to standard manual techniques. Surgeons particularly valued AI assistance during challenging radiation or minimally invasive cases (178).

3.16.3 Adaptive Neural Prosthetics

For individuals with spinal cord injuries or neuromuscular disorders, brain–computer interfaces (BCIs) aim to restore functional ability by decoding neural signals to control assistive devices. However, neural signal patterns can shift over time, causing traditional static decoders to degrade in performance. An adaptive deep learning system developed at Stanford was able to continuously track and recalibrate the neural decoding model in real time based on the user's ongoing feedback. When tested with quadriplegic patients operating robotic arms and computer interfaces via BCIs, this system tripled the practical use time and allowed continuous high-fidelity control over multiple years (179).

3.16.4 AI Echocardiogram Analysis

Echocardiography is widely used to visualize heart anatomy and function, but interpreting echo videos and calculating key metrics like ejection fraction requires extensive expert training. Researchers at MIT and Massachusetts General Hospital developed an automated machine learning system to analyze echo videos and efficiently quantify various structural indicators and functional parameters. When validated on a test set of over 3,000 echoes, the AI matched expert human performance and could precisely calculate metrics like volumes and strain in just a few seconds. This allowed for much faster and more scalable echo analysis to streamline clinical workflow (180).

3.16.5 Closed-Loop Physiological Control

For patients in ICUs, maintaining optimal physiological parameters like blood pressure and glucose levels is critical but challenging due to the need for continual manual monitoring and adjustment of drug dosages. At the University of Pennsylvania, researchers developed a closed-loop AI system that could automatically regulate these physiological variables by modulating drug infusions. In prospective clinical trials across over 200 patients, this automated system kept parameters in the desired ranges significantly more effectively than manual control by human nurses and clinicians. It reduced life-threatening deviations by over 30% while reducing clinical workload. While there are still many challenges around safety, robustness, interpretability, and human-AI interaction, these case studies demonstrate how automated medical devices powered by AI/ML can provide affordable access, enhance precision, reduce errors, streamline clinical workflows, and potentially improve patient outcomes. As the underlying techniques continue advancing, we may see increasing real-world adoption and impact, albeit carefully regulated to ensure ethics and safety. Ongoing multidisciplinary research combining AI/ML, human factors, clinical insight, and domain expertise will be crucial for realizing the full transformative potential of automated medical devices (181–183).

3.16.6 Virtual Patient Monitoring

Virtual medical assistants powered by AI allow healthcare systems to remotely monitor patients outside the clinic. One system developed by Suki integrated electronic health records, wearable data, and conversational AI to enable virtual check-ins with patients recovering from surgeries or managing chronic diseases. In a pilot across 2000 patients over 6 months, over 90% of patients described the virtual assistant as easy to use and reported higher care satisfaction. Meanwhile, clinicians regained over 3 hours per day that would have been spent on patient monitoring. Readmission rates dropped by 15% versus standard care (184).

3.16.7 Robotic Process Automation in Healthcare

While not directly a medical device, robotic process automation (RPA) is having an impact by using software "robots" to automate routine digital tasks in healthcare. At Stanford Health, over 50 different AI bots have been deployed to automate tasks like data entry, prescription handling, scheduling, billing, and reporting. This has helped reduce administrative burdens on staff. Similarly, at UCSF Health, RPA has been used to streamline EHR data migration and automate over 60 routine processes. Such back-office automation can improve productivity and reduce burnout (185).

3.17 CASE STUDIES (LESSONS LEARNED FROM FAILURES)

3.17.1 Unexpected Safety Issues

The IBM Watson for Oncology system, aimed at providing therapeutic recommendations for cancer treatment, had safety issues identified during initial deployment studies. In some cases, it made recommendations that contradicted established clinical practices or missed key evidence, potentially putting patients at risk if followed blindly. This highlighted the need for rigorous real-world testing and human oversight rather than blindly trusting AI systems (186).

3.17.2 Failure to Generalize

Many AI models tend to be "brittle"—they can perform well on test datasets from one hospital, but then fail to generalize when encountering data from a new healthcare system with different equipment, protocols, or patient demographics. For example, a deep learning system for pneumonia detection achieved over 90% accuracy at one hospital but only 65% when evaluated on data from other sites. This reinforces the importance of continual learning, transfer learning, and diverse, representative datasets (187).

3.17.3 Dataset Shift and Distribution Mismatch

Models can degrade when applied to data that deviates from the training distribution. Google's highly touted deep learning system for diabetic retinopathy screening saw a major performance drop from 97% to 75% accuracy in Thailand due to differences in camera models and image characteristics compared to the original U.S. datasets. Such distribution shifts must be continuously monitored (188).

3.17.4 Bias and Unfair Outcomes

If trained on data reflecting societal biases, AI systems can discriminate and perpetuate those biases. A study of a popular commercial AI for reviewing chest X-rays found it was significantly more likely to miss important findings for women and minority subgroups. Issues like selection bias, proxy discrimination, and skewed datasets must be rigorously audited (189).

3.17.5 Human–AI Interaction Challenges

For AI to augment rather than alienate clinicians, interfaces must be designed with human factors in mind. An early electronic triage system at hospitals missed almost 1 in 3 high-risk cases because staff frequently overrode automated risk scores; they didn't understand or trust Interpretability, uncertainty communication, and human-in-the-loop controls become critical (190).

3.17.6 Lack of Real-World Validation

Many AI systems show promising results on curated datasets but stumble when facing more diverse, noisy real-world conditions. An AI for detecting breast cancer missed 10–15% of cancers when deployed prospectively even after strong retrospective performance. More rigorous prospective and external validation is needed before high-stakes clinical use (191).

3.17.7 Regulatory and Liability Challenges

Lack of clarity around evolving AI system behavior makes regulatory approval difficult. A novel AI surgical robot intended to pilot and progressively learn from early human-supervised cases was delayed for years due to questions around how to validate it and assign liability as it became more autonomous. Agile regulatory frameworks aligned with AI's unique properties are required (192).

3.17.8 Unexpected Safety Risks from Lack of Robustness

A major failure mode for AI systems is a lack of robustness to out-of-distribution inputs, noise, or adversarial attacks, which can lead to unexpected and potentially dangerous errors. This was highlighted in a 2019 study by the University of Toronto researchers. They investigated the robustness of a commercial AI system for detecting pneumonia from chest X-rays by introducing different types of corruptions and perturbations. While the model performed with 95% accuracy on clean test images, its performance degraded substantially in the presence of common corruptions like image noise, blurring, contrast changes, rotations, etc. On some perturbations, the accuracy dropped below 20%. Even worse, they found the system could be fooled by carefully crafted adversarial inputs into making wildly incorrect predictions with high confidence. Such lack of robustness under realistic conditions is a major safety hazard if the AI system's outputs are blindly trusted. A key lesson is that testing AI robustness cannot rely solely on independent and identically distributed test sets from the same distribution as training—it requires much more diverse and challenging testing regimes. Techniques like data augmentation, adversarial training, and formal verification methods can help improve robustness but are still limited (193, 194).

3.17.9 Distributional Shift and Domain Gaps

Related to robustness issues, another common pitfall is domain shift or mismatch between training/testing conditions and real-world deployment environments. A striking example comes from a study on automated speech recognition for transcribing medical conversations. While commercially available speech systems achieved around 80–90% accuracy on carefully curated medical recordings, their performance plummeted below 60% accuracy when deployed in the emergency department of a children's hospital. The background noise, non-native accents, colloquial speech, and rapid dialogue defeated models trained primarily on clean adult speech. This failure to translate highlights the importance of explicitly accounting for domain gaps and shifting testing distributions closer to the real use case during AI development. Simply evaluating data from one clinical site or demographic may be insufficient. As analysis showed, even data variations like different imaging equipment can significantly impact performance (195).

3.17.10 Compounding Errors and Feedback Loops

Some of the most challenging failure modes come when individual model errors systematically propagate or compound in problematic ways over time. This is especially risky with continual learning systems intended to automatically update and adapt as new data streams in. Researchers at UChicago Medicine analyzed an AI system for sepsis prediction that was deployed in their ICUs. While initially accurate, they discovered that periods of systemic underestimation of sepsis risk led to cases being systematically missed. This caused patients to experience higher occult sepsis rates, which then fed back into the training data used to further update the model. Over time this created a compounding feedback loop where the model's blindspots became increasingly reinforced and harder to overcome without manual intervention. Similar issues have plagued other systems like automated radiologist triage models reinforcing the same abnormalities. These kinds of insidious feedback loops underscore the need for diligent monitoring, human oversight, and explicit mechanisms to correct errors and distribute the model updates safely. AI systems cannot be treated as autonomous black boxes but require carefully governed deployments (196, 197).

3.17.11 Lack of Reproducibility and Evaluation Standards

Many of the high-profile failures have also revealed deeper systemic issues around lack of reproducibility, insufficient external validation, and the absence of agreed-upon AI evaluation procedures in healthcare. For instance, found shockingly poor reproducibility and lack of generalization when re-implementing and independently testing influential papers on medical imaging AI. Simple things like dataset leakage, different randomization seeds, or minor preprocessing changes could swing results dramatically. Beyond reproducibility, there is the issue of evaluation mismatch. A systematic review found most studies testing medical AI still relied primarily on small, local institution datasets rather than larger, diverse, multi-site benchmarks—leading to systematically inflated performance estimates. This underscores the need for community-driven efforts to establish more robust, standardized, reproducible evaluation practices and open benchmarks that stress-test AI models in more realistic, heterogeneous conditions. Several initiatives are underway like the RSNA AI Data Challenge, DRCRAD, and AIDIP; but broader adoption and coordination is still lacking (198).

3.17.12 Human–AI Teamwork and Interaction Failures

While technical robustness is crucial, many pitfalls have also stemmed from a lack of human-centered design and Poor integration of AI systems into real clinical workflows. A case study at Cedars-Sinai Hospital examined the deployment of an "ambient AI" system using speech recognition to automatically transcribe physician–patient conversations. While touting high accuracy scores, frontline staff experienced many usability frustrations from ambient noise interference to privacy concerns. Poor authentication and lack of customization led to widespread rejection. At Mount Sinai, a predictive AI system correctly anticipated a high influx of flu patients. However, because it was not integrated into scheduling and staffing decision flows, no actions were taken by administrators to boost capacity. User experience gaps rendered the accurate predictions essentially worthless. These examples highlight that even technically robust AI solutions will fail without rigorously studying and designing for the sociotechnical context—how humans actually perceive, trust, and interact with these systems in messy real-world conditions. Participatory design, human factors testing, and qualitative observational research must be core practices (199).

3.17.13 Ethical Issues and Public Backlash

Another key area of lessons learned revolves around upholding ethical principles like fairness, transparency, privacy, and accountability for high-stakes AI systems impacting human health. For instance, a pioneering AI system from Stanford to guide treatment for COVID-19 patients became mired in controversy around both methodology transparency and biased outcomes against certain racial groups. The system was not sufficiently documented or externally validated, yet was thrust into sensitive deployment without inclusive processes to audit for potential harms. A related public backlash occurred around IBM Watson's AI system being used for cancer treatment advisement. After anecdotes of potentially life-threatening errors, investigations raised concerns about lack of accountability, insufficient physician oversight, and conflicts of interest. There was a sense that safety was deprioritized over commercial motives. While the ethical AI research community has made important strides in technical approaches like bias testing and interpretability, the persistent pattern of failures indicates a need for stronger governance, regulation, and public inclusion from the very start. Simply checking off ethics checklist items as an afterthought is inadequate; ethical and community-aligned practices must be fundamentally embedded throughout the entire AI lifecycle. While these examples underscore the challenges, they also highlight valuable lessons that the broader AI in medicine community can learn from to develop more robust, trustworthy, and impactful systems moving forward. Multi-stakeholder collaboration will be key to collectively advancing this sociotechnical complex domain (200, 201).

3.18 CONCLUSION

This chapter provides a comprehensive overview of the role of embedded systems in automating medical devices. It covers a wide range of topics, from basic concepts to specific applications, highlighting the significance of this technology in modern healthcare. Comprehensive Scope: The chapter effectively covers the evolution of medical device technology, key components of embedded systems (both hardware and software), and their impact on various aspects of healthcare, including patient care, therapeutic interventions, and surgical procedures. Clear Structure and Organization: The chapter is well-structured, progressing logically from an introduction to embedded systems to specific examples of their applications in healthcare. The chapter provides numerous examples of how embedded systems are currently being used in medical devices, such as insulin pumps, pacemakers, and robotic surgical systems. This helps to ground the discussion and demonstrate the tangible benefits of this technology. Recognition of Challenges: The chapter acknowledges the importance of cybersecurity and privacy considerations, as well as the need for interoperability and integration in the development and deployment of embedded systems in healthcare. Depth of Technical Discussion: While the chapter provides a good overview, it could benefit from a more in-depth discussion of specific technical challenges and solutions. For example, a deeper dive into RTOS, communication protocols, and cybersecurity measures would be valuable for a technical audience. While the chapter mentions several examples, incorporating more detailed case studies showcasing successful implementations of embedded systems in medical devices would strengthen the discussion and provide valuable insights. The chapter could be further enriched by discussing future trends and emerging technologies in the field of embedded systems for medical devices. This could include topics like AI, machine learning, and the Internet of Medical Things (IoMT). Visual Aids and Diagrams: Incorporating more visual aids, such as diagrams, charts, and illustrations, would enhance the clarity and readability of the chapter, particularly for complex technical concepts.

LIST OF ABBREVIATIONS

ADC	Analog-to-Digital Converter
AI	Artificial Intelligence
AR	Augmented Reality
ARM	Advanced RISC Machines
CAD	Computer-Aided Design
CGM	Continuous Glucose Monitoring
COPD	Chronic Obstructive Pulmonary Disease
CT	Computed Tomography
DAC	Digital-to-Analog Converter
DICOM	Digital Imaging and Communications in Medicine
ECG	Electrocardiograph
EEG	Electroencephalogram
EEPROM	Electrically Erasable Programmable Read-Only Memory
EMG	Electromyogram

FDA	Food and Drug Administration
FMEA	Failure Mode and Effects Analysis
FTA	Fault Tree Analysis
GDPR	General Data Protection Regulation
GHTF	Global Harmonization Task Force
GPIO	General-Purpose Input/Output
GUI	Graphical User Interface
HIL	Hardware-in-the-Loop
HIPAA	Health Insurance Portability and Accountability Act
HL7	Health Level Seven
I2C	Inter-Integrated Circuit
ICD	Implantable Cardioverter-Defibrillator
ICU	Intensive Care Unit
IEC	International Electrotechnical Commission
IHE	Integrating the Healthcare Enterprise
IMDRF	International Medical Device Regulators Forum
IMDRF	International Medical Device Regulators Forum
IoT	Internet of Things
ISO	International Organization for Standardization
LCD	Liquid Crystal Display
LCP	Liquid Crystal Polymer
LED	Light-Emitting Diode
MCDA	Multi-Criteria Decision Analysis
MCDA -	Multi-Criteria Decision Analysis
mHealth	Mobile Health
ML	Machine Learning
MRI	Magnetic Resonance Imaging
PCB	Printed Circuit Board
PHE	Premarket Approval
PID	Proportional-Integral-Derivative
PPG	Photoplethysmogram
QMS	Quality Management Systems
QSR	Quality System Regulation
RAM	Random Access Memory
RTC	Real-Time Clock
SPI	Serial Peripheral Interface
TPM	Trusted Platform Module
UART	Universal Asynchronous Receiver/Transmitter
UI	User Interface
USB	Universal Serial Bus
UX	User Experience
VR	Virtual Reality
WBAN	Wireless Body Area Network
WCAG	Web Content Accessibility Guidelines

REFERENCES

1. Arandia N, Garate JI, Mabe J. Embedded sensor systems in medical devices: Requisites and challenges ahead. *Sensors* [Internet]. 2022 Dec 16 [cited 2024 Jun 4];22(24):9917. Available from: https://www.mdpi.com/1424-8220/22/24/9917/htm
2. Liu B, Zhang H, Zhu S. An incremental V-model process for automotive development. *Proceedings – Asia-Pacific Software Engineering Conference, APSEC*. 2016 Jul 2;225–32.
3. Akbar MA, Sang J, Khan AA, Amin FE, Nasrullah, Hussain S, et al. Statistical analysis of the effects of heavyweight and lightweight methodologies on the six-pointed star model. *IEEE Access*. 2018 Feb 12;6:8066–79.
4. Chari K, Agrawal M. Impact of incorrect and new requirements on waterfall software project outcomes. *Empirical Software Engineering* 2018 Feb 1;23(1):165–85.
5. Arandia N, Garate JI, Mabe J. Medical devices with embedded sensor systems: Design and development methodology for start-ups. *Sensors* [Internet]. 2023 Feb 26 [cited 2024 Jun 4];23(5):2578. Available from: https://www.mdpi.com/1424-8220/23/5/2578/htm
6. Zhao H. Applications of embedded systems in medicine: Challenges and future trends. *Highlights in Science, Engineering and Technology*. 2023 Jul 27;62:31–5.
7. Iniewski K. *Embedded systems: Hardware, design, and implementation*. 1st Edition, John Wiley & Sons, Inc. 2012, 1–386.
8. Valvano JW. *Embedded systems real time operating systems for arm cortex m microcontrollers*. Vol 3, 4th Edition, Createspace Independent Pub, 2021, 1–366.
9. Peckol JK. Embedded systems: for signal integrity, system security, low power, and hardware-software co-design. [cited 2024 Jun 4];1017. Available from: https://books.google.com/books/about/Embedded_Systems.html?id=ummPDwAAQBAJ
10. Kaule S, Bock A, Dierke A, Siewert S, Schmitz KP, Stiehm M, et al. Medical device regulation and current challenges for the implementation of new technologies. *Current Directions in Biomedical Engineering*. 2020 Sep 1;6(3): 1–4.
11. Mohapatra S, Mirza MA, Hilles AR, Zakir F, Gomes AC, Ansari MJ, et al. Biomedical application, patent repository, clinical trial and regulatory updates on hydrogel: An extensive review. *Gels*. 2021 Dec 1;7(4): 1–32.
12. Ravizza A, De Maria C, Di Pietro L, Sternini F, Audenino AL, Bignardi C. Comprehensive review on current and future regulatory requirements on wearable sensors in preclinical and clinical testing. *Frontiers in Bioengineering and Biotechnology*. 2019 Nov 8;7:1–9.
13. Lima FV, Kadiyala V, Huang A, Agusala K, Cho D, Freeman AM, et al. At the crossroads! Time to start taking smartwatches seriously. *American Journal of Cardiology*. 2022 Sep 15;179:96–101.
14. Arandia N, Garate JI, Mabe J. Embedded sensor systems in medical devices: Requisites and challenges ahead. *Sensors (Basel)* [Internet]. 2022 Dec 1 [cited 2024 Jun 4];22(24). Available from: https://doi.org/10.3390/s22249917
15. Zaouiat CEA, Latif A. Internet of things and machine learning convergence: The E-healthcare revolution. *ACM International Conference Proceeding Series* [Internet]. 2017 Nov 14 [cited 2024 Jul 3]; Available from: https://doi.org/10.1145/3167486.3167551
16. Hu L, Li L, Ji J, Sanderson M. Identifying and understanding determinants of high healthcare costs for breast cancer: A quantile regression machine learning approach. BMC Health Services Research [Internet]. 2020 Dec 1 [cited 2024 Jul 3];20(1):1–10. Available from: https://link.springer.com/articles/10.1186/s12913-020-05936-6
17. Bharadwaj HK, Agarwal A, Chamola V, Lakkaniga NR, Hassija V, Guizani M, et al. A review on the role of machine learning in enabling IoT based healthcare applications. *IEEE Access*. 2021;9:38859–90.

18. Ambigavathi M, Sridharan D. Analysis of clustering algorithms in machine learning for healthcare data. *Communications in Computer and Information Science* [Internet]. 2020 [cited 2024 Jul 3];1244 CCIS:117–28. Available from: https://link.springer.com/chapter/10.1007/978-981-15-6634-9_12
19. Chen JH, Verghese A. Planning for the known unknown: Machine learning for human healthcare systems. *American Journal of Bioethics* [Internet]. 2020 Nov 1 [cited 2024 Jul 3];20(11):1–3. Available from: https://www.tandfonline.com/doi/abs/10.1080/15265161.2020.1822674
20. Seguí FL, Aguilar RAE, de Maeztu G, García-Altés A, Cuyàs FG, Walsh S, et al. Teleconsultations between patients and healthcare professionals in primary care in Catalonia: The evaluation of text classification algorithms using supervised machine learning. *International Journal of Environmental Research and Public Health.* 2020 Feb 9 [cited 2024 Jul 3];17(3):1093. Available from: https://www.mdpi.com/1660-4601/17/3/1093/htm
21. Patel HB, Gandhi S. A review on big data analytics in healthcare using machine learning approaches. *Proceedings of the 2nd International Conference on Trends in Electronics and Informatics, ICOEI 2018.* 2018 Nov 29;84–90.
22. Miotto R, Wang F, Wang S, Jiang X, Dudley JT. Deep learning for healthcare: review, opportunities and challenges. Brief Bioinformatics [Internet]. 2018 Nov 27 [cited 2024 Jul 3];19(6):1236–46. Available from: https://doi.org/10.1093/bib/bbx044
23. Rajkomar A, Dean J, Kohane I. Machine learning in medicine. *New England Journal of Medicine* [Internet]. 2019 Apr 4 [cited 2024 Jul 3];380(14):1347–58. Available from: https://www.nejm.org/doi/abs/10.1056/NEJMra1814259
24. Olczak KP, Otto KJ. Coatings for microneural implants: Biological and mechanical considerations. *Handbook of Neuroengineering* [Internet]. 2021 [cited 2024 Jul 3]; 1–38. Available from: https://link.springer.com/referenceworkentry/10.1007/978-981-15-2848-4_132-1
25. Haleem A, Javaid M, Vaishya R. Industry 4.0 and its applications in orthopaedics. *Journal of Clinical Orthopaedics and Trauma.* 2019 May 1;10(3):615–6.
26. Roderick O, Marko N, Sanchez D, Aryasomajula A. Data analysis and machine learning effort in healthcare. *Internet of Things and Data Analytics Handbook* [Internet]. 2017 Feb 17 [cited 2024 Jul 3];295–328. Available from: https://onlinelibrary.wiley.com/doi/full/10.1002/9781119173601.ch18
27. Purushotham S, Meng C, Che Z, Liu Y. Benchmarking deep learning models on large healthcare datasets. *Journal of Biomedical Informatics.* 2018 Jul 1;83:112–34.
28. Ahmadzadeh S, Luo J, Wiffen R. Review on biomedical sensors, technologies and algorithms for diagnosis of sleep disordered breathing: Comprehensive survey. *IEEE Reviews in Biomedical Engineering* 2022;15:4–22.
29. Rodriguez S, Osorio AF, Silva RO, Domingues LR, Onisto HJ, Fonseca GC, et al. Fully configurable real-time ultrasound platform for medical imaging research. *IFMBE Proc* [Internet]. 2022 [cited 2024 Jun 4];83:807–12. Available from: https://link.springer.com/chapter/10.1007/978-3-030-70601-2_122
30. Bastos-Filho TF, Caldeira EM de O, … *XXVII Brazilian Congress on Biomedical Engineering: Proceedings of CBEB 2020, October 26–30, 2020, Vitória, Brazil.* Bastos-Filho TF, de Oliveira Caldeira EM, Frizera-Neto A, editors. 2022 [cited 2024 Jun 4];83. Available from: https://books.google.com/books?hl=en&lr=&id=2-5qEAAAQBAJ&oi=fnd&pg=PR5&dq=taekwondo+machine+learning&ots=-_uDt6LcEH&sig=FvilswYLLRQbzFyFME46EvCFp4I
31. Dere G, Dere G. Biomedical applications with using embedded systems. *Data Acquisition – Recent Advances and Applications in Biomedical Engineering* [Internet]. 2021 Feb 24 [cited 2024 Jun 4]; Available from: https://www.intechopen.com/chapters/75395

32. Khalifa University, Institute of Electrical and Electronics Engineers. *Proceedings of 2016 IEEE Global Engineering Education Conference (EDUCON): date and venue: 10–13 April 2016, Abu Dhabi, UAE.*
33. Polster JM, Winalski CS, Sundaram M, Lieber ML, Schils J, Ilaslan H, et al. Rheumatoid arthritis: Evaluation with contrast-enhanced CT with digital bone masking. *Radiology.* 2009 Jul;252(1):225–31.
34. Noguerol TM, Alcalá AL, Beltrán LS, Cabrera MG, Cabrero JB, Vilanova JC. Advanced MR imaging techniques for differentiation of neuropathic arthropathy and osteomyelitis in the diabetic foot. *Radiographics.* 2017 Jul 1;37(4):1161–80.
35. Lillegraven S, Bøyesen P, Hammer HB, Østergaard M, Uhlig T, Sesseng S, et al. Tenosynovitis of the extensor carpi ulnaris tendon predicts erosive progression in early rheumatoid arthritis. *Annals of the Rheumatic Diseases.* 2011 Nov;70(11):2049–50.
36. Szkudlarek M, Narvestad E, Klarlund M, Court-Payen M, Thomsen HS, Østergaard M. Ultrasonography of the metatarsophalangeal joints in rheumatoid arthritis: Comparison with magnetic resonance imaging, conventional radiography, and clinical examination. *Arthritis Rheumatology*, 2004 Jul;50(7):2103–12.
37. Bokolo AJ. Exploring the adoption of telemedicine and virtual software for care of outpatients during and after COVID-19 pandemic. *Irish Journal of Medical Sciences.* 2021 Feb 1;190(1): 1–10.
38. Hong YR, Lawrence J, Williams D, Mainous A. Population-level interest and telehealth capacity of US hospitals in response to COVID-19: Cross-sectional analysis of Google search and National Hospital Survey Data. *JMIR Public Health Surveillance.* 2020 Apr 1;6(2): e18961.
39. Promila, Jyothi T, Jain S. TPM based Secure Boot in Embedded Systems. *ICSCCC 2023 – 3rd International Conference on Secure Cyber Computing and Communications.* 2023;786–90.
40. Williams PAH, Woodward AJ. Cybersecurity vulnerabilities in medical devices: A complex environment and multifaceted problem. *Med Devices* (Auckl) [Internet]. 2015 Jul 20 [cited 2024 Jun 4];8:305. Available from: https://doi.org/10.2196/18961
41. Khan M, Han K, Karthik S. Designing smart control systems based on Internet of Things and big data analytics. *Wireless Personal Communications.* 2018 Apr 1;99(4):1683–97.
42. Pradhan B, Bhattacharyya S, Pal K. IoT-based applications in healthcare devices. *Journal of Healthcare Engineering* [Internet]. 2021 [cited 2024 Jun 4];2021. Available from: https://doi.org/10.1155/2021/6632599
43. Heneghan C, Thompson M, Billingsley M, Cohen D. Medical-device recalls in the UK and the device-regulation process: Retrospective review of safety notices and alerts. BMJ Open. 2011;1(1):e000155.
44. Jefferys DB. The regulation of medical devices and the role of the Medical Devices Agency. *British Journal of Clinical Pharmacology, Supplement.* 2001;52(3):229–35.
45. Arandia N, Garate JI, Mabe J. Embedded sensor systems in medical devices: Requisites and challenges ahead. *Sensors (Basel)* [Internet]. 2022 Dec 1 [cited 2024 Jun 4];22(24). Available from: https://doi.org/10.3390/s22249917
46. McCarthy AD, Lawford PV. Standalone medical device software: The evolving regulatory framework. *Journal of Medical Engineering & Technology.* 2015 Oct 3;39(7):441–7.
47. Gehr S, Russmann C. Shaping the future of cardiovascular medicine in the new era of wearable devices. *Nature Reviews Cardiology.* 2022 Aug 1;19(8):501–2.
48. Ben-Menahem SM, Nistor-Gallo R, Macia G, von Krogh G, Goldhahn J. How the new European regulation on medical devices will affect innovation. *Nature Biomedical Engineering.* 2020 Jun 1;4(6):585–90.
49. Takei K, Honda W, Harada S, Arie T, Akita S. Toward flexible and wearable human-interactive health-monitoring devices. *Advanced Healthcare Materials* 2015 Mar 1;4(4):487–500.

50. Kaule S, Bock A, Dierke A, Siewert S, Schmitz KP, Stiehm M, et al. Medical device regulation and current challenges for the implementation of new technologies. *Current Directions in Biomedical Engineering*. 2020 Sep 1;6(3):1–4.
51. Mohapatra S, Mirza MA, Hilles AR, Zakir F, Gomes AC, Ansari MJ, et al. Biomedical application, patent repository, clinical trial and regulatory updates on hydrogel: An extensive review. *Gels*. 2021 Dec 1;7(4):1–32.
52. Jennings D, Little MM, Johnson-Jennings M. Developing a tribal health sovereignty model for obesity prevention. *Program Community Health Partnership*. 2018 Sep 1;12(3):353–62.
53. Chui KT, Alhalabi W, Pang SSH, de Pablos PO, Liu RW, Zhao M. Disease diagnosis in smart healthcare: Innovation, technologies and applications. *Sustainability (Switzerland)*. 2017 Dec 18;9(12): 1–23.
54. Seçkin M, Seçkin AÇ, Gençer Ç. Biomedical sensors and applications of wearable technologies on arm and hand. *Biomedical Materials & Devices*. 2023 Mar;1(1):443–55.
55. Carroll N, Richardson I. Software-as-a-medical device: Demystifying connected health regulations. *Journal of Systems and Information Technology*. 2016;18(2):186–215.
56. Ahmadzadeh S, Luo J, Wiffen R. Review on biomedical sensors, technologies and algorithms for diagnosis of sleep disordered breathing: Comprehensive survey. *IEEE Reviews in Biomedical Engineering*. 2022;15:4–22.
57. Troisi J. Artificial intelligence in medicine: Disease diagnosis, drug development and treatment personalization. *Current Medical Chemistry*. 2021 Oct 20;28(32):6509–11.
58. Mansour RF, Amraoui El A, Nouaouri I, Diaz VG, Gupta D, Kumar S. Artificial intelligence and Internet of Things enabled disease diagnosis model for smart healthcare systems. *IEEE Access*. 2021;9:45137–46.
59. Ravizza A, De Maria C, Di Pietro L, Sternini F, Audenino AL, Bignardi C. Comprehensive review on current and future regulatory requirements on wearable sensors in preclinical and clinical testing. *Frontiers in Bioengineering and Biotechnology*. 2019 Nov 8;7.
60. Wang L, Alexander CA. Big data analytics in medical engineering and healthcare: Methods, advances and challenges. *Journal of Medical Engineering & Technology* 2020 Aug 17;44(6):267–83.
61. Ruan K, Wu Z, Xu Q. Smart cleaner: A new autonomous indoor disinfection robot for combating the covid-19 pandemic. *Robotics*. 2021 Sep 1;10(3): 1–16.
62. Wani SUD, Khan NA, Thakur G, Gautam SP, Ali M, Alam P, et al. Utilization of Artificial Intelligence in disease prevention: Diagnosis, treatment, and implications for the healthcare workforce. *Healthcare (Switzerland)*. 2022 Apr 1;10(4): 1–17.
63. Chen PT, Lin CL, Wu WN. Big data management in healthcare: Adoption challenges and implications. *International Journal of Information Management*. 2020 Aug 1;53: 1–11.
64. Lima FV, Kadiyala V, Huang A, Agusala K, Cho D, Freeman AM, et al. At the crossroads! Time to start taking smartwatches seriously. *American Journal of Cardiology*. 2022 Sep 15;179:96–101.
65. Petretto DR, Pili R. Ageing and COVID-19: What is the role for elderly people? *Geriatrics (Switzerland)*. 2020 Jun 1;5(2): 1–4.
66. Sqalli MT, Al-Thani D. On how chronic conditions affect the patient-AI interaction: A literature review. *Healthcare (Switzerland)*. 2020;8(3):1–26.
67. Fouad H, Hassanein AS, Soliman AM, Al-Feel H. Analyzing patient health information based on IoT sensor with AI for improving patient assistance in the future direction. *Measurement (London)*. 2020 Jul 15;159: 1–11.
68. Gillespie BM, Gillespie J, Boorman RJ, Granqvist K, Stranne J, Erichsen-Andersson A. The impact of robotic-assisted surgery on team performance: A systematic mixed studies review. *Human Factors* [Internet]. 2021 Dec 1 [cited 2024 May 29];63(8):1352–79. Available from: https://pubmed.ncbi.nlm.nih.gov/32613863/

69. Mehta A, Cheng Ng J, Andrew Awuah W, Huang H, Kalmanovich J, Agrawal A, et al. Embracing robotic surgery in low- and middle-income countries: potential benefits, challenges, and scope in the future. *Annals of Medicine and Surgery (London)*. 2022 Dec 1;84; 1–5.
70. Chatterjee S, Das S, Ganguly K, Mandal D. Advancements in robotic surgery: innovations, challenges and future prospects. *Journal of Robotic Surgery* [Internet]. 2024 Dec 1 [cited 2024 Jun 4];18(1):1–11. Available from: https://link.springer.com/article/10.1007/s11701-023-01801-w
71. Sinha A, Dolz J. Multi-scale self-guided attention for medical image segmentation. *IEEE Journal of Biomedical and Health Informatics* 2021 Jan 1;25(1):121–30.
72. Schork NJ. Artificial Intelligence and personalized medicine. *Cancer Treatment and Research*. 2019;178:265–83.
73. Popescu D, Stanciulescu A, Pomohaci MD, Ichim L. Decision support system for liver lesion segmentation based on advanced convolutional neural network architectures. *Bioengineering*. 2022 Sep 1;9(9):1–28.
74. Ghaffar Nia N, Kaplanoglu E, Nasab A. Evaluation of artificial intelligence techniques in disease diagnosis and prediction. *Discover Artificial Intelligence*. 2023 Dec 1;3(5):1–14.
75. Uddin M, Wang Y, Woodbury-Smith M. Artificial intelligence for precision medicine in neurodevelopmental disorders. *NPJ Digital Medicine*. 2019 Dec 1;2(112):1–10.
76. Hashimoto DA, Rosman G, Rus D, Meireles OR. Artificial Intelligence in surgery: Promises and perils. *Annals of Surgery*. 2018 Jul 1;268(1):70–6.
77. Sarmet M, Kabani A, Coelho L, dos Reis SS, Zeredo JL, Mehta AK. The use of natural language processing in palliative care research: A scoping review. *Palliative Medicine*. 2023 Feb 1;37(2):275–90.
78. Altini N, Brunetti A, Puro E, Taccogna MG, Saponaro C, Zito FA, et al. NDG-CAM: Nuclei detection in histopathology images with semantic segmentation networks and Grad-CAM. *Bioengineering*. 2022 Sep 1;9(9): 1–19.
79. Bobrow TL, Golhar M, Vijayan R, Akshintala VS, Garcia JR, Durr NJ. Colonoscopy 3D video dataset with paired depth from 2D-3D registration. *Medical Image Analysis*. 2023 Dec 1;90: 1–10.
80. Roodschild M, Gotay Sardiñas J, Will A. A new approach for the vanishing gradient problem on sigmoid activation. *Progress in Artificial Intelligence*. 2020 Dec 1;9(4):351–60.
81. Al-Hammuri K, Gebali F, Kanan A, Chelvan IT. Vision transformer architecture and applications in digital health: A tutorial and survey. *Visual Computing for Industry, Biomedicine, and Art*. 2023 Dec 1;6(14):1–28.
82. Alowais SA, Alghamdi SS, Alsuhebany N, Alqahtani T, Alshaya AI, Almohareb SN, et al. Revolutionizing healthcare: The role of artificial intelligence in clinical practice. *BMC Medical Education*. 2023 Dec 1;23(1):1–15.
83. Pinto-Coelho L. How Artificial Intelligence is shaping medical imaging technology: A survey of innovations and applications. *Bioengineering* [Internet]. 2023 Dec 1 [cited 2024 Jun 4];10(12). Available from: https://doi.org/10.3390/bioengineering10121435
84. Kumar Y, Koul A, Singla R, Ijaz MF. Artificial intelligence in disease diagnosis: A systematic literature review, synthesizing framework and future research agenda. *Journal of Ambient Intelligence and Humanized Computing*. 2023 Jul 1;14(7):8459–86.
85. Uemura T, Näppi JJ, Ryu Y, Watari C, Kamiya T, Yoshida H. A generative flow-based model for volumetric data augmentation in 3D deep learning for computed tomographic colonography. *International Journal of Computer Assisted Radiology and Surgery*. 2021 Jan 1;16(1):81–9.
86. van de Sande D, Sharabiani M, Bluemink H, Kneepkens E, Bakx N, Hagelaar E, et al. Artificial intelligence based treatment planning of radiotherapy for locally advanced breast cancer. *Physics and Imaging in Radiation Oncology*. 2021 Oct 1;20:111–6.

87. Hosny A, Parmar C, Quackenbush J, Schwartz LH, Aerts HJWL. Artificial intelligence in radiology. *Nature Reviews Cancer*. 2018 Aug 1;18(8):500–10.
88. Waldstein SM, Seeböck P, Donner R, Sadeghipour A, Bogunović H, Osborne A, et al. Unbiased identification of novel subclinical imaging biomarkers using unsupervised deep learning. *Scientific Reports*. 2020 Dec 1;10(1):1–9.
89. Lengua CAG. History of rapid prototyping. *Rapid Prototyping in Cardiac Disease: 3D Printing the Heart* [Internet]. 2017 Apr 26 [cited 2024 Jun 5];3–7. Available from: https://link.springer.com/chapter/10.1007/978-3-319-53523-4_1
90. Najjar R. Redefining radiology: A review of artificial intelligence integration in medical imaging. *Diagnostics*. 2023 Sep 1;13(17):1–25.
91. Khalifa M, Albadawy M. AI in diagnostic imaging: Revolutionising accuracy and efficiency. *Computer Methods and Programs in Biomedicine Update*. 2024 Jan 1;5:100146.
92. Vaghasiya JV, Mayorga-Martinez CC, Pumera M. Wearable sensors for telehealth based on emerging materials and nanoarchitectonics. *npj Flexible Electronics* [Internet]. 2023 Jun 2 [cited 2024 Jun 5];7(1):1–14. Available from: https://www.nature.com/articles/s41528-023-00261-4
93. Aneziris ON, Nivolianitou Z, Konstandinidou M, Mavridis G, Plot E. A total safety management framework in case of a major hazards plant producing pesticides. *Safety Science*. 2017 Dec 1;100:183–94.
94. Ab Rahim MS, Reniers G, Yang M, Bajpai S. Risk assessment methods for process safety, process security and resilience in the chemical process industry: A thorough literature review. *Journal of Loss Prevention in the Process Industries*. 2024 Apr 1;88:105274.
95. Amin MT, Khan F, Halim SZ, Pistikopoulos S. A holistic framework for process safety and security analysis. *Computers & Chemical Engineering*. 2022 Sep 1;165: 107963.
96. Ebrahimi SM, Norouzi F, Dastres H, Faieghi R, Naderi M, Malekzadeh M. Sensor fault detection and compensation with performance prescription for robotic manipulators. *Journal of the Franklin Institute*. 2024 May 1;361(7):1–39.
97. Gordon WJ, Stern AD. Challenges and opportunities in software-driven medical devices. *Nature Biomedical Engineering* [Internet]. 2019 Jul 5 [cited 2024 Jun 4];3(7):493–7. Available from: https://www.nature.com/articles/s41551-019-0426-z
98. Parikh RB, Kakad M, Bates DW. Integrating predictive analytics into high-valuecare the dawn of precision delivery. *JAMA*. 2016 Feb 16;315(7):651–2.
99. Bates DW, Saria S, Ohno-Machado L, Shah A, Escobar G. Big data in health care: Using analytics to identify and manage high-risk and high-cost patients. Health Affairs. 2014;33(7):1123–31.
100. Jiang F, Jiang Y, Zhi H, Dong Y, Li H, Ma S, et al. Artificial intelligence in healthcare: Past, present and future. Stroke and Vascular Neurology. 2017 Dec 1;2(4):230–43.
101. Schaeffer NE, Parks LJ, Verhoef ET, Morgan CA, Stal M. Insulin pumps and remote software updates: A new way forward. *Journal of Diabetes Science and Technology*. 2015 Mar 1;10(2):453–6.
102. Ghassemi M, Celi LA, Stone DJ. State of the art review: The data revolution in critical care. *Critical Care*. 2015 Dec 14;19(1):573–586.
103. Ram S, Zhang W, Williams M, Pengetnze Y. Predicting asthma-related emergency department visits using big data. *IEEE Journal of Biomedical and Health Informatics*. 2015 Jul 1;19(4):1216–23.
104. Bhatia R. Emerging health technologies and how they can transform healthcare delivery. https://doi.org/101177/0972063421995025 [Internet]. 2021 Feb 28 [cited 2024 Jun 4];23(1):63–73. Available from: https://journals.sagepub.com/doi/full/10.1177/0972063421995025

105. Human factors & usability engineering: Designing for humans | Coursera [Internet]. [cited 2024 Jun 4]. Available from: https://www.coursera.org/specializations/human-factors-and-usability-engineering-designing-for-humans
106. What is user centered design (UCD)? – updated 2024 | IxDF [Internet]. [cited 2024 Jun 4]. Available from: https://www.interaction-design.org/literature/topics/user-centered-design
107. Bitkina OV, Kim HK, Park J. Usability and user experience of medical devices: An overview of the current state, analysis methodologies, and future challenges. *International Journal of Industrial Ergonomics* 2020 Mar 1;76:102932.
108. The crucial role of UI/UX in cybersecurity products – UX Parrot [Internet]. [cited 2024 Jun 4]. Available from: https://uxparrot.com/the-crucial-role-of-ui-ux-in-cybersecurity-products/
109. Flannery D, Jarrin R. Building a regulatory and payment framework flexible enough to withstand technological progress. *Health Affairs* 2018 Dec 1;37(12):2052–9.
110. Gordon WJ, Landman A, Zhang H, Bates DW. Beyond validation: Getting health apps into clinical practice. *npj Digital Medicine*. 2020 Dec 1;3(1):1–6.
111. Patel NA, Butte AJ. Characteristics and challenges of the clinical pipeline of digital therapeutics. *npj Digital Medicine* 2020 Dec 1;3(1):1–5.
112. Morse KE, Bagely SC, Shah NH. Estimate the hidden deployment cost of predictive models to improve patient care. *Nature Medicine*. 2020 Jan 1;26(1):18–9.
113. Marwaha JS, Landman AB, Brat GA, Dunn T, Gordon WJ. Deploying digital health tools within large, complex health systems: key considerations for adoption and implementation. *npj Digital Medicine* [Internet]. 2022 Jan 27 [cited 2024 Jun 4];5(1):1–7. Available from: https://www.nature.com/articles/s41746-022-00557-1
114. Manu M, Anand G. A review of medical device regulations in India, comparison with European Union and way-ahead. *Perspectives in Clinical Research* [Internet]. 2022 Jan 1 [cited 2024 Jun 4];13(1):3-11. Available from: https://doi.org/10.4103/picr.PICR_222_20
115. Stoumpos AI, Kitsios F, Talias MA. Digital transformation in healthcare: Technology acceptance and its applications. *International Journal of Environmental Research and Public Health* [Internet]. 2023 Feb 1 [cited 2024 Jun 4];20(4). Available from: https://doi.org/10.3390/ijerph20043407
116. Tettey F, Parupelli SK, Desai S. A review of biomedical devices: Classification, regulatory guidelines, human factors, software as a medical device, and cybersecurity. *Biomedical Materials & Devices* [Internet]. 2023 Aug 1 [cited 2024 Jun 4];2(1):316–41. Available from: https://link.springer.com/article/10.1007/s44174-023-00113-9
117. IMDRF SaMD Working Group. Software as a medical device (SaMD): Application of Quality Management System. IMDRF International Medical Device Regulators Forum2015:1-34.
118. Helmold M. Audits and quality management systems (QMS). 2023 [cited 2024 Jun 4];75–86. Available from: https://link.springer.com/chapter/10.1007/978-3-031-30089-9_7
119. Carayon P, Hoonakker P. Human factors and usability for health information technology: Old and new challenges. *Yearbook of Medical Informatics* [Internet]. 2019 Aug 1 [cited 2024 Jun 4];28(1):71-77. Available from: https://doi.org/10.1055/s-0039-1677907
120. Parry E. Medical products: Packing and labeling requirements. 2023 [cited 2024 Jun 5];1–27. Available from: https://link.springer.com/referenceworkentry/10.1007/978-3-030-98743-5_7-1
121. Judd T. Post-market surveillance (PMS) of medical devices: From a clinical engineering perspective. 2024 [cited 2024 Jun 5];93–114. Available from: https://link.springer.com/chapter/10.1007/978-3-031-43444-0_5
122. Xu M, Zhang L, Feng X, Zhang Z, Huang Y. Regulatory reliance for convergence and harmonisation in the medical device space in Asia-Pacific. *BMJ Global Health* [Internet]. 2022 Aug 19 [cited 2024 Jun 5];7(8):9798. Available from: https://doi.org/10.1136/bmjgh-2022-009798

123. Mennella C, Maniscalco U, De Pietro G, Esposito M. Ethical and regulatory challenges of AI technologies in healthcare: A narrative review. *Heliyon*. 2024 Feb 29;10(4):e26297.
124. Lee A, Baker TS, Bederson JB, Rapoport BI. Levels of autonomy in FDA-cleared surgical robots: a systematic review. *npj Digital Medicine* [Internet]. 2024 Apr 26 [cited 2024 Jun 5];7(1):1–8. Available from: https://www.nature.com/articles/s41746-024-01102-y
125. And H. Sciences communications I S. Shaping the future of AI in healthcare through ethics and governance. *Humanities and Social Sciences Communications* [Internet]. 2024 Mar 15 [cited 2024 Jun 5];11(1):1–12. Available from: https://www.nature.com/articles/s41599-024-02894-w
126. Stoumpos AI, Kitsios F, Talias MA. Digital transformation in healthcare: Technology acceptance and its applications. *International Journal of Environmental Research and Public Health* [Internet]. 2023 Feb 1 [cited 2024 Jun 5];20(4). Available from: https://doi.org/10.3390/ijerph20043407
127. International Organization for Standardization (ISO) I Definition I Britannica [Internet]. [cited 2024 Jun 5]. Available from: https://www.britannica.com/topic/International-Organization-for-Standardization
128. International Electrotechnical Commission (IEC). [cited 2024 Jun 5]; Available from: https://doi.org/10.1787/9789264244047-en
129. Or CK, Holden RJ, Valdez RS. Human factors engineering and user-centered design for mobile health technology: Enhancing effectiveness, efficiency, and satisfaction. 2023 [cited 2024 Jun 5];97–118. Available from: https://link.springer.com/chapter/10.1007/978-3-031-10788-7_6
130. Imdrf. IMDRF/SaMD WG/N23 FINAL: 2015 – Software as a medical device (SaMD): Application of quality. 2015.
131. Gübitz B, Klinger U. Risk management for medical devices in compliance with EN ISO 14971. 2023 [cited 2024 Jun 5];89–120. Available from: https://link.springer.com/referenceworkentry/10.1007/978-3-031-22091-3_6
132. Bailey R. Applying design principles to instructional materials. *Applied Human Factors in Medical Device Design*. 2019 Jan 1; 1:139–62.
133. International Medical Device Regulators Forum (IMDRF) I International Medical Device Regulators Forum [Internet]. [cited 2024 Jun 5]. Available from: https://www.imdrf.org/
134. Stasevych M, Zvarych V. Innovative robotic technologies and artificial intelligence in pharmacy and medicine: Paving the way for the future of health care – A review. *Big Data and Cognitive Computing* [Internet]. 2023 Aug 30 [cited 2024 Jun 5];7(3):147. Available from: https://www.mdpi.com/2504-2289/7/3/147/htm
135. Process I of M (US) C on the PHE of the F 510(k) C, Wizemann T. The global framework for regulation of medical devices. 2010 [cited 2024 Jun 5]; Available from: https://www.ncbi.nlm.nih.gov/books/NBK209785/
136. And H, Sciences Communications I S. Shaping the future of AI in healthcare through ethics and governance. *Humanities and Social Sciences Communications* [Internet]. 2024 Mar 15 [cited 2024 Jun 5];11(1):1–12. Available from: https://www.nature.com/articles/s41599-024-02894-w
137. Mennella C, Maniscalco U, De Pietro G, Esposito M. Ethical and regulatory challenges of AI technologies in healthcare: A narrative review. *Heliyon*. 2024 Feb 29;10(4):e26297.
138. Mennella C, Maniscalco U, De Pietro G, Esposito M. Ethical and regulatory challenges of AI technologies in healthcare: A narrative review. *Heliyon*. 2024 Feb 29;10(4):e26297.
139. Mittermaier M, Raza MM, Kvedar JC. Bias in AI-based models for medical applications: Challenges and mitigation strategies. *npj Digital Medicine*. 2023 Jun 14 [cited 2024 Jun 5];6(1):1–3. Available from: https://www.nature.com/articles/s41746-023-00858-z

140. Jawad LA. Security and privacy in digital healthcare systems: Challenges and mitigation strategies. https://doi.org/101177/09702385241233073 [Internet]. 2024 Mar 28 [cited 2024 Jun 5]; Available from: https://journals.sagepub.com/doi/full/10.1177/09702385241233073
141. Bracciale L, Loreti P, Bianchi G. Cybersecurity vulnerability analysis of medical devices purchased by national health services. *Scientific Reports* [Internet]. 2023 Nov 9 [cited 2024 Jun 5];13(1):1–12. Available from: https://www.nature.com/articles/s41598-023-45927-1
142. Jongsma KR, Sand M, Milota M. Why we should not mistake accuracy of medical AI for efficiency. *npj Digital Medicine* [Internet]. 2024 Mar 4 [cited 2024 Jun 5];7(1):1–3. Available from: https://www.nature.com/articles/s41746-024-01047-2
143. Eldakak A, Alremeithi A, Dahiyat E, El-Gheriani M, Mohamed H, Abdulrahim Abdulla MI. Civil liability for the actions of autonomous AI in healthcare: An invitation to further contemplation. *Humanities and Social Sciences Communications* [Internet]. 2024 Feb 23 [cited 2024 Jun 5];11(1):1–8. Available from: https://www.nature.com/articles/s41599-024-02806-y
144. And H, Sciences Communications I S. Shaping the future of AI in healthcare through ethics and governance. *Humanities and Social Sciences Communications* [Internet]. 2024 Mar 15 [cited 2024 Jun 5];11(1):1–12. Available from: https://www.nature.com/articles/s41599-024-02894-w
145. And H, Sciences Communications I S. Shaping the future of AI in healthcare through ethics and governance. *Humanities and Social Sciences Communications* [Internet]. 2024 Mar 15 [cited 2024 Jun 5];11(1):1–12. Available from: https://www.nature.com/articles/s41599-024-02894-w
146. Albahri AS, Duhaim AM, Fadhel MA, Alnoor A, Baqer NS, Alzubaidi L, et al. A systematic review of trustworthy and explainable artificial intelligence in healthcare: Assessment of quality, bias risk, and data fusion. *Information Fusion*. 2023 Aug 1;96:156–91.
147. Anderson TO, Nunes F, Wilcox L, Coiera E, Rogers Y. Introduction to the special issue on human-centred AI in healthcare: Challenges appearing in the wild. *ACM Transactions on Computer-Human Interaction*. 2023 Jun 1;30(2):1–11.
148. Hong AS, Levin D, Parker L, Rao VM, Ross-Degnan D, Wharam JF. Trends in diagnostic imaging utilization among medicare and commercially insured adults from 2003 through 2016. *Radiology*. 2020;294(2):342–50.
149. McGenity C, Clarke EL, Jennings C, Matthews G, Cartlidge C, Freduah-Agyemang H, et al. Artificial intelligence in digital pathology: A systematic review and meta-analysis of diagnostic test accuracy. *npj Digital Medicine* [Internet]. 2024 May 4 [cited 2024 Jun 5];7(1):1–19. Available from: https://www.nature.com/articles/s41746-024-01106-8
150. Bayoumy K, Gaber M, Elshafeey A, Mhaimeed O, Dineen EH, Marvel FA, et al. Smart wearable devices in cardiovascular care: where we are and how to move forward. *Nature Reviews Cardiology* [Internet]. 2021 Mar 4 [cited 2024 Jun 5];18(8):581–99. Available from: https://www.nature.com/articles/s41569-021-00522-7
151. Fairag M, Almahdi RH, Siddiqi AA, Alharthi FK, Alqurashi BS, Alzahrani NG, et al. Robotic revolution in surgery: Diverse applications across specialties and future prospects review article. *Cureus* [Internet]. 2024 Jan 12 [cited 2024 Jun 5];16(1). Available from: https://doi.org/10.7759/cureus.52148
152. Batson S, Herranz A, Rohrbach N, Canobbio M, Mitchell SA, Bonnabry P. Automation of in-hospital pharmacy dispensing: A systematic review. *European Journal of Hospital Pharmacy* [Internet]. 2021 Mar 1 [cited 2024 Jun 5];28(2):58. Available from: https://doi.org/10.1136/ejhpharm-2019-002081

153. Laut J, Porfiri M, Raghavan P. The present and future of robotic technology in rehabilitation. *Current Physical Medicine and Rehabilitation Reports* [Internet]. 2016 Dec 1 [cited 2024 Jun 5];4(4):312-319. Available from: https://doi.org/10.1007/s40141-016-0139-0
154. Zhou Y, Holets SR, Li M, Cortes-Puentes GA, Meyer TJ, Hanson AC, et al. Etiology, incidence, and outcomes of patient–ventilator asynchrony in critically-ill patients undergoing invasive mechanical ventilation. *Scientific Reports* [Internet]. 2021 Jun 11 [cited 2024 Jun 5];11(1):1–9. Available from: https://www.nature.com/articles/s41598-021-90013-z
155. Spatz ES, Ginsburg GS, Rumsfeld JS, Turakhia MP. Wearable digital health technologies for monitoring in cardiovascular medicine. *New England Journal of Medicine* [Internet]. 2024 Jan 25 [cited 2024 Jun 5];390(4):346–56. Available from: https://www.nejm.org/doi/full/10.1056/NEJMra2301903
156. Ajjan RA, Battelino T, Cos X, Del Prato S, Philips JC, Meyer L, et al. Continuous glucose monitoring for the routine care of type 2 diabetes mellitus. *Nature Reviews Endocrinology* [Internet]. 2024 Apr 8 [cited 2024 Jun 5];1–15. Available from: https://www.nature.com/articles/s41574-024-00973-1
157. Kaptoge S, Pennells L, De Bacquer D, Cooney MT, Kavousi M, Stevens G, et al. World Health Organization cardiovascular disease risk charts: revised models to estimate risk in 21 global regions. *Lancet Global Health* [Internet]. 2019 Oct 1 [cited 2024 Jun 5];7(10):e1332–45. Available from: http://www.thelancet.com/article/S2214109X19303183/fulltext
158. Abd-Alrazaq A, AlSaad R, Shuweihdi F, Ahmed A, Aziz S, Sheikh J. Systematic review and meta-analysis of performance of wearable artificial intelligence in detecting and predicting depression. *NPJ Digital Medicine*. 2023 Dec 1;6(1):84.
159. Gibson PG, Simpson JL. The overlap syndrome of asthma and COPD: What are its features and how important is it? *Thorax*. 2009;64(8):728–35.
160. Vudathaneni VKP, Lanke RB, Mudaliyar MC, Movva KV, Kalluri LM, Boyapati R. The impact of telemedicine and remote patient monitoring on healthcare delivery: A comprehensive evaluation. *Cureus* [Internet]. 2024 Mar 5 [cited 2024 Jun 5];16(3): e55534. Available from: https://doi.org/10.7759/cureus.55534
161. Caulfield B, Reginatto B, Slevin P. Not all sensors are created equal: A framework for evaluating human performance measurement technologies. *NPJ Digital Medicine*. 2019 Dec 1;14(2):7. https://doi.org10.1038/s41746-019-0082-4
162. Hilty DM, Armstrong CM, Edwards-Stewart A, Gentry MT, Luxton DD, Krupinski EA. Sensor, wearable, and remote patient monitoring competencies for clinical care and training: Scoping review. *Journal of Technology in Behavioral Science* [Internet]. 2021 Jun 1 [cited 2024 Jun 5];6(2):252-277. Available from: https://doi.org/10.1007/s41347-020-00190-3
163. Busso M, Gonzalez MP, Scartascini C. On the demand for telemedicine: Evidence from the COVID-19 pandemic. *Health Economics* [Internet]. 2022 Jul 1 [cited 2024 Jun 5];31(7):1491–1505. Available from: https://doi.org/10.1002/hec.4523
164. Onitiu D, Wachter S, Mittelstadt B. How AI challenges the medical device regulation: patient safety, benefits, and intended uses. *The Journal of Law and the Biosciences* [Internet]. 2024 Apr 9 [cited 2024 Jun 5]; Available from: https://doi.org/10.1093/jlb/lsae007
165. Henry KE, Kornfield R, Sridharan A, Linton RC, Groh C, Wang T, et al. Human–machine teaming is key to AI adoption: clinicians' experiences with a deployed machine learning system. *npj Digital Medicine* [Internet]. 2022 Jul 21 [cited 2024 Jun 5];5(1):1–6. Available from: https://www.nature.com/articles/s41746-022-00597-7
166. Acosta JN, Falcone GJ, Rajpurkar P, Topol EJ. Multimodal biomedical AI. *Nature Medicine* [Internet]. 2022 Sep 15 [cited 2024 Jun 5];28(9):1773–84. Available from: https://www.nature.com/articles/s41591-022-01981-2

167. Sharma A, Lysenko A, Jia S, Boroevich KA, Tsunoda T. Advances in AI and machine learning for predictive medicine. *Journal of Human Genetics* [Internet]. 2024 Feb 29 [cited 2024 Jun 5];1–11. Available from: https://www.nature.com/articles/s10038-024-01231-y
168. Varoquaux G, Cheplygina V. Machine learning for medical imaging: Methodological failures and recommendations for the future. *NPJ Digital Medicine*. 2022 Dec 1;5(1):48.
169. Chen H, Gomez C, Huang CM, Unberath M. Explainable medical imaging AI needs human-centered design: Guidelines and evidence from a systematic review. *NPJ Digital Medicine*, 2022 Dec 1;5(1):156.
170. McNamara SL, Yi PH, Lotter W. The clinician-AI interface: Intended use and explainability in FDA-cleared AI devices for medical image interpretation. *npj Digital Medicine* [Internet]. 2024 Mar 26 [cited 2024 Jun 5];7(1):1–5. Available from: https://www.nature.com/articles/s41746-024-01080-1
171. van der Velden BHM, Kuijf HJ, Gilhuijs KGA, Viergever MA. Explainable artificial intelligence (XAI) in deep learning-based medical image analysis. *Medical Image Analysis*. 2022 Jul 1;79:102470.
172. Silcox C, Zimlichmann E, Huber K, Rowen N, Saunders R, McClellan M, et al. The potential for artificial intelligence to transform healthcare: Perspectives from international health leaders. *npj Digital Medicine* [Internet]. 2024 Apr 9 [cited 2024 Jun 5];7(1):1–3. Available from: https://www.nature.com/articles/s41746-024-01097-6
173. Zharima C, Griffiths F, Goudge J. Exploring the barriers and facilitators to implementing electronic health records in a middle-income country: A qualitative study from South Africa. *Frontiers in Digital Health*. 2023;5:1207602.
174. Lee AR, Koo D, Kim IK, Lee E, Kim HH, Yoo S, et al. Identifying facilitators of and barriers to the adoption of dynamic consent in digital health ecosystems: A scoping review. *BMC Medical Ethics*. 2023 Dec 1;24(1):107.
175. Hamm P, Klesel M, Coberger P, Wittmann HF. Explanation matters: An experimental study on explainable AI. *Electronic Markets* [Internet]. 2023 Dec 1 [cited 2024 Jun 5];33(1):1–21. Available from: https://link.springer.com/article/10.1007/s12525-023-00640-9
176. Kaissis GA, Makowski MR, Rückert D, Braren RF. Secure, privacy-preserving and federated machine learning in medical imaging. *Nature Machine Intelligence* [Internet]. 2020 Jun 8 [cited 2024 Jun 5];2(6):305–11. Available from: https://www.nature.com/articles/s42256-020-0186-1
177. Dai L, Wu L, Li H, Cai C, Wu Q, Kong H, et al. A deep learning system for detecting diabetic retinopathy across the disease spectrum. *Nature Communications* [Internet]. 2021 May 28 [cited 2024 Jun 5];12(1):1–11. Available from: https://www.nature.com/articles/s41467-021-23458-5
178. Varghese C, Harrison EM, O'Grady G, Topol EJ. Artificial intelligence in surgery. *Nature Medicine* [Internet]. 2024 May 13 [cited 2024 Jun 5];30(5):1257–68. Available from: https://www.nature.com/articles/s41591-024-02970-3
179. Young MJ, Lin DJ, Hochberg LR. Brain-computer interfaces in neurorecovery and neurorehabilitation. *Seminars in Neurology* [Internet]. 2021 Apr 1 [cited 2024 Jun 5];41(2):206-216. Available from: https://doi.org/10.1055/s-0041-1725137
180. Ghorbani A, Ouyang D, Abid A, He B, Chen JH, Harrington RA, et al. Deep learning interpretation of echocardiograms. *npj Digital Medicine* [Internet]. 2020 Jan 24 [cited 2024 Jun 5];3(1):1–10. Available from: https://www.nature.com/articles/s41746-019-0216-8
181. Prabhakar H, Singhal V, Zirpe KG, Sapra H, editors. Principles and practice of neurocritical care. 2024 [cited 2024 Jun 5]; Available from: https://link.springer.com/10.1007/978-981-99-8059-8

182. Bissett B, Leditschke IA, Green M, Marzano V, Collins S, Van Haren F. Inspiratory muscle training for intensive care patients: A multidisciplinary practical guide for clinicians. *Australian Critical Care*. 2019 May 1;32(3):249–55.
183. Aggarwal R, Dua V, Sachdev HS. Physiotherapeutic management in neurocritical care. *Principles and Practice of Neurocritical Care* [Internet]. 2024 [cited 2024 Jun 5];561–78. Available from: https://link.springer.com/chapter/10.1007/978-981-99-8059-8_42
184. Jeddi Z, Bohr A. Chapter 9 Remote patient monitoring using artificial intelligence. *Artificial Intelligence in Healthcare*. 2020 Jan 1;203–234.
185. Dhatterwal JS, Kaswan KS, Kumar N. Robotic process automation in healthcare. *Smart Innovation, Systems and Technologies* [Internet]. 2023 [cited 2024 Jun 5];335:157–75. Available from: https://link.springer.com/chapter/10.1007/978-981-19-8296-5_7
186. Jie Z, Zhiying Z, Li L. A meta-analysis of Watson for Oncology in clinical application. *Scientific Reports* [Internet]. 2021 Mar 11 [cited 2024 Jun 5];11(1):1–13. Available from: https://www.nature.com/articles/s41598-021-84973-5
187. Choudhary K, DeCost B, Chen C, Jain A, Tavazza F, Cohn R, et al. Recent advances and applications of deep learning methods in materials science. *npj Computational Materials* [Internet]. 2022 Apr 5 [cited 2024 Jun 5];8(1):1–26. Available from: https://www.nature.com/articles/s41524-022-00734-6
188. Kim BC, Kim B, Hyun Y. Investigation of out-of-distribution detection across various models and training methodologies. *Neural Networks*. 2024 Jul 1;175:106288.
189. Chen Z. Ethics and discrimination in artificial intelligence-enabled recruitment practices. *Humanities and Social Sciences Communications* [Internet]. 2023 Sep 13 [cited 2024 Jun 5];10(1):1–12. Available from: https://www.nature.com/articles/s41599-023-02079-x
190. Henry KE, Kornfield R, Sridharan A, Linton RC, Groh C, Wang T, et al. Human–machine teaming is key to AI adoption: Clinicians' experiences with a deployed machine learning system. *npj Digital Medicine* [Internet]. 2022 Jul 21 [cited 2024 Jun 5];5(1):1–6. Available from: https://www.nature.com/articles/s41746-022-00597-7
191. Feng J, Phillips RV, Malenica I, Bishara A, Hubbard AE, Celi LA, et al. Clinical artificial intelligence quality improvement: towards continual monitoring and updating of AI algorithms in healthcare. *npj Digital Medicine* [Internet]. 2022 May 31 [cited 2024 Jun 5];5(1):1–9. Available from: https://www.nature.com/articles/s41746-022-00611-y
192. de Almeida PGR, dos Santos CD, Farias JS. Artificial Intelligence regulation: A framework for governance. *Ethics and Information Technology* [Internet]. 2021 Sep 1 [cited 2024 Jun 5];23(3):505–25. Available from: https://link.springer.com/article/10.1007/s10676-021-09593-z
193. Novelli C, Taddeo M, Floridi L. Accountability in artificial intelligence: What it is and how it works. *AI & Society*. 2024;39:1871–1882. https://doi.org/10.1007/s00146-023-01635-y
194. Lin YT, Hung TW, Huang LTL. Engineering equity: How AI can help reduce the harm of implicit bias. *Philosophy & Technology*. 2020 Nov 1;34:65–90.
195. Guo LL, Pfohl SR, Fries J, Johnson AEW, Posada J, Aftandilian C, et al. Evaluation of domain generalization and adaptation on improving model robustness to temporal dataset shift in clinical medicine. *Scientific Reports* [Internet]. 2022 Feb 17 [cited 2024 Jun 5];12(1):1–10. Available from: https://www.nature.com/articles/s41598-022-06484-1
196. Buhl D, Lanquillon C. Challenges of machine failure prediction with product data – A case study. 2024 [cited 2024 Jun 5];308–22. Available from: https://link.springer.com/chapter/10.1007/978-3-031-60611-3_22
197. Degen H, Ntoa S, editors. Artificial Intelligence in HCI. 2024 [cited 2024 Jun 5];14735. Available from: https://link.springer.com/10.1007/978-3-031-60611-3

198. Köbis NC, Doležalová B, Soraperra I. Fooled twice: People cannot detect deepfakes but think they can. *iScience* [Internet]. 2021 Nov 11 [cited 2024 Jun 5];24(11):103364. Available from: https://doi.org/10.1016/j.isci.2021.103364
199. Tocchetti A, Corti L, Balayn A, Yurrita M, Lippmann P, Brambilla M, et al. A.I. robustness: A human-centered perspective on technological challenges and opportunities. *ACM Computing Surveys* [Internet]. 2024 May 27 [cited 2024 Jun 5]; Available from: https://dl.acm.org/doi/10.1145/3665926
200. Fjeld J, Achten N, Hilligoss H, Nagy A, Srikumar M. Principled artificial intelligence: Mapping consensus in ethical and rights-based approaches to principles for AI. *SSRN Electronic Journal*. 2020 Feb 9. 2020(1):1–39. http://doi.org/10.2139/ssrn.3518482
201. Hickok M. Lessons learned from AI ethics principles for future actions. *AI and Ethics*. 2020 Oct 6 [cited 2024 Jun 5];1(1):41–7. Available from: https://link.springer.com/article/10.1007/s43681-020-00008-1

4 Embedded Systems in Developing Imaging Devices

Sündüz Alemdar and Nursel Pekel Bayramgil

4.1 INTRODUCTION

Access to high-quality, affordable, and appropriate health products is crucial for maintaining a healthy population, resolving medical emergencies, and achieving universal health care. Medical gadgets are important for carrying out normal medical treatments, such as the treatment of an injured ankle, the detection of HIV/AIDS, the implantation of an artificial hip, or the performance of any surgical operation. In a variety of settings, medical devices are used for screening, prevention, and palliative care. This includes households with no medical background, outpatient clinics with paramedical staff and clinicians, dental offices with optometrists and dentists, and hospitals with highly trained medical workers. These medical technologies are used to diagnose and treat both acute and chronic illnesses, as well as to monitor medical procedures and aid those with disabilities. There are around 2 million unique types of medical devices currently available worldwide, spanning across more than 7000 generic device categories. A medical device is defined as any item, such as a tool, machine, or software, that is intended to be used for medical reasons, either on its own or in combination with other items [1]. An imaging device is any gadget that can take and store still or moving pictures. Examples of such gadgets include digital or other cameras, video cameras, cell phones that can take and record videos, and more. "Medical imaging" encompasses several technologies that allow for the visualization of the human body for the purpose of diagnosing, tracking, or treating medical disorders. Different information regarding potential diseases, injuries, and the efficacy of medical treatments is provided by each type of technology concerning the body part being investigated or treated [2].

What we call "embedded systems" are electronic gadgets designed to do certain jobs. Almost all modern electronic tools and devices, including cell phones, car engines, and security systems, contain embedded software. Embedded systems enable a medical equipment to perform a variety of tasks, including hardware operation, wireless data transmission and reception, patient data tracking, and recording. For example, smartwatches have embedded systems that use wireless connectivity, sensors, and microprocessors to track health information, show alerts, and communicate with smartphones. Fitness trackers, like smartwatches, use

 DOI: 10.1201/9781003508199-4

embedded technologies to detect heart rate, routines for sleep, and physical activity, giving individuals important health information. Pacemakers equipped with embedded systems keep an eye on cardiac activity and pulse electrically to maintain cardiac rhythm and proper operation. In response to user choices and external factors, embedded systems in hearing aids modify settings, filter out background noise, and boost sound. Vital signs and activity levels are tracked by wearable health monitors using embedded systems, which also give users feedback on their health.

Innovations in technology have paved the way for the creation of more intelligent medical devices. Modern embedded systems have greatly facilitated the combination of Internet of Things, machine learning, and artificial intelligence into the design of medical devices. Because of their exceptional adaptability, embedded sensor systems are becoming increasingly important in the advancement of innovative medical equipment. Thanks to them, state-of-the-art diagnostic and patient monitoring devices that can be utilized in both healthcare facilities and private residences can be developed [3]. These advancements in technology have made it possible to constantly and daily check and maintain patients' health. By reducing size, increasing processing power, and incorporating programmed automatic technologies, medical-standard embedded technologies are regularly enhanced to provide patients with better treatments and medications. There is a scarcity of doctors in rural places, but medical systems connected to the internet could help. These devices' operating system interfaces and fast processors can speed up the diagnosis and treatment processes for patients.

4.2 MEDICAL IMAGING

Medical imaging is a valuable way employed to provide graphic representations of the anatomical structures within the body that are examined and treated for medical purposes, as well as visual depictions of the functioning of certain organs or tissues. These images are utilized for the purpose of diagnosing, monitoring, or treating medical disorders by offering intricate insights that cannot be observed from external examination. This activity is conducted for medical treatments and academic study to comprehend the anatomy and physiology of the body, both in its healthy state and when affected by disease. Radiology is an essential part of biological imaging and involves the use of various imaging technologies such as X-ray radiography, MRI, X-ray CT, ESI, digital mammography, endoscopy, PET, IR imaging, SPECT, and US imaging [4]. Figure 4.1 shows the traditional and modern imaging systems used in the medical field. Imaging technologies are essential for the diagnosis of nearly all serious medical ailments and disorders, including problems with the brain, heart disorders, trauma diseases, cancers, and many more [5]. They are an advanced visual aid that physicians use to better understand the situations of their patients [6, 7]. Scientists, researchers, and medical specialists have been working together for years to create the greatest equipment on the market. CT scanners, MRI machines, X-ray machines, ECG machines, and other equipment are examples of modern medical devices that incorporate embedded technology [8].

A detailed presentation of medical-standard embedded systems-based imaging devices is provided in the upcoming sections.

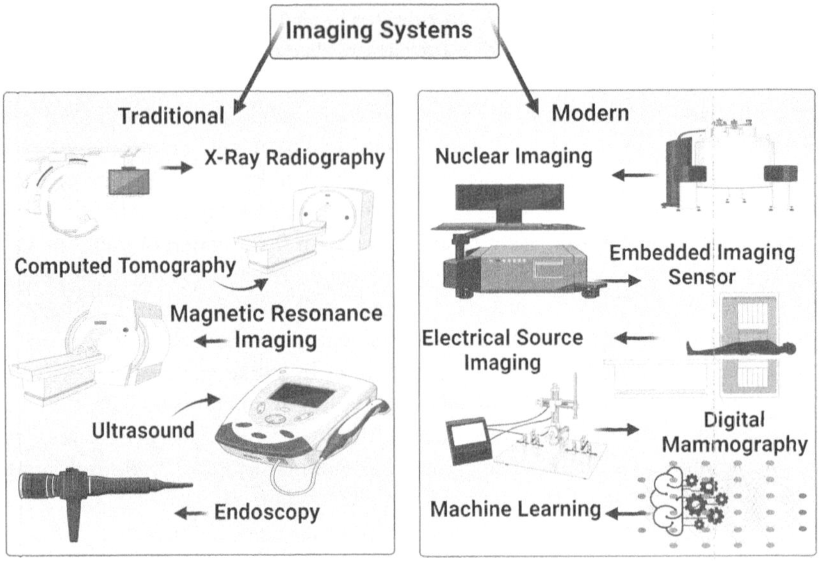

FIGURE 4.1 Traditional and modern imaging systems in medicine.

4.2.1 Embedded Sensor Systems in Imaging Devices

Radiology is essential in today's healthcare as it offers non-invasive imaging techniques to diagnose and monitor various medical disorders. Classical imaging strategies, such as X-ray, MRI, CT scan, and ultrasound, have made substantial progress. Nevertheless, the incorporation of embedded sensors has enhanced their capabilities, leading to more precise and efficient diagnostics [9]. These sensors are used in a wide range of radiological imaging techniques. Embedded sensors in MRI machines provide the monitoring of patient vital signs, including heart rate and respiration, during the scanning process. Besides, they assist in monitoring movement, enabling the rectification of any irregularities in patient mobility. CT scanners are equipped with embedded sensors that improve the quality of images by providing immediate input on the distribution of radiation exposure. Additionally, they assist in the alignment of patients and monitoring their movements, hence reducing the necessity for doing scans multiple times. Conical beam CT, panoramic, and cephalometric imaging are just a few of the dental radiology applications that have benefited from Teledyne Technological Company's CMOS-based image sensor technology. CMOS sensors have many advantages over their conventional counterparts. For example, they have radiation-resistant pixels, which prolong the sensor's life, and a packaging approach that makes them immune to harsh conditions, shocks, and impacts [10].

The integration of sensors into X-ray equipment enhances the management of radiation dosage and the quality of the images produced. They contribute to the process of dynamic imaging, such as fluoroscopy, by offering information on exposure settings and patient location. Xineos X-Ray Image Reconstruction Technology, created by Teledyne Technology Company, captures high-resolution panoramic images,

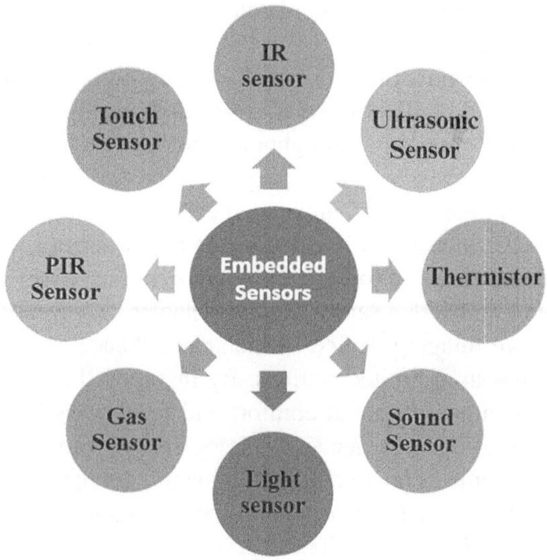

FIGURE 4.2 Embedded sensors used in imaging.

allowing users to bypass traditional limitations. A 3-D tomographic volume, including crucial human anatomy, is acquired using the method, which employs rapid frame-based CMOS detectors [10]. An article detailing a straightforward and dependable technique for utilizing a device was released in the Review of Scientific Instruments. One theory behind this approach is that X-ray photons can build up an electric charge in a chip based on a charge-linked device, allowing for a quick and accurate reading [11].

Embedded sensors provide instant monitoring of the location and orientation of the ultrasonic probe, hence improving image-guided procedures and minimizing differences in performance across operators. The utilization of sensors in nuclear imaging systems enhances the ability to precisely determine the location of radiopharmaceuticals, hence increasing the precision of diagnostic and therapeutic treatments. Figure 4.2 displays embedded sensors used in imaging.

Real-time feedback from embedded sensors enables the optimization of imaging parameters, resulting in higher-quality images with reduced artifacts. Continuous monitoring of vital signs and radiation dose ensures patient safety during imaging procedures. Automation of certain processes, such as patient positioning and motion correction, reduces scan time and enhances workflow efficiency. Embedded sensors enable precise localization and tracking of anatomical structures and medical devices, leading to more accurate diagnosis and treatment planning. Thanks to advancements in connectivity across digital health systems, remote monitoring of imaging parameters and patient data is now within reach. This further improves the usefulness of telemedicine and online consultations. Since radiological equipment with integrated sensor systems could have greater initial costs, a thorough return on investment analysis is required. There is a risk of incompatibility when integrating new sensors into older imaging equipment or connecting them to legacy systems. Data security and privacy legislation compliance are legitimate concerns regarding the transmission and storage of sensitive patient data collected by embedded sensors. Adherence to regulatory standards and guidelines for radiation safety and medical devices is critical for ensuring the safe and successful use of embedded sensor systems in radiology.

The use of sensor technology throughout radiology has the potential to open up numerous fascinating new avenues of inquiry. With the development of smaller, more sensitive, and multi-mode sensors, embedded sensor systems will gain power. The use of artificial intelligence algorithms for image reconstruction, analysis, and decision support will pave the way for novel and tailored diagnostic imaging solutions. Reducing the size of embedded sensor systems enables the invention of easily transportable point-of-care imaging devices, which can enhance the availability of diagnostic imaging in resource-limited settings. By incorporating sensors into imaging techniques, we may enhance patient comfort and feedback systems, which in turn improves the whole patient experience. Radiologists are witnessing a sea change as embedded sensor systems improve diagnostic imaging, image quality, patient safety, and workflow efficiency. The future of radiological imaging is bright, thanks to ever-improving sensor technology and its integration with artificial intelligence (AI). However, there will always be challenges with pricing, interoperability, and legal compliance. The majority of bioimaging sensors fall into one of two categories: quantum sensors or silicon sensors. A brief summary of each is given in the following sections.

4.2.1.1 Quantum Sensors

The integration of quantum sensors with imaging systems holds tremendous potential for applications such as monitoring the environment, healthcare imaging, and security systems. These sensors employ quantum mechanical principles to enhance the sensitivity, resolution, and accuracy of images. Detecting signals as faint as individual photons is within the capabilities of quantum sensors. When imaging in low-light situations or with partially or completely opaque materials, for example, the ability to detect tiny signals is critical, and thus high sensitivity is ideal for such tasks. When compared to classical sensors, quantum ones are able to achieve far higher resolutions. Advanced imaging methods, such as quantum enhanced and quantum ghost imagings, are made possible by quantum sensors. In addition, they possess outstanding metrological capabilities, allowing for precise measurement of many physical parameters such as electric fields, magnetic fields, temperature, and pressure. With these abilities built into imaging systems, high-tech features like sensitivity- and resolution-boosting magnetic resonance imaging (MRI) are within reach. Early disease detection, personalized medical treatments, and cutting-edge brain research are all areas that stand to benefit greatly from this development. These technologies have the potential to reduce radiation emissions while providing remarkably clear images of biological tissues. Because of this, they are very important in the fields of medicine and treatment planning. The promising applications of quantum sensors, especially Quantum Dots (QDs), in areas such as medical imaging, biological sensing, and drug delivery, have piqued the curiosity of scientists worldwide [12, 13]. Quantum dots are semiconductor particles with distinct optical, electrical, and other physicochemical properties that vary depending on their size. Their surface functionalization characteristics and biocompatibility are exceptional. Quantum dots have been extensively studied for a diverse range of biomedical purposes, such as illness diagnosis, medication administration, biosensing, bioimaging, and many therapeutic uses [12, 14, 15].

Metal nanocavities can generate intensified light-up conversion signals when stimulated by ultrashort pulses. These properties make them highly beneficial for various applications, including medical imaging, sensing, and integrated photonics. A study was conducted by researchers from Virginia Tech to investigate the improvement of light-up conversion. Their measurements indicated the disparities and associations between the plasmon-enhanced ASPL and SHG phenomena under different modal and ultrashort pulsed laser stimulation conditions, including incident flow, wavelength, and polarization [16].

Lately, improvements in quantum metrics, communicating, and the integration and interfaces between tailored biologically active chemicals have resulted in a very precise study of immediate biological events. These technologies are anticipated to offer the capability to measure and document fluctuations in varied pressure, temperature, and electromagnetic fields at quantum levels [17].

4.2.1.2 Silicon Sensors

Silicon-based sensors are widely used in biomedical applications due to their high sensitivity, stability, and compatibility with electronics [18–20]. Silicon nanomaterials, including silicon nanoparticles and silicon nanoneedles, are of great interest because of their ability to break down into molecules that can be eliminated by the kidneys, specifically silicic acid, without causing harm to living organisms [18]. These sensors are utilized in a range of analytical applications, such as very sensitive biomolecular detection and real-time biological imaging analysis. Porous Silicon (PSi) optical-biosensors are a type of silicon-based sensors employed in bioimaging. PSi is an attractive substrate for biosensing purposes due to its cost-effective production procedure, high internal surface area, variable pore size, and photonic features [19].

A novel X-ray medical image sensor made on amorphous silicon (Si) was recently created by Wiesfield *et al.* [21]. This new discovery exemplifies the remarkable strides that medical imaging science is currently making. A series of a-Si solar cells are used in conjunction with an X-ray fluorescent screen to detect natural light, and a-Si semiconductor thin-film transistors link the solar cells to electrical components for external output. These imaging devices capture images quickly and can be easily connected to a standard personal computer.

4.2.2 Embedded Systems in X-ray Radiography

Embedded systems are integral in X-ray radiography for diagnosing and treating patients. However, X-ray radiography itself is primarily a diagnostic imaging modality used to visualize internal structures of the body. It's not typically used for curing patients directly. That said, embedded systems are crucial for guaranteeing the efficacy and safety of X-ray operations, which indirectly contributes to patient care and treatment. During X-ray operations, embedded technologies keep an eye on radiation dosage levels to minimize radiation exposure while guaranteeing that patients obtain the essential diagnostic information. By controlling the X-ray tube parameters and monitoring dose levels in real-time, embedded systems help reduce the risk of radiation-related side effects. These systems ensure that diagnostic images are of sufficient quality for accurate interpretation by healthcare professionals by adjusting factors such as exposure time, tube current, and filtration. While X-ray radiography is mostly used for diagnostic purposes, the obtained images can also be crucial for treatment planning in certain cases, such as radiation therapy. Embedded systems enable the seamless integration of X-ray images into treatment planning software, thereby improving the accuracy of radiation targeting and delivery to malignant tumors while reducing harm to healthy tissues. To summarize, X-ray radiography itself does not directly treat patients, but the integrated systems within X-ray equipment play a vital role in safeguarding patient well-being, enhancing the accuracy of diagnostic images, and optimizing operational efficiency. These elements jointly contribute to the efficient provision of patient care and treatment.

Currently, COVID-19 poses the most significant danger to humanity. Scientists have suggested a design for an embedded system that can be utilized at the entrance of airports, train terminals, and subway stations. The system utilizes X-ray imaging technology to compare the X-ray image of a passenger with the X-ray image of a COVID-19 patient which is currently recorded in the SD card. Upon detecting a resemblance between the two X-ray images, audible alarms and visual indicators will be triggered. This approach has the potential to effectively limit the transmission of COVID-19 [22].

Chest X-rays play a crucial role in assessing affected patients in the worldwide battle against this infection. Therefore, the implementation of diverse technologies that provide swift identification of COVID-19 can provide health professionals with a high level of precision in detecting the virus, enabling them to make informed judgments. Researchers are attempting to utilize the current advancements in deep-learning to improve the capabilities of medical imaging equipment, namely in X-ray detection. However, their efforts have been met with minimal success. A scholarly article presented a resilient and efficient network that achieves accurate classification results in diagnosing COVID-19 by analyzing chest X-rays. For the first time, this research presents a refined model for an embedded system that is both power efficient and better at detecting threats [23]. A different research study introduced a comprehensive deep neural network that utilizes contextual representations of words to provide medically valuable radiological outputs from chest X-ray (CXR) images. The network presented, referred to as RadioBERT, utilizes DistilBERT for representing words in context and takes advantage of transfer learning. Furthermore, the network recognizes the significance of atypical data in comparison to regular ones. In order to emphasize outstanding descriptions, the network rearranges the generated phrases through sentiment analysis, placing atypical descriptions at the start of the resulting report. The proposed methodology significantly enhanced the performance metrics, surpassing the present cutting-edge by an immense range. The study demonstrates a considerable improvement in the performance of hierarchical long short-term memory in producing clinical reports when using word embeddings generated by DistilBERT [24].

4.2.3 Embedded Systems in Computed Tomography (CT)

Computed Tomography (CT) has become a renowned medical imaging technology because of its extraordinary ability to provide detailed and precise images of anatomical structures with high spatial and temporal resolution [25]. The essential component of these devices is their embedded systems, which facilitate the seamless integration of sensors, data collection modules, and processing units, allowing for fast and accurate analysis of complex medical data [26]. CT scanners are highly dependent on embedded technologies for their functioning. These scanners utilize embedded systems to carry out several duties, including: Embedded systems are responsible for managing the whole operation of the CT scanner. This involves regulating the motion of the X-ray source and detector around the patient, overseeing the timing and synchronization of data gathering, and coordinating the various subsystems engaged in the scanning procedure. After gathering data, CT scanners employ complex algorithms to generate cross-sectional images from the acquired raw data. Embedded devices effectively execute these algorithms to produce high-resolution photos in real-time or close to real-time. Embedded systems are employed to handle and examine reconstructed images. This entails the use of image enhancement techniques, performing picture segmentation to identify organs or tissues, and monitoring various parameters for diagnostic purposes. Embedded systems provide the user interface for controlling the CT scanner, including setting scan parameters, initiating scans, and displaying images and diagnostic information to the operator [27]. Embedded systems implement safety features and interlocks to ensure patient safety during scanning, such as monitoring radiation dose levels, detecting motion artifacts, and automatically halting the scan if any abnormal conditions are detected.

The applications of CT devices with embedded systems are vast and continue to grow with advancements in technology. A few notable applications found in literature are given following paragraphs:

A method for detecting COVID-19 using deep learning has been suggested and tested on embedded edge-computing devices [28]. In a separate study, CT scans have been used to identify COVID-19, pneumonia, and normal people. In order to accomplish classification, two models are utilized. These models are often employed for jobs involving picture classification. In order to assess the efficacy of the suggested technique, a widely used method (k-fold cross-validation) for estimating the performance of deep learning models was chosen. The system is trained and confirmed using a four-fold cross-validation approach, with an average accuracy of 98.83% [29].

CT imaging has become a primary tool in various fields of medicine [30]. The growing prevalence of exams utilizing this method, along with the implementation of new procedures conducted with the guidance of CT scans in clinical practice, has spurred research into novel uses in this context. If it's to be summarized, the use of embedded systems in CT devices has greatly improved patient care, enhanced healthcare professionals' performance, and reduced healthcare costs. As technology continues to advance, the use of these systems in CT devices is expected to become even more sophisticated and integral to the field of medicine.

4.2.4 Embedded Systems in Endoscopy

Embedded systems are essential in modern endoscopy as they enable precise control, visualization, and management of data during diagnostic and therapeutic procedures. The integration of these devices with endoscopic instruments enhances the efficiency, safety, and efficacy of gastrointestinal, respiratory, and other endoscopic treatments. They guarantee that healthcare personnel get maximum clarity and precision in visualizing the interior of organs and tissues during medical procedures. Embedded systems govern the illumination system of the endoscope, overseeing the adjustment of brightness and color temperature to improve vision within the bodily cavity being examined. Furthermore, they have the potential to incorporate features like as adaptive lighting, which enhances contrast and minimizes glare. These technologies provide the transmission of video and image data from the endoscope to external display monitors or recording devices. The endoscopic system can offer support for several transmission protocols, such as HDMI, USB, or wireless connectivity, according to its individual requirements.

In recent years, powerful endoscopy has experienced notable technological breakthroughs, with embedded systems playing a vital part in this progress [31, 32]. Endoscopic devices have been improved by the addition of sensors, actuators, and computers, which boost their diagnostic and therapeutic capacities. Embedded systems can be utilized in modern endoscopic treatments to manage supplementary instruments that are included in the endoscope, such as biopsy forceps, snares, or cautery devices. This allows for accurate manipulation and intervention within the bodily cavity while directly observing the process. The potential uses of advanced endoscopy with embedded systems are extensive and expanding as technology progresses. Here are some noteworthy examples of applications discovered in literature: Robotic flexible endoscopes have been developed to overcome the limitations of current flexible endoscopes. They enhance the accuracy of diagnosis and improve the effectiveness of treatment, resulting in increased skill, precision, and ergonomic benefits. The integration of biorobotics and computer help in clinical practice will revolutionize diagnostic endoscopy for both doctors and patients [32]. The scientific community has increasingly focused on AI in recent years. AI allows robots to analyze information in a way that resembles human thinking, perhaps with significantly greater efficiency. AI has the potential to completely transform endoscopic diagnosis [33]. Imaging techniques have progressed from using ordinary white light endoscopes to employing high-definition resolution endoscopes and other color enhancement techniques [34]. This literature review intended to comprehensively summarize the latest breakthroughs in the realm of sophisticated gastrointestinal endoscopy. Data from various sources on the patient's anatomy is combined with massive volumes of data by endoscopic navigators. They are used to control the mobility of medical endoscopes and surgical equipment, as well as provide guidance to surgeons during endoscopic procedures [35].

The wireless capsule endoscope (WCE) is a significant innovation that has been launched in the field of biomedical technology. The process is ingesting a compact, disposable video capsule that captures photographic images while traversing the gastrointestinal (GI) tract. WCE enables clinicians to visually examine and diagnose illnesses that affect the whole GI tract. While WCE can yield valuable images of the gastrointestinal tract, it does not provide a clear indication of the precise site of the identified disease. Accurate data is crucial in determining the suitable medical solution for a diagnosed ailment, whether it necessitates surgery or focused medicine administration. The future utilization of Wireless Capsule Endoscopy relies heavily on the accurate surveillance of the capsule [36].

These potential answers, along with a better knowledge of what they can do, will allow modern endoscopy to be used in a variety of therapeutic contexts in a safe and effective manner. Finally, embedded systems in advanced endoscopy have decreased healthcare expenses, improved the performance of healthcare workers, and substantially improved patient care. The integration of these systems into advanced endoscopy is anticipated to grow in sophistication and significance within the medical industry as technology progresses.

4.2.5 Embedded Systems in Magnetic Resonance Imaging (MRI)

One of the most useful medical imaging modalities, magnetic resonance imaging (MRI) allows for precise and non-invasive observation of anatomical structures inside the body [37]. Magnetic resonance imaging devices rely on embedded systems for control, functioning, and safety. Motion correction, artifact removal, and dynamic image reconstruction are only a few examples of real-time image processing tasks that few MRI embedded systems are capable of. With these improvements, cutting-edge imaging methods are made possible, and MRI images are of higher quality. The following is a selection of publications on embedded systems utilized in magnetic MRI.

Magnetic resonance imaging might make extensive use of functional nanoparticles because of their versatility and their capacity to bind selectively to specific sites inside living organisms. This article presents a thorough examination of MRI concepts, contrast agent classification, manufacture, and surface modification techniques, and their clinical applications. The goal is to provide guidance for the creation of novel contrast agents and ways to improve their existing effectiveness. The text highlights the promising future of functional nanomaterials in the field of biomedicine and emphasizes the importance of making major advancements in clinical translation [38].

When different modalities are used together, they can provide more information and work together more effectively than when they are used alone. Dual modality probes that combine fluorescent imaging (FI) with MRI connect the sensitivity of FI with the spatial and temporal resolution and ability to penetrate deep tissues of MRI. Cellular marking, enzyme activity measurement, tumor diagnosis and treatment, and real-time monitoring during surgery are just a few of the many biological applications of these probes [39].

Contrast agents (CAs) enhance the specificity and dependability of MRI in illness detection. However, their imaging signals persist regardless of whether they contact with the desired tissues or cells. Scientists have offered a brief synopsis of the most recent advances in the principles and methods of design for activable MR contrast agents (MR CAs), which include ion alteration, self-assembly, and dismantling. Comparing the results obtained with these methods to those of conventional MR contrast agents, they also assessed the benefits of these approaches in biological settings, including in vitro detection and in vivo disease diagnosis. In addition, they deliberated on the potential constraints, proposed remedies, and forthcoming opportunities associated with these activatable contrast agents [40]. A recent study presented a smart theranostic probe, called DMCR, which was specifically developed to enable simultaneous imaging using CT, MR, and FL techniques, as well as to provide chemo/photothermal synergistic therapy. Gadolinium and iodine-doped carbon nanodots (referred to as Gd/I-CDs) are successfully manufactured utilizing a simple one-step solvent thermal method. These nanodots are meant to function as a highly effective trimodal imaging component for fluorescence, magnetic resonance, and computed tomography in the context of DMCR. The incorporation of DOX into MPDA enhances the subsequent DMCR for the combined chemo/photothermal treatment of tumors. Efforts reveal that DMCR is highly effective in using three different imaging techniques (fluorescence, magnetic resonance, and computed tomography) to detect cancers [41].

4.2.6 Embedded Systems in Fluoroscopy

Medical fluoroscopy is a dynamic imaging technique employed in various diagnostic and interventional procedures, such as angiography, orthopedic surgeries, and gastrointestinal studies. It provides real-time visualization of internal structures, aiding physicians in making accurate diagnoses and guiding surgical interventions. Embedded systems have revolutionized fluoroscopy by integrating sophisticated hardware and software components into compact, efficient, and reliable platforms. Medical fluoroscopy involves the projection of X-ray images onto a fluorescent screen or digital detector in real-time. It requires continuous X-ray exposure and image processing to produce dynamic visuals of anatomical structures and physiological processes. Traditional fluoroscopy systems relied on bulky analog components, limiting mobility and flexibility. Embedded systems have transformed these systems into compact, high-performance devices with enhanced functionalities. Embedded systems serve as the backbone of modern fluoroscopy platforms, facilitating various critical functions like real-time image processing, radiation dose optimization, user interface and control, interoperability with ultrasound and MRI modalities, and remote monitoring and telemetry.

Biplane fluoroscopic imaging methods are widely recognized as the most precise and accurate tools for investigating the movement of joints in living animals. Researchers compared various methods of biplane fluoroscopy calibration. This involved assessing a novel approach that employs a distinctive nested optimization mechanism. This method is preferred due to its faster speed and similar accuracy compared to the revolutionary nested-optimization method [42].

4.2.7 Embedded Systems in Ultrasound (US) Imaging

Ultrasound (US) imaging is an efficient, non-invasive, method for medical diagnosis. Embedded systems play a pivotal role in enhancing the functionality, portability, and efficiency of medical ultrasound devices. Applications of embedded systems in medical ultrasound are diagnostic imaging, monitoring fetal development and health, assessing heart structure and function, evaluating blood vessels and circulation, and guiding needle insertions and other interventions.

US Doppler systems are frequently used to diagnose cardiovascular issues. The decision to send single-tone bursts or more intricate waveforms through a piezoelectric transducer toward the targeted area is contingent upon the particular use case. The procedure for gathering Doppler data from echoes reflected by circulating blood cells normally entails periodic demodulation and subsequent sorting of the input signal, followed by an appropriate analysis module. The researchers introduced an embedded US Doppler system that has been developed as an open research platform. This system may be programmed to implement various tactics for both transmitting and receiving signals [43].

In photoacoustic tomography (PAT), the identification of ultrasound is often accomplished by using ultrasonic transducers that are in direct contact with the biological tissue through an interface medium. This is a significant limitation for critical potential uses, such as surgery. A distant optical approach, based on industrial laser ultrasonics, has been utilized to detect ultrasound in tissues. Optical and auditory differences were seen in inclusions that originated from within the chicken breast and calf brain specimens, as well as those that came from external sources. Inclusions as small as 0.3 mm were found at depths greater than 1 cm. The approach has the potential to broaden the range of photoacoustic and US applications in in-vivo biological settings when physical contact is not feasible [44].

Point-of-Care Ultrasound: POCUS devices have brought ultrasound technologies to the bedside, transforming patient care. Healthcare providers can swiftly evaluate patients in a variety of clinical settings with the help of these small, inexpensive, and user-friendly handheld gadgets. In settings where resources are scarce, such as in emergency medicine or critical care, point-of-care ultrasound (POCUS) devices are invaluable. They are useful for making quick diagnoses, providing direction during procedures, and keeping tabs on interventions in real time [45, 46].

4.2.8 Embedded Systems in Magnetic Resonance Spectroscopy and Hyperspectral Imaging

MR spectroscopy (MRS) is a valuable technique for assessing metabolic metabolism in human organs and tissues without intrusive procedures. However, its adoption in clinical settings has been gradual and primarily confined to specialist institutes or hospitals with MRS experts. The quantity of 3-T clinical MR scanners is now on the rise, which presents a significant possibility for advancing the utilization of clinical MRS [47]. A study was conducted where researchers introduced a novel method to simulate and reproduce spectroscopic signals. This was achieved by acquiring a nonlinear low-dimensional representation of the overall MR spectra through learning. They trained a deep neural network to recognize the low-dimensional manifold that contains the high-dimensional spectroscopic signals. A regularization approach is suggested to efficiently combine the acquired model and physics-based data collection model for MRSI reconstruction, while also allowing for the inclusion of additional restrictions related to space and spectrum characteristics. A highly effective numerical technique was devised to handle the optimization challenge associated with back-propagating the trained network. The trained model's representation power and the proposed formulation's ability to produce SNR-enhancing reconstruction from practical MRSI data were demonstrated through simulation and experimental results [48].

Embedded systems play a crucial role in MRS imaging, where they are responsible for controlling various aspects of the imaging process, acquiring data, and processing signals. Embedded systems govern the execution of pulse sequences in MRS imaging. These sequences determine the timing and parameters of RF pulses, gradient pulses, and other modulation schemes necessary for spatial encoding and spectroscopic acquisition. Embedded systems acquire raw data from the MR scanner's receiver coils. They digitize the received signals and preprocess them to remove noise, correct for artifacts, and optimize signal-to-noise ratio (SNR) for accurate spectroscopic measurements. In recent times, MRI and MRS have become highly promising techniques for detecting prostate cancer. Nevertheless, the significant disparities in dimensionality between MR imaging and spectral information have posed a considerable obstacle in effectively combining T_2-weighted MRI (T_2w MRI) with MRS to enhance prostate cancer detection [49].

Multi-spatial MRS Imaging is a valuable imaging modality that integrates imaging and spectroscopic methodologies. MRSI has proven to be advantageous in various clinical contexts within the field of neurology, specifically in neuro-oncology, multiple sclerosis, stroke, and epilepsy. Nevertheless, a significant obstacle with traditional MRSI is the increased duration of data collecting necessary to get sufficient signal. Performing rapid MRS imaging of the brain in a living organism is an alternate method to decrease the duration of scanning and enhance the therapeutic applicability of MRSI. Whole brain rapid spectroscopic techniques have clinical applications that can aid in evaluating neurochemical alterations in the human brain, specifically in the context of multiple sclerosis. These techniques also contribute to our comprehension of the functions these changes have in the disease [50].

Hyperspectral imaging is a method used to obtain a greater amount of spectral data from an image. It uncovers more bands and expands beyond the range of wavelengths that can be seen with the naked eye. The acquisition of hyperspectral information is highly valuable for enhancing our comprehension of the world. Almost all materials possess a distinct "spectral signature", even if they appear identical to the human eye. The capacity to perceive accurate hues has transformative possibilities in various fields, including precision agriculture, earth monitoring, art analysis, and medicine [51]. Hyperspectral imaging is a technology that is both safe and user-friendly, providing advantages to medical professionals and researchers. Hyperspectral video cameras provide real-time information to surgeons that is imperceptible to the unaided eye.

4.2.9 Embedded Systems in Positron Emission Tomography (PET) and Single Photon Emission Computed Tomography (SPECT)

Embedded systems play a significant role in various applications, including those in PET (Positron Emission Tomography) imaging devices. In PET systems, embedded systems are crucial for controlling and coordinating various components such as detectors, data acquisition units, signal processing units, and image reconstruction algorithms. Attenuation and scatter adjustments are essential procedures in PET systems to achieve precise quantitative modeling of the radiopharmaceutical distribution. Recent advancements in deep learning have sparked the development of numerous algorithms that utilize convolutional neural networks. These algorithms aim to automatically reduce the effects of attenuation and scatter, hence enhancing the performance of PET scanners that do not have CT or MR capabilities. This is particularly beneficial in mitigating artifacts associated with CT imaging. An established attribute of PET imaging is the presence of diverse tracer uptake levels among different patients and/or anatomical locations. Nevertheless, current deep learning algorithms employ a consistent model for various subjects and anatomical locations during the inference process, potentially leading to inaccurate outputs. A unique deep learning-based approach has been described in literature for directly reconstructing attenuation and scatter-adjusted PET images from non-attenuation-corrected images, even in the lack of structural information. A new model was presented to address variances in PET imaging caused by differences between subjects and within subjects. This model uses convolution kernels to filter the data in a way that takes into account the contextual coherence between surrounding slices, allowing for subject- and region-specific filtering. In this manner, the context-aware convolution can direct the formation of intermediate features to prioritize the regression of tracer uptakes that are dependent on the input and/or peculiar to certain regions. Qualitative assessments in experimental investigations demonstrated that the suggested CT-free technique has the ability to generate corrected PET images that closely resemble ground truth images adjusted using CT scans [52].

Single Photon Emission Computed Tomography (SPECT): Cancer, heart disease, and neurological disorders are just some of the many diseases that can be diagnosed with the help of SPECT scans, a nuclear medicine imaging technique that uses gamma-ray emitting radiotracers to provide three-dimensional pictures of the body's physiological processes. The SPECT method is based on the gamma rays released into the patient's bloodstream by radiotracers. A gamma camera picks up on these rays and records the information needed to create 3D pictures. Data acquisition, signal processing, picture reconstruction, and system control are just a few of the many functions performed by the embedded systems included in SPECT devices. The use of nuclear medicine to evaluate functional capacity in both healthy and diseased subjects has long been considered the gold standard in the field. By providing 3D images of tracer distribution in the body, single photon emission computed tomography (SPECT) greatly enhances this assessment. But to get the most out of the technology, we need to be able to picture the ever-changing metabolic and flow processes in living things. It is necessary to consider tissue mobility and deformation as well. The ability to precisely measure the exact amount of these changing processes occurring in the body has the potential to enhance the accuracy of diagnosis. Advancements in multi-resolution spatiotemporal techniques now allow for the estimation of kinetic parameters in partition models of dynamic processes utilizing data obtained from a single camera head with a slow traverse rotation. By directly estimating kinetic parameters from projection measurements, bias and variance are reduced compared to the traditional approach of reconstructing 3D dynamic images first, producing time–activity curves from specific regions of interest, and then estimating kinetic parameters from the time–activity curves produced. While the complete utilization of SPECT for imaging dynamic processes in clinical settings has not yet been achieved, recent advancements have shed light on the promise of SPECT for dynamic imaging. These advancements allow for the direct assessment of dynamic processes from prediction measurements [53, 54].

4.2.10 Embedded Systems in Infrared (IR) Radiology (Thermal Imaging or Thermography)

Infrared (IR) radiology, also known as thermal imaging or medical thermography, a non-invasive imaging technique, involves the use of infrared radiation to create images of the body's internal structures based on variations in temperature. It has gained significant attention in recent years due to its potential in detecting various medical conditions by capturing and analyzing temperature distributions on the body's surface. Embedded systems, consisting of hardware and software components integrated into imaging devices, play a crucial role in advancing medical thermography by facilitating real-time data acquisition, processing, interpretation, and ensuring the accuracy and safety of imaging procedures. Applications in medical diagnosis, including breast cancer detection, inflammation assessment, vascular disease diagnosis, and pain management.

Nanotechnology-based medical devices utilized in Infrared (IR) applications might be employed for diagnostic purposes, therapeutic purposes, or a combination of both, commonly known as theranostics. Various techniques have been investigated to create medical devices with nanoparticles, tailored to the specific requirements of individual patients [55]. Quantum dots are renowned for their exceptional photostability and robust tissue-penetrating capabilities, making them a more advantageous choice for near IR (NIR) fluorescence applications as compared to conventional organic dyes. Moreover, the minute dimensions of nanoparticles make them highly advantageous in the field of drug administration, as they exhibit improved solubility and better ability to reach specific cells, tissues, or organs at this particular size [55]. Various nanomaterials have been utilized as contrast agents in different imaging techniques, including X-ray, CT, MRI, and optical or fluorescence imaging, due to their great sensitivity, and included to enhance their visibility under X-ray imaging.

Prompt and precise identification of breast cancer is an essential component of the approach to diminish the illness and death rates linked to this prevalent condition. Although current guidelines suggest using mammography for screening, the accuracy of mammograms, in terms of sensitivity and specificity, is still suboptimal, particularly for people with dense breast tissue. Thermography has previously been investigated as a substitute for mammography. The accuracy of thermography has been greatly improved by the development of advanced infrared (IR) cameras for obtaining thermal images of the breast, as well as the use of computational tools to predict heat transfer within the breast with precision. A compelling study assessed the advancements in utilizing thermal imaging for breast cancer detection over the last thirty years and highlights areas that require more improvement in order to establish it as a dependable diagnostic tool for breast cancer. The paper discusses recent advancements and proposes future directions in the field, such as employing sophisticated simulation techniques, inverse modeling, imaging procedures, and artificial neural networks to enhance the accuracy of tumor localization prediction [56].

4.2.11 Embedded Systems in Electrical Source Imaging (ESI)

Neuroimaging applications of electrical source imaging (ESI) include the localization of brain electrical activity sources as assessed by electroencephalography (EEG) or magnetoencephalography (MEG). When it comes to electroencephalogram (EEG) and magnetoencephalogram (MEG) systems, embedded systems are crucial since they manage data collection, signal processing, and system control. Electrical source imaging makes use of embedded systems in the following ways: The embedded system coordinates the collection of EEG or MEG signals from various sensors or electrodes positioned on or near the head, ensures that the signals are sampled at the same time across channels, preprocesses the raw data to remove noise and improve signal quality, and controls the storage and transfer of the data, keeping both the raw and processed signals for subsequent analysis. They also provide visualization and display capabilities for EEG or MEG data, allowing researchers and clinicians to visualize brain activity patterns.

In recent years, cortex source localization has been routinely used to understand complicated brain functions by combining the EEG's high temporal resolution with the estimated sources' high spatial estimation. The text discusses the new dimensions for analyzing brain processes in terms of clinical and intellectual ESI applications. It also addresses the obstacles and restrictions associated with these dimensions and provides perspectives for future approaches that could help overcome methodological and technical drawbacks [57].

4.2.12 Embedded Systems in Mammography

Embedded systems play a critical role in modern mammography, contributing to the development of advanced imaging that aids in on-time detection and diagnosis of breast cancer. Integration of embedded systems with mammography modalities are digital mammography (how embedded systems improve image acquisition, processing, and display in digital mammography systems), tomosynthesis (role of embedded systems in reconstructing 3D breast images from multiple 2D projections), and Molecular Breast Imaging (MBI) and Positron Emission Mammography (PEM) (utilization of embedded systems for image acquisition and analysis in molecular imaging modalities). Advanced applications of embedded systems in mammography are how embedded systems support AI and ML algorithms for automated detection of suspicious lesions, integration of embedded systems for combining data from multiple imaging modalities to improve diagnostic accuracy, and real-time image processing.

Breast cancer screening is now more accessible than ever before, thanks to mobile mammography programs, which also guarantee participation from outlying locations without permanent centers. However, there are limitations to the speed and accuracy of analysis and diagnosis that even highly trained radiologists encounter. In order to improve mobile mammography, some papers suggest combining digital mammography (X-ray) equipment with smart transducer interface and network-capable application processor information modules. Breast cancer screening and detection can now be done remotely thanks to the proposed paradigm's vendor-and network-agnostic transducer interfaces [58].

In a subsequent study, the tactile sensing and palpation techniques used by physicians to identify abnormal masses in the breast were examined. A simplified model of the tissue containing a mass, and utilized contact elements to analyze the functionality of the tactile sensor was proposed. Through the application of the finite element method, we observed the impact of the mass on the surface of the tissue. This occurred as a result of applying mechanical force to the surface of the simulated tissue. The next step was the development and construction of a tactile sensing device called the "tactile tumor detector". By physically touching the surfaces of the models, this device may detect anomalies inside the virtual models. In order to carry out a series of exacting studies, a robot armed with a touch probe was employed. To avoid dynamic effects, the probe moves at a slow enough linear velocity that the tissue stays in the linear elastic range. The highest stress value served as the basis for the comparison criterion selection. The study looked at how this criterion changed in response to changes in the mass parameter and discovered that experimental and numerical results were highly correlated [59].

4.2.13 Embedded Systems in Electrical Impedance Tomography (EIT)

A non-invasive imaging technique known as Electrical Impedance Tomography (EIT) utilizes surface measurements of electrical impedance to generate a comprehensive picture of an object's or body's interior conductivity distribution. Because they allow for the gathering, processing, and display of real-time data, embedded systems are vital in EIT applications. Some examples of medical imaging's many uses include examining the lungs, keeping tabs on the brain, and even finding breast cancer. Because it is a radiation-free, wearable, real-time way to track a person's vitals, EIT has garnered a lot of interest [60].

EIT is a useful method for examining the brain and lungs, among other areas of medicine and industry. The article presents the introduction of an embedded system (ES) for the development of a portable, dependable, and low-cost EIT system for image reconstruction. The main innovation of this study lies in the creation of a cost-effective EIT system, including hardware development, along with the implementation of three straightforward and effective algorithms on ES. The suggested EIT method shows promise for use in mechanical ventilation, the food sector, and structural health monitoring [61].

4.3 EMBEDDED SYSTEMS USING INTERNET OF THINGS (IOT), MACHINE LEARNING (ML), AND ARTIFICIAL INTELLIGENCE (AI)

As we move toward the information society, every aspect of our existence is quickly transitioning to the digital realm. Education, health, citizenship procedures, and social life are all interconnected within the digital cyber world. Smart cities, smart networks, and smart factories, which are essential for social life, have now been connected to both intranet and internet to enhance efficiency, speed, and enable remote maintenance and management. In addition to this procedure, these systems have encountered new areas of vulnerability. Embedded systems are a crucial component in the functioning of these systems. These systems make a substantial contribution to the efficient functioning of critical infrastructures [62]. The recent progress in Internet of Things (IoT), cloud computing, and Artificial Intelligence (AI) has revolutionized the traditional healthcare system, turning it into a smart healthcare system. By integrating essential technologies like the Internet of Things (IoT) and Artificial Intelligence (AI), medical services can be enhanced. The integration of Internet of Things (IoT) with Artificial Intelligence (AI) has several prospects in the healthcare industry [63].

The Internet of Things (IoT) has transformed the functionality of embedded systems by facilitating communication and data interchange across objects. For example, in the field of healthcare, Internet of Things (IoT) embedded systems facilitate the ability to remotely monitor patients and track medical equipment in real-time. The growing use of embedded control systems in the Internet of Things (IoT) and cloud has led to a significant interest in real-time control of time-sensitive systems in industrial settings [64, 65].

Embedded systems have incorporated Machine Learning to augment their functionalities. TensorFlow Lite Micro is an open-source machine learning inference framework designed specifically for executing deep-learning models on embedded computers. Embedded machine learning (EML) finds its applications in several fields such as computer vision, speech recognition, healthcare, robotics, and more [66].

Artificial intelligence (AI) has been integrated into embedded systems to facilitate intelligent decision-making. The development of AI algorithms and models, together with the integration of embedded device support, has made it possible to address the problem of high-level of energy usage and low level of support that arises when using embedded devices to install AI networks and models. Embedded AI is applied in several fields such as manufacturing, IoT, cloud and control systems, mechatronics and robotics, healthcare services, and others [67].

As a result, the integration of IoT, ML, and AI into embedded systems has greatly enhanced their capabilities, leading to the development of smarter and more efficient devices. Embedded artificial intelligence has emerged as a new area of study made possible by these developments. As technology continues to advance, the use of these systems in various fields is expected to become even more sophisticated and integral to our daily lives.

4.4 IMAGING TECHNOLOGY INTEGRATED INTO WEARABLES

The use of imaging technology has greatly improved the speed and accuracy of patient diagnostics. On the other hand, symptoms could get better or get worse with time. Wearable tools, especially due to their ability to monitor in real-time, are well-suited for extended usage of gadgets. Constructing a long-lasting, secure, and pleasant product that delivers accurate data is one of the most difficult tasks. Emerging imaging technology is diminishing in size, augmenting in speed, and enhancing efficiency [68]. So, it is not surprising that efforts are underway to incorporate image technology into wearables. Furthermore, these devices not only collect a greater range of physiological data but also promote prompt patient intervention. The integration of imaging technology into mobile phones is another aspect of the future of imaging. This will allow pregnant women to do their examinations through an app if necessary. This technology will not ever be able to take the position of human doctors, but it will provide them with better data to work with.

4.4.1 Wearable Brain Imaging Tool

It is crucial to monitor a patient's activity across a variety of tasks and environments when assessing brain function. Brain imaging sometimes requires expensive equipment and significant time commitments, which frequently makes this endeavor challenging. In the end, brain imaging is currently seeing a significant transformation following the development of wearable imaging tools, such as a cap that is capable of capturing images of the brain. Consequently, patients can be observed throughout their normal activities, leading to the collection of more genuine and dependable data. In addition, it works equally well for imaging younger patients as it does for older ones. The hat is making progress, but it still has a way to go before it can be mass-produced. Patients should be constantly monitored on a daily basis as they engage in their daily activities and socialize with others [69].

4.4.2 Wearable Device Integrates Ultrasound Sensor

A wearable electronic gadget that provides ultrasonic imaging even during physical exercise is another instance of wearable electronics. You can record cardiac ultrasounds with this wearable device, and it can stay on your body all day long. Because of its portability and ease of use, this device represents a significant departure from previous wearable imaging technology. On top of that, this gadget uses AI to measure the heart's blood pumping rate, which is helpful for diagnosis and therapy. Furthermore, the patient can use this wearable gadget while moving, which gives them information on their heart's reaction to stress and exercise [70]. Patients requiring long-term monitoring without invasive treatments can benefit from this wearable imaging device. In addition, by allowing doctors to get up-to-the-minute assessments of a patient's cardiac health, this technology improves the diagnostic process.

4.4.3 The Promising Future of Wearable Scanners

Improvements in portability, durability, and usability are common goals for medical device manufacturers. Due to their common usage in the treatment of prolonged and persistent diseases, these medications must possess sufficient durability to withstand various patient conditions. Therefore, although encountering similar obstacles as medical devices, wearable technology plays a crucial role in providing extended monitoring to patients. In the future, wearable technology will incorporate compact imaging devices capable of rapidly capturing scans. Also, these gadgets may sync with smartphone apps and record a plethora of data that doctors can utilize to craft personalized treatment regimens. Wearable imaging tools must possess affordability and user-friendliness, with none of these aspects being obstructive [71]. In order to enhance clinical results, wearable imaging devices need to integrate advanced technologies such as AI, cloud computing, online medical care, and other related advancements.

4.5 RESULTS AND PERSPECTIVES ON EMBEDDED SYSTEMS IN MEDICAL IMAGING

Embedded systems have revolutionized the field of medical imaging, leading to significant advancements in diagnosis and treatment. The following text presents significant findings and potential future directions derived from recent scholarly publications.

The utilization of tracking and diagnostic medical devices has revolutionized the delivery of medical care by improving diagnoses, patient monitoring, and controlling illnesses. Wearable devices, advanced imaging technologies, point-of-care ultrasound, and telemonitoring systems have revolutionized healthcare by providing real-time data, improving accuracy, and enabling remote monitoring and interventions. With the continuous advancement of technology, the ability to monitor and image medical equipment will increasingly enhance the capabilities of healthcare providers, enhance patient results, and influence the trajectory of medicine.

Future progress in the development of medical imaging sensors will take place along two separate trajectories. The initial pathway is related to neural circuits, microprocessors, and smart software setup. The second factor is the phenomenon of miniaturization. With the advancement of nano-processing technology, sensor's progress will shift from micro-sensors to nano-sensors. A new era of electronic medical device design is on the horizon, poised to revolutionize healthcare. For instance, wearable devices have the capability to administer medication to patients following their specific medical condition. The complexity of electronic and embedded software in medical equipment is increasing. Ensuring the security of personal data collected by IoT devices is crucial in order to safeguard patient privacy. In order to ensure the delivery of high-quality solutions with little risk and compliance with the highest medical certification criteria, it is imperative for development teams to possess the appropriate level of expertise.

Furthermore, as the Internet of Things (IoT) continues to grow, these devices are becoming more and more networked, enabling the seamless exchange of real-time data and the ability to operate them remotely. This contributes to a substantial improvement in the capabilities of medical devices and the quality of patient treatment. Machine learning and artificial intelligence are essential techniques that allow for intelligent robotic picture gathering, specifically tailored to patients and processes, taking into account motion and distortion. Future research on autonomous robotic ultrasound acquisitions could be regarded as equally significant and indispensable as the advancements achieved in the examination of robotic ultrasound itself. Subsequent investigations are expected to prioritize artificial intelligence and virtual/augmented reality in order to enhance picture comprehension and optimize ergonomics. Embedded systems in the medical profession will evolve toward more intelligence, miniaturization, and personalization in the future. As technology advances and embedded systems develop, the medical industry will undergo significant changes to help society.

REFERENCES

1. https://www.who.int/health-topics/medical-devices
2. https://www.fda.gov/radiation-emitting-products/radiation-emitting-products-and-procedures/medical-imaging
3. https://www.ncbi.nlm.nih.gov/pmc/articles/PMC9781231/
4. Kasban H, El-Bendary MAM, Salama DH. A comparative study of medical imaging techniques. *International Journal of Information Science and Intelligent System.* 2015;4(2):37–58.
5. Laal M. Innovation process in medical imaging. *Procedia-Social and Behavioral Science*. 2013;81:60–64.
6. National Research Council. *Mathematics and Physics of Emerging Biomedical Imaging*. National Academies Press; 1996.
7. Flower MA. *Webb's Physics of Medical Imaging*. CRC Press; 2012.
8. Hussain S, Mubeen I, Ullah N, Shah SSUD, Khan BA, Zahoor M, Ullah R, Khan FA, Sultan MA. Modern diagnostic imaging technique applications and risk factors in the medical field: A review. *Biomed Research Interantional.* 2022 Jun 6;2022:5164970.
9. Arandia N, Garate JI, Mabe J. Embedded sensor systems in medical devices: Requisites and challenges ahead. *Sensors (Basel).* 2022 Dec 16;22(24):9917.
10. https://www.teledynedalsa.com/en/home/
11. Zhao W and Sakurai K. CCD camera as feasible large-area-size X-ray detector for X-ray fluorescence spectroscopy and imaging. *Review of Scientific Instruments.* 2017;88(6):063703.
12. Mondal S, Pan A. Quantum dots in biosensing, bioimaging, and drug delivery. In: Barik P, Mondal S. (eds) *Application of Quantum Dots in Biology and Medicine*. Springer, Singapore 2022.
13. Rajamanickam K. *Application of Quantum Dots in Bio-Sensing, Bio-Imaging, Drug Delivery, Anti-Bacterial Activity, Photo-Thermal, Photo-Dynamic Therapy, and Optoelectronic Devices*. IntechOpen, 2023.
14. Aslam N, Zhou H, Urbach EK. et al. Quantum sensors for biomedical applications. *Nature Review Physics* 2023;5:157–169.
15. Degen CL, Reinhard F & Cappellaro P. Quantum sensing. *Reviews of Modern Physics.* 2017;89:035002.
16. Safiabadi Tali SA, Mudiyanselage RRHH, Qian Y, Smith NWG, Zhao Y, Morral A, Song J, (…), Zhou W. Dual-modal nanoplasmonic light upconversion through anti-stokes photoluminescence and second-harmonic generation from broadband multiresonant metal nanocavities. *ACS Nano*. 2023;17(12):11362–11373.
17. Vibhas C, Basu A, Kaushik A, Basu AK. Progression in quantum sensing/bio-sensing technologies for healthcare. *ECS Sensors Plus*. 2023;2:015001.
18. Xiaoyuan J, Houyu W, Bin S, Binbin C, Yao H. Silicon nanomaterials for biosensing and bioimaging analysis. *Frontiers in Chemistry*. 2018;6:38.
19. Moretta R, De Stefano L, Terracciano M, Rea I. Porous silicon optical devices: Recent advances in biosensing applications. *Sensors*. 2021;21:1336.
20. Xu Y, Hu X, Kundu S, Nag A, Afsarimanesh N, Sapra S, Mukhopadhyay SC, Han T. Silicon-based sensors for biomedical applications: A review. *Sensors*. 2019;19:2908.

21. Weisfield RL, Hartney MA, Street RA and Apte RB. New amorphous-silicon image sensor for X-ray diagnostic medical imaging applications. *Proceedings of SPIE - The International Society for Optical Engineering* 1998;3336:444–452.
22. Nasir S, & Verma A. Role of embedded system for X-ray comparison of lungs to detect a COVID-19 affected person at the entry point of aerodromes, railway stations and metro stations in perspective of India. *SAMRIDDHI: A Journal of Physical Sciences, Engineering and Technology*. 2022;14(1):108–111.
23. Sanida T, Sideris A, Tsiktsiris D & Dasygenis M. Lightweight neural network for COVID-19 detection from chest X-ray images implemented on an embedded system. *Technologies*. 2022; 10(2):37.
24. Kaur N, Mittal A. RadioBERT: A deep learning-based system for medical report generation from chest X-ray images using contextual embeddings. *Journal of Biomedical Informatics* 2022;135:104220.
25. Hashem N, Pryor M, Haas D, Hunter J. Design of a computed tomography automation architecture. *Applied Sciences*. 2021;11:2858.
26. https://blog.boston-engineering.com/embedded-systems-med-devices
27. https://www.medicaldevice-network.com/buyers-guide/embedded-technology/
28. Lou L, Liang H, Wang Z. Deep-learning-based COVID-19 diagnosis and implementation in embedded edge-computing device. *Diagnostics*. 2023;13:1329.
29. Ulutas H, Sahin ME, Karakus MO. Application of a novel deep learning technique using CT images for COVID-19 diagnosis on embedded systems. *Alexandria Engineering Journal*. 2023;*74*:345–358.
30. Liguori C, Frauenfelder G, Massaroni C, Saccomandi P, Giurazza F, Pitocco F, Marano R, Schena E. Emerging clinical applications of computed tomography. *Med Devices (Auckl)*. 2015;8:265–278.
31. Alian, A, Zari, E, Wang, Z, Franco, E, Avery, JP, Runciman, M, ... & Mylonas, G. Current Engineering Developments for Robotic Systems in Flexible Endoscopy https://doi.org/10.1016/j.tige.2022.11.006
32. Rodríguez-Luna MR, Pizzicannella M, Perretta S. Robotic flexible endoscopes. In: Horgan S, Fuchs KH. (eds) *Innovative Endoscopic and Surgical Technology in the GI Tract*. Springer; 2021.
33. Foerster F, Neumann H. Advanced endoscopic imaging methods. In: Horgan, S, Fuchs, KH. (eds) *Innovative Endoscopic and Surgical Technology in the GI Tract*. Springer; 2021.
34. Sinonquel, P, Vermeire, S, Maes, F, & Bisschops, R. Advanced Imaging in Gastrointestinal Endoscopy: A Literature Review of the Current State of the Art https://doi.org/10.1159/000527083
35. Luo X, Mori K, Peters TM. Advanced endoscopic navigation: Surgical big data, methodology, and applications. *Annual Review of Biomedical Engineering*. 2018;4(20):221–251.
36. Mateen H, Basar R, Ahmed AU, Ahmad MY. Localization of wireless capsule endoscope: A systematic review. *IEEE Sensors Journal*. 2017;*17*(5):1197–1206.
37. Koptyug I, Kovtunov K, Svyatova A. Magnetic resonance imaging (MRI). In: Wachs IE, Bañares MA. (eds) *Springer Handbook of Advanced Catalyst Characterization*. Springer Handbooks. Springer; 2023.
38. Huang R, Zhou X, Chen G, Su L, Liu Z, Zhou P, Min Y. Advances of functional nanomaterials for magnetic resonance imaging and biomedical engineering applications. *Wiley Interdisciplinary Reviews: Nanomedicine and Nanobiotechnology*. 2022;14(4):e1800.
39. Deng Y, Xu A, Yu Y, Fu C, Liang G. Biomedical applications of fluorescent and magnetic resonance imaging dual-modality probes. *ChemBioChem*. 2019;20(4):499–510.
40. Jin X, Yang W, Xu Y, Bian K, Zhang B. Emerging strategies of activatable MR imaging probes and their advantages for biomedical applications. *View*. 2021;2(5):20200141.

41. Zhao J, Dai D, Zhou L, Yu Z, Ma J, Yang M, Yi C. A tumor microenvironment responsive mesoporous polydopamine theranostic probe embedded with Gd/I-doped carbon nanodots for CT/MR/FL imaging and chemo/photothermal synergistic therapy. *Carbon*. 2024;224:119065.
42. Kaptein BL, Shelburne KB, Torry MR, Giphart JE. A comparison of calibration methods for stereo fluoroscopic imaging systems. *Journal of Biomechanics*. 2011;44(13):2511–2515.
43. Ricci S, Dallai A, Boni E, Bassi L, Guidi F, Cellai A, Tortoli P. Embedded system for real-time digital processing of medical ultrasound Doppler signals. *EURASIP Journal on Advances in Signal Processing*. 2008;418235: 1–7.
44. Rousseau G, Gauthier B, Blouin A, Monchalin JP. Non-contact biomedical photoacoustic and ultrasound imaging. *Journal of Biomedical Optics*. 2012;*17*(6):061217.
45. Koratala A, Kazory A. Point of care ultrasonography for objective assessment of heart failure: Integration of cardiac, vascular, and extravascular determinants of volume status. *Cardiorenal Medicine*. 2021;11(1):5–17.
46. Koratala A, Kazory A. An introduction to point-of-care ultrasound: Laennec to lichtenstein. *Advances in Chronic Kidney Disease*. 2021;28(3):193–199.
47. Tomiyasu M, Harada M. In vivo human MR spectroscopy using a clinical scanner: Development, applications, and future prospects. *Magnetic Resonance in Medical Sciences*. 2022;21(1):235–252.
48. Lam F, Li Y, Peng X. Constrained magnetic resonance spectroscopic imaging by learning nonlinear low-dimensional models. *IEEE Transactions on Medical Imaging*. 2019;39(3):545–555.
49. Tiwari P, Viswanath S, Kurhanewicz J, Sridhar A, Madabhushi A. Multimodal wavelet embedding representation for data combination (MaWERiC): Integrating magnetic resonance imaging and spectroscopy for prostate cancer detection. *NMR in Biomedicine*. 2012;25(4):607–619.
50. Al-Iedani O, Lechner-Scott J, Ribbons K, Ramadan S. Fast magnetic resonance spectroscopic imaging techniques in human brain-applications in multiple sclerosis. *Journal of Biomedical Science* 2017;*24*:1–19.
51. Sowmya V, Soman KP, Hassaballah M. Hyperspectral image: Fundamentals and advances. In Hassaballah M, Hosny KM. (eds) *Recent Advances in Computer Vision: Theories and Applications*. Studies in Computational Intelligence. Springer International Publishing; 2019:401–424.
52. Izadi S, Shiri I, Uribe CF, Geramifar P, Zaidi H, Rahmim A, Hamarneh G. Enhanced direct joint attenuation and scatter correction of whole-body PET images via context- aware deep networks. *Zeitschrift für Medizinische Physik*. 2024. https://doi.org/10.1016/j.zemedi.2024.01.002
53. Koua KMC, Panier S, Arpin L, Njejimana L, Bouziri H, Abidi M, Fontaine R. A fully integrated pulse charge generator embedded in a 64-channel readout ASIC dedicated to a PET/CT detector module. Paper presented at the *2012 IEEE International Conference on Electronics Design, Systems and Applications (ICEDSA)*.
54. Gullberg GT, Reutter BW, Sitek A, Maltz JS, Budinger TF. Dynamic single photon emission computed tomography—basic principles and cardiac applications. *Physics in Medicine & Biology*. 2010;*55*(20):R111.
55. San Valentin EMD, Barcena AJR, Klusman C, Martin B, Melancon MP. Nano-embedded medical devices and delivery systems in interventional radiology. *Wiley Interdisciplinary Reviews: Nanomedicine and Nanobiotechnology*. 2023 Jan;15(1):e1841.
56. Kandlikar SG, Perez-Raya I, Raghupathi PA, Gonzalez-Hernandez JL, Dabydeen D, Medeiros L, Phatak P. Infrared imaging technology for breast cancer detection–Current status, protocols and new directions. *International Journal of Heat and Mass Transfer*. 2017;108:2303–2320.

57. Zorzos I, Kakkos I, Ventouras EM, Matsopoulos GK. Advances in electrical source imaging: A review of the current approaches, applications and challenges. *Signals*. 2021;*2*(3):378–391.
58. Bhateja V, Urooj S, Misra M. Technical advancements to mobile mammography using nonlinear polynomial filters and IEEE 21451-1 NCAP information model. *IEEE Sensors Journal*. 2014;15(5):2559–2566.
59. Hosseini SM, Kashani SMT, Najarian S, Panahi F, Naeini SMM, Mojra A. A medical tactile sensing instrument for detecting embedded objects, with specific application for breast examination. *The International Journal of Medical Robotics and Computer Assisted Surgery*. 2010;6(1):73–82.
60. Wu Y, Hanzaee FF, Jiang D, Bayford RH, Demosthenous A. Electrical impedance tomography for biomedical applications: Circuits and systems review. *IEEE Open Journal of Circuits and Systems*. 2021;2:380–397.
61. Zamora-Arellano F, López-Bonilla OR, García-Guerrero EE, Olguín-Tiznado JE, Inzunza-González E, López-Mancilla D, Tlelo-Cuautle E. Development of a portable, reliable and low-cost electrical impedance tomography system using an embedded system. *Electronics*. 2020;10(1):15.
62. Alnıacik F, Yıldırım F, Gönen S, Alhan B, Barışkan MA, Sayan HH & Yılmaz EN. Artificial intelligence supported detection systems on embedded devices. *El-Cezeri*. 2023;*11*(1):109–119.
63. Mansour RF, El Amraoui A, Nouaouri I, Díaz VG, Gupta D, Kumar S. Artificial intelligence and internet of things enabled disease diagnosis model for smart healthcare systems. *IEEE Access*. 2021;9:45137–45146.
64. https://robots.net/tech/what-is-iot-embedded-system/
65. Giannoutakis KM, Filelis-Papadopoulos CK, Gravvanis GA, Tzovaras D. On the optimization of self-organization and self-management hardware resource allocation for heterogeneous clouds. *Computers*. 2021;10:147. https://doi.org/10.3390/computers10110147
66. Ajani TS, Imoize AL, Atayero AA. An overview of machine learning within embedded and mobile devices–optimizations and applications. *Sensors*. 2021;21:4412.
67. Zhang Z, Li JA. Review of artificial intelligence in embedded systems. Micromachines. *Micromachines* 2023;14:897.
68. https://www.aa.com.tr/en/health/wearable-tech-and-portable-imaging-devices-to-revolutionize-medical-sector/2688677
69. https://medicine.wustl.edu/news/wearable-light-based-brain-imaging-tech-to-be-commercialized-with-aid-of-nih-grant/
70. https://today.ucsd.edu/story/cardiac-imaging-on-the-go
71. https://www.theguardian.com/science/2022/jul/28/stick-on-ultrasound-patch-revolution-medical-imaging

5 Deep Learning of Telecommunication Technology for the Efficient Utilization of Embedded Systems

Gulcicek Dere

5.1 INTRODUCTION

5.1.1 EMBEDDED SYSTEMS

An embedded system is a combination of software and hardware designed to perform a specific function. Unlike general-purpose computers, which are utilized to execute complex applications, embedded systems are hardware platform and function-specific. Software on embedded systems is usually real-time, semi-permanent, and called firmware. Industrial, automotive, home appliances, biomedical, and telecommunications sectors are all industries that utilize embedded systems [1–10]. This section of the book will discuss telecommunications applications, as well as their crossovers with various other topics. The basic structure of an embedded system includes sensors, A-D and D-A converters, a processor, memory, and actuators for detecting, processing, storing, and executing tasks mentioned in Figure 5.1.

Embedded systems are comprised of three fundamental components that are specialized for performing out a particular task: a processor, memory, and input/output modules [11].

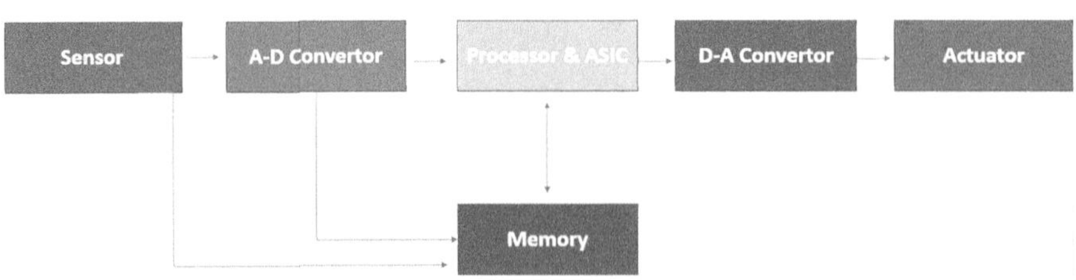

FIGURE 5.1 Basic structure of embedded system.

DOI: 10.1201/9781003508199-5

5.1.2 Embedded Operating Systems

- ECos (open source, free, real time, 2MB RAM)
- FreeRTOS (real-time, user code off, kernel open)
- Embedded Linux (designed for Linux un CepT, PDA, MediaO)
- JavaOS (written with Java)
- LynxOS (especially aviation, space, military industry, telecommunications)
- Mobilinux (for Linux-based power consumption on mobile devices)
- Nucleus RTOS (Mentor Graphics' real-time system)
- Palm OS (PalmOS, by PalmSource (for PDAs))
- Prex (real-time distributed under the Prex BSD License)
- VxWorks (Unix-based, real-time)
- Windows CE (OS developed by Windows for small systems)
- Windows XP Embedded (Reduced Windows Xp)

Embedded Communication Systems (EcoSys) utilizes the disciplines of electronics and telecommunications to provide services such as measurement, characterization, and modeling; algorithms and protocols; signal processing; and fast prototyping [12].

The performance of communication systems, baseband and Radiofrequency (RF) hardware platforms, and propagation medium are all characterized via measurement processes. Physical layer approaches like as MIMO (multiple-input and multiple-output), filter bank modulation, and ultra-wide band systems are used in the development of wireless communications [13]. MAC (Message Authentication Code) algorithms are used to allocate resources and enhance energy efficiency [14]. The study focuses on the factors that enable the convergence of the network layer in heterogeneous networks. Power line communications is a dynamic area of study that focuses on developing communication methods that are both efficient in terms of exploiting the available frequency spectrum and dependable while transmitting data over existing electrical lines [15]. Applications include a wide range of uses, including those inside the house, outdoors, and in vehicles. Electronics and signal processing are used in several sectors such as energy, power management, smart automotive systems, and industrial control [16]. Embedded systems are often integrated into bigger devices that fulfill a particular function, such as the Gibson Robot Guitar, which features an embedded system for tuning strings, although the ultimate objective is to play music. In automobiles, embedded systems provide specific functions as subsystems. Firmware, the program instructions for embedded systems, is stored in read-only memory or flash memory chips and runs with limited hardware resources, such as little memory or a small keyboard or screen [17]. These are merely a few instances of embedded systems outside of the field of telecommunications.

"Remote control" is an example of embedded systems' telecommunications applications. One example of the system focuses on how a simple SMS from a mobile phone can control a remote device, hardware requirements, compatible software, and potential applications [18]. Home security, factory remote automation, remote recording, and controllers include a communication interface with this system [19].

Embedded systems in telecommunications equipment, including microcontrollers and microprocessors, enhance communication through protocol handling, data routing, and signal processing, ensuring seamless connectivity and security. Embedded systems are commonly used in the field of healthcare in specialized disciplines such as Biomedical Imaging, Device Technology, and others, as well as big data, similar to their use in other technical applications [20, 21].

5.2 DEEP LEARNING

Deep Learning is a potent technology used in telecommunication-embedded systems to enhance signal processing, allocate resources, mitigate interference, anticipate wireless channels, sense spectrum, ensure security, optimize networks, and facilitate edge computing [22]. Neural networks provide the ability to acquire intricate patterns in data, resulting in enhanced efficiency and precision in processing. In addition, they have the capability to enhance the efficiency of resource distribution in wireless networks by facilitating the adaptive allocation of bandwidth and power to users according to their specific requirements. Deep learning may aid in reducing interference in wireless communication by identifying and suppressing interference signals, resulting in improved signal quality and increased data throughput [23–25].

Additionally, it has the capability to forecast wireless channel conditions by analyzing past data, enabling the adjustment of transmission parameters in real time. Furthermore, it has the capability to improve the process of detecting and analyzing available radio frequencies in cognitive radio systems, therefore allowing for a more effective use of the spectrum and the simultaneous operation of several wireless systems. It also has the capability to improve network performance by acquiring knowledge of network traffic patterns and user behavior [26].

Deep Learning has the potential to significantly revolutionize certain aspects of telecommunications in embedded systems. It can be used in speech recognition, speaker identification, and audio processing, enabling hands-free operation and voice-controlled interfaces. Moreover, it possesses the potential to improve network administration tasks such as detecting errors, overseeing performance, and examining data flow. Modifying settings in real-time can optimize the quality of service (QoS), resulting in enhanced user satisfaction and increased network performance [27, 28]. Through the examination of equipment data, it can also help with predictive maintenance by predicting faults and proactively planning repair tasks. It also forecasts network traffic patterns using historical data, which helps with traffic management and congestion [29]. Further uses include RF fingerprinting, device authentication and location, and enhancing security. Additionally, it has the ability to optimize the energy consumption of both the network and devices. Better system dependability and faster problem-solving can also come from its ability to help detect errors [30–32].

5.3 BIOMEDICAL APPLICATIONS

In antiquity, our understanding of the functioning of the human brain was nonexistent. EEG (electroencephalography) research recorded brain impulses, but they were unable to provide complete information about connection [33]. Prior to the advent of methods such as fMRI (functional Magnetic Resonance Imaging), the brain was

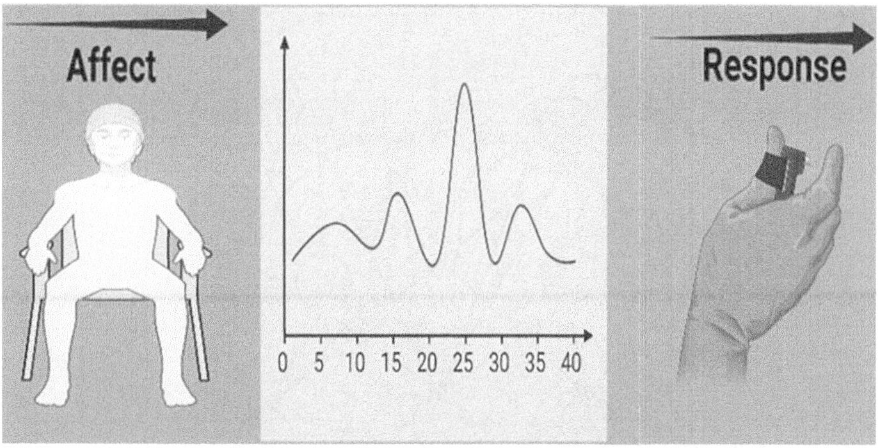

FIGURE 5.2 Affect-response example scheme.

often shown as an enclosed entity. The operations occurring inside this opaque enclosure, situated between an input and an output, proved to be challenging to comprehend. The fMRI investigations specifically focused on examining the connections, synapses, and pathways in the brain, particularly in relation to the effects of stimulants. Upon input, it was feasible to monitor the activation of specific regions and neural connections in the brain in response to an alert [34]. The EEG analysis of the brain waves within the stimulus and response box is depicted in Figure 5.2.

Functional connection networks were determined by integrating the time series data and brain activation pictures of the areas. Neuropsychologist Donald Hebb originated the well-known term to explain the connections in the brain: "Neurons that fire together, wire together". The CNN structure has a significant position in the field of artificial intelligence (AI), drawing inspiration from the neural networks present in the human brain [35, 36].

Figure 5.3 shows a schematic drawing of the connectivity in the brain.

The use of holistic image classification techniques or pixel-based segmentation approaches has not been postponed in the biomedical domain. Critical contributions were made to the field in 1998 through his collaboration with Yann Lecun on the LeNet model analysis of numerical images [37, 38]. Building upon CNN's architecture (Figure 5.4(a)), AlexNet introduced the Unet model in 2015 for analyzing biological pictures. This approach involves downsampling the image, upsampling it, and then using maxpooling to create a U-shaped structure (Figure 5.4(b)). Unet is currently expanding with the development of newer versions, including nnUnet and connected Unet. Diff-UNet may be used in the embedded system of the widely used Unet model for image processing, and SqueezeNet to the widely used AlexNet model for the embedded system. These architectures have coders and decoders in the modules mentioned [39].

These architectures are the infrastructure of the Deep Learning model, a subset of machine learning. Deep Learning with big data necessitates a substantial storage capacity. Users currently use a cloud-based supercomputer to do this task [40].

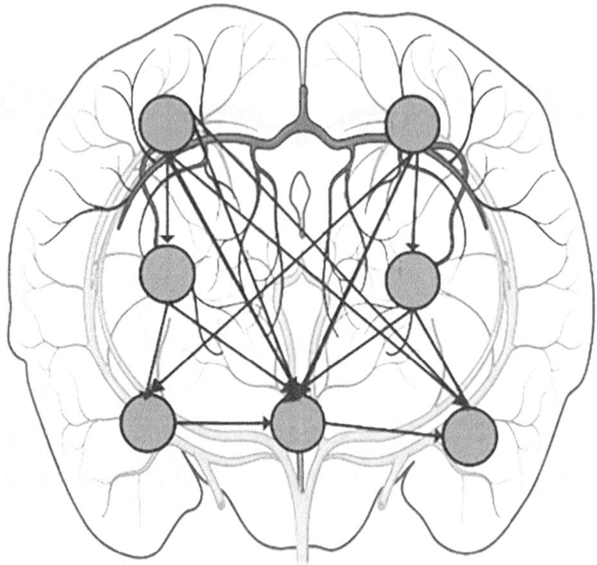

FIGURE 5.3 Anotomic image of brain connectivity example.

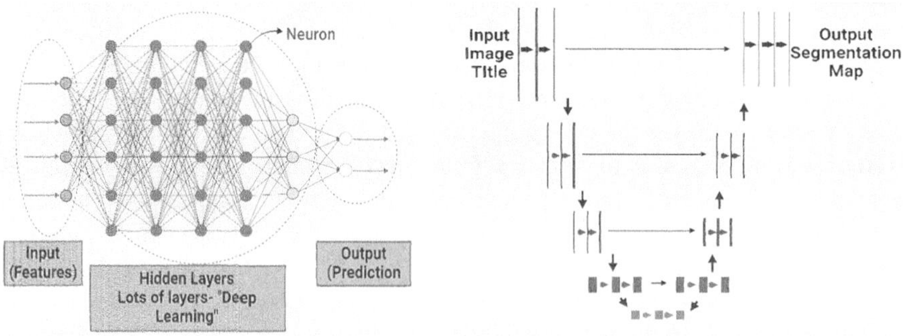

(a) (b)

FIGURE 5.4 (a) General CNN architecture. (b) Typically UNet architecture.

Deep Learning algorithms enable the comprehensive analysis of large volumes of raw data and facilitate the identification and management of diseases.

Regarding production, we may discuss generative AI, which is a subset of deep learning, often referred to as productive AIe. Generative AI refers to an artificial intelligence system capable of creating many forms of information, including voice, text, video, and graphics. Generative AI utilizes algorithms to harness acquired knowledge and extensive datasets in order to generate completely novel content. A Generative Adversarial Network (GAN) model, which is an AI system, created and commercially distributed the first picture. The picture was created by training AI using the works of renowned artists [41].

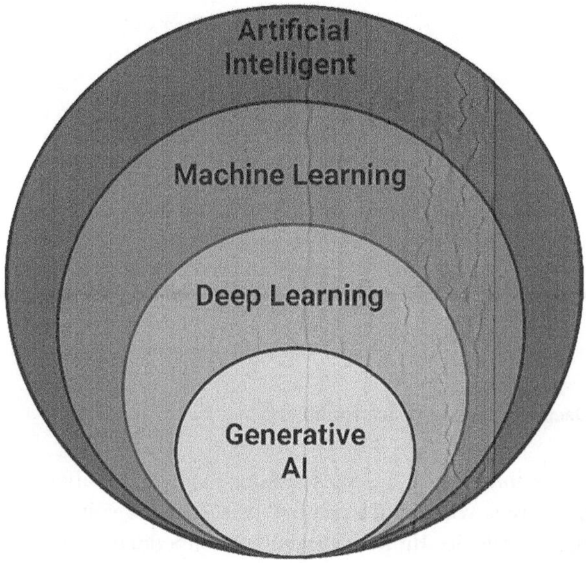

FIGURE 5.5 Unraveling AI complexity: a comparative view of AI, machine learning, deep learning, and generative AI.

An appropriate model in the field of Generative AI algorithms is the Variational Autoencoder (VAE). The Variational Autoencoder (VAE) is capable of properly representing several forms of data, facilitating the extraction of information from actual data. The main duties of a VAE are generating accurate and simple data, converting data into a clear and comprehensible structure, and managing data storage and retrieval. Using TensorFlow, a well-liked deep learning framework, VAEs are utilized to discern between regular and aberrant data points and comprehend the significance of real-world applications in order to build practical abilities [42]. Figure 5.5 compares AI, machine learning, deep learning, and generative AI, highlighting their hierarchical progression and increasing complexity.

Virtual assistants, which are Natural Language Processing (NLP) algorithms, are apps that simplify everyday and professional tasks. Language processing techniques, using a fundamental framework called diction, surpass the scope of simple data analysis. Emerging technologies have the capability to analyze an individual's emotional or physical well-being based on the tone of their voice. Embedded systems are broadening the range of applications for these NLP tools by decreasing their size. The data gathered for language processing is of an appropriate magnitude for deep learning [43]. Figure 5.6 shows the deep learning approach for NLP, highlighting the layered processing of text data to generate meaningful outputs.

Several companies use AI software as a user-friendly tool to record photos into their software architecture while doing reconstruction and analysis.

Genetic mapping plays a crucial role in the management and prevention of illnesses by facilitating the identification of genetic predispositions. Genetic datasets

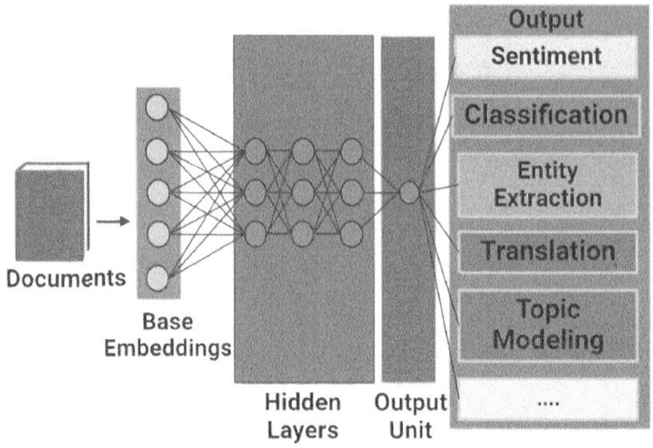

FIGURE 5.6 Deep learning approach for NLP [55].

are therefore accessible. We use deep learning methods to effectively handle and analyze these databases, which once again consist of large volumes of data [44, 45].

Telemedicine, despite its limited number of embedded system applications, is among the numerous fields that have been profoundly impacted by AI on account of its versatility and adaptability. Medical imaging, echocardiography, speech pattern analysis, emotion recognition, teleradiology, and teledermatology have all been enhanced by AI models. These technologies enhance workflow, reduce expenses, and improve prognoses [46].

Teleradiology enhances workflow efficiency and circumvents financial limitations through the transmission of digital radiological images across international boundaries. The objective of teledermatology is to mitigate disparities in the provision of healthcare and tackle the concerning prevalence of emotional disorders, suicide, and burnout. Telemedicine, a global healthcare delivery infrastructure combining Machine Learning, Robotics, Telecom, computational neuroscience, and cloud computing, considers distance and accessibility in healthcare services [47].

5.4 CONCLUSION

Telecommunication technology for embedded systems integrates communication capabilities into small, resource-constrained devices, commonly used in The Internet of Things (IoT), industrial automation, and remote monitoring. Key aspects include wireless communication, protocols, security, power efficiency, real-time communication, integration with sensors and actuators, scalability and interoperability, development tools, testing, and validation. Emerging technologies like 5G, NB-IoT, and edge computing are influencing this field [48–50].

IoT is a network of physical objects embedded with sensors and software that connects and exchanges data with other devices and systems over the internet. In telecommunication-embedded systems, IoT plays a crucial role in enabling various applications and services. It relies on various connectivity options like Wi-Fi, Bluetooth, Zigbee, cellular networks, and LPWAN technologies. IoT devices collect real-time data from sensors and devices, enabling monitoring, analytics, and decision-making. They also enable remote control and automation of devices and systems, such as industrial equipment and smart home devices. IoT devices often integrate with cloud services for data storage, processing, and analysis. Security measures, scalability, and energy efficiency are essential for IoT devices [51–53].

AI is generating high hopes for the future. Future applications of AI are expected to be significant not just in the arts but also in the realms of technology and health. Deep dreaming is providing robots with algorithms capable of simulating the dreaming process in human neural networks. These little visual artworks exemplify the capacity of AI to exceed human imagination. Embedded systems devices provide compact and efficient solutions, as opposed to bulky computers. This indicates that the potential for using AI without spatial limitations might reach highly advanced levels in many aspects of life.

Deep Learning Embedded Systems consist of digital devices, such as processors, GPUs, memory, and I/O devices, that facilitate deep learning applications. They are capable of operating as inference engines for other deep learning applications or training neural networks. By facilitating the deployment of deep learning applications, enhancing performance, and serving as a foundation for future AI-based technologies, these systems can be advantageous to organizations.[54] An organization must have a comprehensive understanding of various plans and benefits prior to implementing deep learning embedded systems. The adaptability, scalability, and speed and accuracy with which Deep Learning Embedded Systems can analyze massive volumes of data are driving their rising popularity and making them a great fit for businesses looking to grow.

REFERENCES

1. LeCun, Y., Bengio, Y., & Hinton, G. (2015). Deep Learning. *Nature*, 521(7553), 436–444.
2. Jiasi C., Xukan R. (2019). Deep learning with edge computing: A review. *IEE Explore*, 107(8), 1655–1674.
3. Al-Fuqaha, A., Guizani, M., Mohammadi, M., Aledhari, M., & Ayyash, M. (2015). Internet of Things: A survey on enabling technologies, protocols, and applications. *IEEE Communications Surveys & Tutorials*, 17(4), 2347–2376.
4. Sze, V., Chen, Y. H., Yang, T. J., & Emer, J. S. (2017). Efficient processing of deep neural networks: A tutorial and survey. *Proceedings of the IEEE*, 105(12), 2295–2329.
5. Wang, W., Zhu, M., Zeng, X., Ye, X., & Sheng, Y. (2020). Deep learning for smart industry: Efficient manufacture inspection system with fog computing. *IEEE Transactions on Industrial Informatics*, 14(10), 4665–4673.
6. Zhang, Z., & Li, J. A. (2023). Review of artificial intelligence in embedded systems. *Micromachines*, 14, 897.
7. Haigh, K. Z., Mackay, A. M., Cook, M. R., & Lin, L. G. (2015) Machine learning for embedded systems: A case study. *BBN Technologies: Cambridge, MA, USA*., 8571, 1–2.
8. Pode, D. A., & Kale, P. S. (2012). Embedded system in communication information. *Science and Technology*, 2, (1), 28–30.
9. Türk, F., & Lüy, M. (2021). Embedded systems and application areas in engineering. *International Journal of Engineering Research and Development*, 13(3), 256–265. https://doi.org/10.29137/umagd.1053602

10. Chiuchisan, I., & Geman, O. (2016). Trends in embedded systems for e-Health and biomedical applications. *2016 International Conference and Exposition on Electrical and Power Engineering (EPE)*, 304–308.
11. Gurunlu B., *Embedded Systems Presentation*. Accessed from http://blog.gurunlu.com/dokumanlar/gomulu-sistemler-sunum.pdf (Release Date: May 2008)
12. Tonello, Andrea M. *Embedded Communication Systems*. Accessed from https://nes.aau.at/?page_id=6067
13. Akesson, B., Nasri, M., Nelissen, G., Altmeyer, S., & Davis, R. I. (2022). A comprehensive survey of industry practice in real-time systems. *Real-Time Systems*, 58(3), 358–398.
14. Angueira, P., et al. (2022). A survey of physical layer techniques for secure wireless communications in industry. *IEEE Communications Surveys and Tutorials*, 24(2), 810–838
15. Pavlidou, Fotini-Niovi, et al. (2003). Power line communications: State of the art and future trends. *IEEE Communications Magazine*, 41(4), 34–40.
16. Harvie, Lance. (2023). Digital signal processing (DSP) in embedded systems, *Medium*. https://medium.com/@lanceharvieruntime/digital-signal-processing-dsp-in-embedded-systems-68b4649ff441
17. Planet Analog. (2008). Under the hood: Robot guitar embeds autotuning. *Embedded Systems Design*. https://www.planetanalog.com/under-the-hood-robot-guitar-embeds-autotuning/
18. Pode, D. A., & Kale, P. S. (2012). Embedded system in communication. *Information Science and Technology*, 2(1), 28.
19. Miramontes Meza, R., Escamilla del Río, L. V., & Aquino Santos, R. T. (2013). Mobile remote control for home automation. *International Journal of Interactive Mobile Technologies (IJIM)*, 7(4), 21.
20. Mane, Shreya. (2023). Theoretical study on embedded processor and networking. *International Journal of Engineering Technology and Management Sciences*, 7(3), 861–867. https://doi.org/10.46647/ijetms.2023.v07i03.131
21. Zhu, Y., & Hou, K. (2024). Development and implementation of an FPGA-embedded multimedia remote monitoring system for information technology server room management. *International Journal of Digital Multimedia Broadcasting*, 2024(1), 4420578.
22. Dai, L., et al. (2020). *Deep Learning for Wireless Communications: An Emerging Interdisciplinary Paradigm*. Tohoku University Scholar.
23. Voghoei, S., Tonekaboni, N. H., Wallace, J. G., & Arabnia, H. R. (2018). Deep learning at the edge. In *2018 International Conference on Computational Science and Computational Intelligence (CSCI)* (pp. 895–901). IEEE.
24. Lansky, J., Ali, S., Mohammadi, M., Majeed, M. K., Karim, S. H., Rashidi, S., Hosseinzadeh, M., & Rahmani, A. M. (2021). Deep learning-based intrusion detection systems: A systematic review. *IEEE Access*, 14(9), 101574–101599.
25. Li, R., Zhao, Z., Sun, Q., Chih-Lin, I., Yang, C., Chen, X., Zhao, M., & Zhang, H. (2018). Deep reinforcement learning for resource management in network slicing. *IEEE Access*, 18(6), 74429–74441.
26. Joo, J., Park, M. C., Han, D. S., & Pejovic, V. (2019). Deep learning-based channel prediction in realistic vehicular communications. *IEEE Access*, 7, 27846–27858. https://doi.org/10.1109/ACCESS.2019.2901710
27. Bharati, S., & Podder, P. (2022). Machine and deep learning for IoT security and privacy: Applications, challenges, and future directions. *Security and Communication Networks*, 2022(1), 8951961.
28. Ertarğın, M., Gürgenç, T., Yıldırım, Ö., & Orhan, A. (2023). A deep learning approach for motor fault detection using mobile accelerometer data. *European Journal of Technique (EJT)*, 13(2), 224–228.

29. Gao, J., Yi, X., Zhong, C., Chen, X., & Zhang, Z. (2019). Deep learning for spectrum sensing. *IEEE Wireless Communications Letters*, 8(6), 1727–1730.
30. Ureten, O., & Serinken, N. (2007). Wireless security through RF fingerprinting. *Canadian Journal of Electrical and Computer Engineering*, 32(1), 27–33.
31. Hasan, A., & Khan, B. M. (2023). Deep learning aided wireless interference identification for coexistence management in the ISM bands. *Wireless Networks*, 29(7), 3311–3331.
32. Hu, Q., Gao, F., Zhang, H., Jin, S., & Li, G. Y. (2021). Deep learning for channel estimation: Interpretation, performance, and comparison. *IEEE Transactions on Wireless Communications*, 20(4), 2398–2412.
33. Britton, J. W., Frey, L. C., Hopp, J. L., Korb, P., Koubeissi, M. Z., Lievens, W. E., Pestana-Knight, E. M., & St Louis, E. K. (2016). Electroencephalography (EEG): An introductory text and atlas of normal and abnormal findings in adults, children, and infants. American Epilepsy Society; 2016. PMID: 27748095.
34. Chen, J. E., & Glover, G. H. (2015). Functional magnetic resonance imaging methods. *Neuropsychology Review*, 25, 289–313.
35. Saon, G., Soltau, H., Emami, A., & Picheny, M. (2014). Unfolded Recurrent Neural Networks for Speech Recognition. *Interspeech*, 2014, 343–347.
36. Cooper, Steven J. (2005). Donald O. Hebb's synapse and learning rule: A history and commentary. *Neuroscience & Biobehavioral Reviews*, 28(8), 851–874.
37. Cheema, M. A., Sarwar, M. Z., Gogineni, V. C., Cantero, D., Rossi, P. S. (2024). Computationally-efficient structural health monitoring using graph signal processing. *IEEE Sensors Journal*, 24(7), 11895–11905.
38. Alzubaidi, L., Zhang, J., Humaidi, A. J. et al. (2021). Review of deep learning: Concepts, CNN architectures, challenges, applications, future directions. *Journal of Big Data*, 8, 53.
39. Yin, X. X., Sun, L., Fu, Y., Lu, R., & Zhang, Y. (2022). [Retracted] U-net-based medical image segmentation. *Journal of Healthcare Engineering*, 2022(1), 4189781.
40. O'Shea, T., & Hoydis, J. (2017). An introduction to deep learning for the physical layer. *IEEE Transactions on Cognitive Communications and Networking*, 3, 563–575.
41. Wu, A. N., Stouffs, R., & Biljecki, F. (2022). Generative adversarial networks in the built environment: A comprehensive review of the application of GANs across data types and scales. *Building and Environment*, 1(223), 109477.
42. Diederik, P. (2019). An introduction to variational autoencoders. *Foundations and Trends® in Machine Learning*, 12(4), 307–392.
43. Sarikaya, Ruhi. (2017). The technology behind personal digital assistants: An overview of the system architecture and key components. *IEEE Signal Processing Magazine*, 34(1), 67–81.
44. Fernandes, N., & Buchan, J. R. (2020). RPS28B mRNA acts as a scaffold promoting cis-translational interaction of proteins driving P-body assembly. *Nucleic Acids Research*, 48(11), 6265–6279.
45. Zhang, H., & Xu, X. (2018). Protein acetylation: An important mechanism in actinobacteria. *Bioscience Reports*, 38(2), BSR20170851.
46. Collins Oguine, O., & Jane Oguine, K. (2022). AI in telemedicine: An appraisal on deep learning-based approaches to virtual diagnostic solutions (VDS), 229–243. https://doi.org/10.5121/csit.2022.121320
47. Cheng, F. C., Chen, M. H., Hu, C. C., Tang, L. H., Liou, Y. de, Tsai, P. F., & Chiang, C. P. (2023). Overview of dental radiology education for medical radiology students in Taiwan. *Journal of Dental Sciences*, 18(1), 295–303.
48. Del Vecchio, A., Salerno, S., Barbagallo, M., Chirico, G., Campoleoni, M., Cannatà, V., Genovese, E., Granata, C., Magistrelli, A., & Tomà, P. (2020). Italian inter-society expert panel position on radiological exposure in neonatal intensive care units. *Italian Journal of Pediatrics*, 46, 1.

49. Wolf, M. H., Putnam, S. M., James, S. A., & Stiles, W. B. (1978). The medical interview satisfaction scale: Development of a scale to measure patient perceptions of physician behavior. *Journal of Behavioral Medicine*, 1, 391–401.
50. Visscher, K. L., & Faden, L. (2018). Designing a comprehensive undergraduate medical education radiology curriculum using the 5C's of radiology education framework. In *Canadian Association of Radiologists Journal* (Vol. 69, Issue 4, pp. 362–366). Canadian Medical Association.
51. Usama, M., et al. (2019). Unsupervised machine learning for networking: Techniques, applications and research challenges. *IEEE Access*, 7, 65579–65615. https://doi.org/10.1109/ACCESS.2019.2916648
52. Gillis, A. S. (2021). What is internet of things (IoT). *IoT Agenda*, 17(17), 2024.
53. Shafiq, M., Gu, Z., Cheikhrouhou, O., Alhakami, W., & Hamam, H. (2022). The rise of "Internet of Things": review and open research issues related to detection and prevention of IoT-based security attacks. *Wireless Communications and Mobile Computing*, 2022(1), 8669348.
54. Chen, Y., Zheng, B., Zhang, Z., Wang, Q., Shen, C., & Zhang, Q. (2020). Deep learning on mobile and embedded devices: State-of-the-art, challenges, and future directions. *ACM Computing Surveys (CSUR)*, 53(4), 1–37.
55. https://s3.amazonaws.com/aylien-main/misc/blog/images/nlp-language-dependence-small.png

6 Role of Embedded Systems in Diagnosis and Decision-Making for Better Treatment

Shristy Verma, Rishabha Malviya, and Sathvik Belagodu Sridhar

6.1 INTRODUCTION

Over the past few years, the medical device industry has undergone constant evolution. On the one hand, there are brand-new healthcare issues that are coming up, like COVID-19 or the issue of an aging population. However, the speed at which technology is developing is enabling the advancement of existing medical technologies and solutions. COVID-19, a disease caused by the novel coronavirus known as SARS-CoV-2, was discovered in Wuhan, China on December 31, 2019 [1–5]. Despite its global spread, COVID-19 also introduced technological innovation to the healthcare sector. Before COVID-19, in-person doctor visits were commonplace; telemedicine is here to stay. On the other hand, the failure of health systems has led to the global development of mobile applications and patient care information systems [6–10]. Similarly, examples of the technological advancements brought about by this pandemic include inexpensive oximeters for home use, robots that can disinfect objects, and tools that track temperature in public areas. New technical advancements have also surfaced in tandem with the emergence of new industry challenges [11, 12]. Many cutting-edge medical technologies are now feasible as a result of technical developments in areas like artificial intelligence (AI) and the Internet of Things (IoT). Consequently, the healthcare sector has witnessed the introduction of novel instruments and resolutions that facilitate (i) the avoidance of ailments or traumas, (ii) the identification of ailments or distinct circumstances, (iii) the observation of the patient's state, (iv) supporting the cure and convalescence of ailments, and (v) furnishing attention and optimizing the recuperation procedure for patients [13–18].

Leading medical companies' research and development (R&D) strategies show how current technology needs to be further developed. Because of their extraordinary versatility, embedded sensor systems have emerged as a crucial component of medical device advancements. They make it possible to develop state-of-the-art diagnostic and patient monitoring tools that can be used in both hospital and home environments. Numerous wearable health monitoring systems have been proposed.

DOI: 10.1201/9781003508199-6

However, wearable sensor systems, like most embedded devices, are geared toward a particular use due to budgetary limitations, technological constraints, and user convenience issues. These are usually used for alerting medical staff to impending patient conditions and for the straightforward, deterministic monitoring of patient's biometric data. Numerous systems showcase advancements in hardware, including novel technologies for wireless networking and on-body sensing [19]. There are now many physiological sensors that can be used as tiny wearable sensors that are embedded in clothing or attached to the body. Utilizing the most recent developments in microelectromechanical systems (MEMS) technology, some of these sensors have been reduced in size. These sensors include, but are not limited to, accelerometers, gyroscopes, magnetometers, piezoelectric sensors, electrocardiogram (ECG), electromyography (EMG), electroencephalography (EEG), skin conductance, body temperature, location (indoor/outdoor), respiration, foot pressure, voice, and others [20, 21]. The development of wireless sensing infrastructures represents a noteworthy breakthrough in the field of wearable systems. Before WBAN was developed, sensors were wired to the wearable computer from various locations on the patient's body. Researchers tried to lessen this by covering the sensors with clothing. These early systems are unsuitable for applications in patient health monitoring due to wearer inconvenience, but they provide reliable sensing platforms for user context detection and context-aware computing research [22].

The R&D initiatives of prominent medical corporations highlight the necessity for additional advancement of existing technology. Embedded sensor systems are crucial in the progress of medical devices because of their high level of adaptability. They enable the creation of cutting-edge diagnostic and patient monitoring devices that are suitable for use in both medical facilities and residential settings. They offer extensive system integration to enhance production procedures and optimize the consumption of products and services. In the context of embedded systems, the customary elements are firmware, software, and hardware. Hardware refers to the physical and electrical components that are necessary to complete the functioning of an embedded system (ES). Because embedded systems offer so many significant benefits, their application in the medical field has gained a lot of interest. Because each application typically requires a custom design for both the hardware and software, these systems are regarded as being extremely controllable and customizable [23, 24]. Embedded systems are now essential parts of the medical device industry, changing the way that healthcare is delivered. These systems are seamlessly integrated into a variety of medical devices to improve their capabilities, efficiency, and precision. They are distinguished by their small size and specialized functionality [25]. Fundamentally, an embedded system in a medical device is a specialized computing platform intended to reliably and efficiently carry out particular tasks, frequently in real time. Vital signs like blood pressure, temperature, and heart rate are monitored and collected by wearable devices that are outfitted with embedded systems [26]. Healthcare providers can continuously monitor the health of their patients due to this real-time data, which enables prompt interventions and individualized treatment plans. In addition, through the utilization of complex algorithms, embedded systems in imaging devices enhance the precision and efficiency of medical imaging operations and facilitate sophisticated diagnostics. Fundamentally, an embedded system in a medical device is a specialized computing platform intended to carry out particular tasks reliably and effectively, frequently in real time. These systems are integrated into a variety of medical devices, from straightforward wearable monitors to sophisticated imaging apparatus and implantable devices that can save lives. Their functions include data processing and analysis, device control, and intercom component communication [27, 28].

6.2 FOUNDATION OF DIAGNOSIS AND DECISION-MAKING

Embedded systems play a crucial role in decision-making and disease diagnostics across various healthcare domains. These systems, consisting of specialized hardware and software components, have transformed the medical business by providing real-time monitoring, analysis, and decision assistance. At the heart of this change is the integration of embedded systems into medical devices, which encompass a wide spectrum of advanced imaging equipment and portable diagnostic instruments [29]. Embedded systems are specifically built to record, process, and interpret biological signals and data, enabling healthcare practitioners to make prompt and precise judgments. Embedded systems are mostly utilized in illness diagnosis for point-of-care (POC) testing. These compact and portable devices are designed to deliver rapid diagnostic outcomes directly at the patient's bedside or in remote areas with restricted availability of traditional laboratory facilities. Handheld devices equipped with embedded biosensors can rapidly detect specific biomarkers associated with various disorders, such as cancer cells, cardiac indicators, or infectious pathogens, within a matter of minutes. These systems enhance the results for patients by using integrated processing units, sensor technologies, and microfluidics to enable early identification and timely intervention [30, 31].

In recent years, embedded systems have revolutionized the healthcare sector. A growing number of smart devices make it possible to continuously monitor things like glucose levels and vital signs. The authors [32] examine various embedded methods for tracking vital signs. It offers several solutions built around smartwatches or even sensors built into clothing or lenses. It is now simpler to gather and send this data to healthcare facilities due to these smaller, networked devices. The authors describe how low-cost, secure communication interfaces for healthcare services are provided by smart embedded systems. AI diagnostic algorithms can be used to post-process data to improve diagnosis outcomes when a significant amount of data is collected [33]. To reduce side effects and improve patient compliance, these algorithms forecast treatment outcomes, identify drug interactions, analyze large datasets, and optimize dosage schedules. They achieve this by employing embedded algorithms and machine-learning approaches. Embedded systems enable continuous observation and monitoring of patients in various healthcare settings, including homes, clinics, and hospitals. Real-time physiological data monitoring is done with wearable devices that have built-in sensors, such as accelerometers, and heart rate monitors, along with electrocardiogram (ECG) sensors. These sensors offer significant data regarding patients' well-being and the advancement of diseases. Embedded systems transmit this data wirelessly to centralized monitoring stations or cloud-based platforms, enabling medical experts to analyze it, detect abnormalities, activate alarms, and respond accordingly [34–37].

Embedded systems' role in disease diagnosis and decision-making is further expanded by their integration with telemedicine platforms. Telemedicine solutions make use of embedded devices to facilitate virtual examinations, remote patient monitoring, and remote consultations. Examples of these devices include wearable sensors, smartphones, and telehealth carts. Embedded systems allow real-time audio-visual communication between patients and medical professionals, enabling remote evaluation, planning of treatment, and follow-up care, especially in underserved or remote areas with no access to specialized healthcare services [38]. Furthermore, embedded systems empower patients to actively participate in the management of their healthcare through self-monitoring and health-tracking apps. Mobile health (mHealth) apps for smartphones and wearable technology collect and analyze user-generated data, such as exercise, eating habits, and medication adherence, to support preventive care and lifestyle modifications. Embedded technologies facilitate the identification of trends, establishment of health goals, and informed decision-making for patients and physicians by either analyzing the data locally or sending it to cloud-based platforms [39–42]. This ultimately improves overall well-being.

Embedded systems play a crucial role in decision-making processes in critical care settings through the use of closed-loop control systems and decision-support algorithms. Embedded systems in intensive care units (ICUs) utilize pre-established algorithms and feedback loops to oversee patients' vital signs and administer critical treatments such as mechanical breathing and intravenous medicine infusions. These systems enhance the effectiveness of treatment while reducing the likelihood of problems by constantly adapting treatment parameters based on the patient's changing state. In addition, embedded technologies provide medical practitioners with practical insights and suggestions based on evidence, assisting them in making clinical decisions at the POC. This is known as clinical decision support (CDS) [43, 44]. Decision support systems integrate clinical standards, medical knowledge bases, and patient-specific data to assist clinicians in diagnosing illnesses, selecting the optimal treatment, and predicting patient outcomes. Embedded algorithms enable real-time analysis of patient data, enhancing diagnostic precision and treatment efficacy. These algorithms identify potential dangers, suggest alternative diagnoses, and alert medical personnel to relevant clinical guidelines and best practices [45]. Hence, embedded systems play a crucial role in several elements of decision-making and sickness diagnosis across the entire healthcare spectrum. These systems enable healthcare providers to provide patients with individualized, efficient care by providing them with real-time data, actionable insights, and decision-support tools. These services range from POC testing and medical imaging to remote monitoring and therapeutic interventions. The incorporation of embedded systems into healthcare systems and devices will spur innovation and revolutionize the provision of healthcare services globally as technology develops [46, 47].

Modern ESs are the engine behind several complex technologies, including mobile industrial robotics and autonomous technologies. The ES is susceptible to anomalies or disturbances, especially in these kinds of natural circumstances. The effects operate in a non-stationary environment and vary over time. The reliability of a sensor, for instance, is dependent upon its environment. Furthermore, internal states—such as determining the current location of a mobile robot—may become increasingly unpredictable and unreliable. Operating the system thus becomes riskier [48]. On the other hand, safe operation is crucial, especially when people are involved. Therefore, the likelihood of errors and odd behavior increases with the requirements for embedded systems. The former is primarily caused by living in an increasingly complex, disruptive, and unpredictable environment, as well as by relying more and more on sensory input. In addition to these hardware problems, the programs used in data flow also cause problems because of the inherent ambiguity in their outputs. Even worse, these uncertainties fluctuate over the lifetime of the system due to various factors, such as fading and drifting impacts [49]. These contradictions seriously impair safe functioning by adding ambiguity and confusion and casting doubt on fundamental knowledge. The idea of trust—or trustworthiness—is crucial in this case because an embedded system's decisions are based on data it has sensed and analyzed, which in turn influences the device's overall security and how it interacts with its surroundings. Therefore, appropriate methods for handling the uncertainties or dependability as required must be developed. IoT and ES are the new domains of autonomous data transmission and collection. It is defined as a network of linked objects that are embedded with sensors, computers, and control mechanisms [50]. Science advances led to the development of IoT technology. Applications for ES and IoT are growing in frequency across practically all industries. Applications for the IoT enable smarter homes and cities, enhance logistics and transportation, support healthcare apps, and keep an eye on public safety and the environment. Embedded system applications include those in the automotive, aerospace, networks and communications, and industrial robot industries [51].

6.3 EMBEDDED SYSTEM IN MEDICAL IMAGING

Because it greatly improves diagnostic efficiency and accuracy, medical image segmentation—which aims to make anatomical or pathological structure changes in images more visible—is an essential part of computer-aided diagnosis and smart medicine. It is crucial to segment some significant organs and targets in abdominal medical images and gather features from segmented targets to assist clinicians in making accurate diagnoses [52]. In particular, it is more difficult to extract discriminating features from medical images than from regular RGB images because they often have issues with noise, blur, low contrast, etc. Due to its superior performance, deep learning—and particularly the U-shaped encoder-decoder network—has been applied widely to medical image segmentation in recent years [53]. These networks achieve high segmentation accuracy, but because of their many parameters and high memory usage, they are challenging to deploy on mobile devices. Convolutional neural networks have demonstrated considerable success in the segmentation of medical images (CNNs). However, their high parameter requirements also make it challenging to use CNNs on low-resource hardware, such as embedded systems and mobile devices [54]. An increasing amount of medical images from hospitals, medical schools, and libraries have been processed and saved in digital formats that are different from common images as computer and electronic technology advances. The concept of a system-on-chip (SoC) was used in the development of the embedded system chip to help researchers and medical professionals quickly retrieve the needed images from image databases and to allow medical expert systems to quickly and accurately diagnose patients. For the chip to communicate with other parts of medical equipment, it must also be low-power and simple to program [55].

Image processing is a technique for improving image quality by removing extraneous image data. A great deal of pointless and irrelevant content can be found in medical images. Certain preprocessing techniques are required to remove these sections from an image. Enhancing the quality of the images in the dataset is the aim of image preprocessing, as this improves the outcomes of feature extraction and segmentation methods [56]. The preprocessing techniques applied in the studies that were reviewed are described in this section. Filtering is an essential technique for improving medical images and removing noise. Instead of just copying the original minor class samples, the authors created synthetic ones using the synthetic minority over-sampling technique. They also used the method of changing the perspective of images to expand the size of the dataset. To produce new images, computer vision techniques like smoothing, gray scaling, sharpening, reducing noise, blurring, and boosting contrast were applied [57]. Image processing has been widely used to diagnose a variety of diseases in humans, animals, and plants, assisting medical professionals in making the best decision. Image processing techniques are critical to the diagnosis of human illness. They can be applied in molecular research to visualize the structure of tissues through microscope images, or they can be used to identify disease symptoms (on the skin, for example). Disease diagnosis systems consist of phases and diagnostic techniques [58, 59].

6.4 ROLE OF EMBEDDED SYSTEMS IN MEDICAL DEVICES FOR TREATMENT

The potential applications of biosensor studies for clinical treatment, pharmaceuticals, biomedical, and healthcare are receiving a lot of attention. Biosensors have demonstrated potential in the diagnosis, treatment, prevention, and rehabilitation of diseases, as well as in the monitoring of patient health. Moreover, pathogenic, bacterial, and viral microorganisms can be recognized by biosensors [60, 61]. Step trackers and physical activity help people form and improve healthier habits. Biosensors offer fine-grained mechanical information about biological structures at the molecular level. Numerous industries, including pharmaceuticals, healthcare, food, agriculture, environmental technology, and biological process research, can benefit from the extensive applications of these analytical tools. Due to this understanding, several techniques for locating biomolecules that are essential for drug discovery, gene therapy, virus and microbe detection, and other biotechnology procedures have been developed. The market for biosensors is expanding quickly as a result of their widespread application in medicine and healthcare. Furthermore, there is a strong development underway for biosensors, which will be useful in several fields such as disease identification, human health management, patient health monitoring, and diagnosis [62]. The potential of wearable biosensors to deliver continuous and real-time physiological data has sparked a lot of interest. With the use of these sensors, non-invasive measurements of the biochemical markers found in biofluids like saliva, tears, sweat, and interstitial fluid can be made. Recent developments have focused on

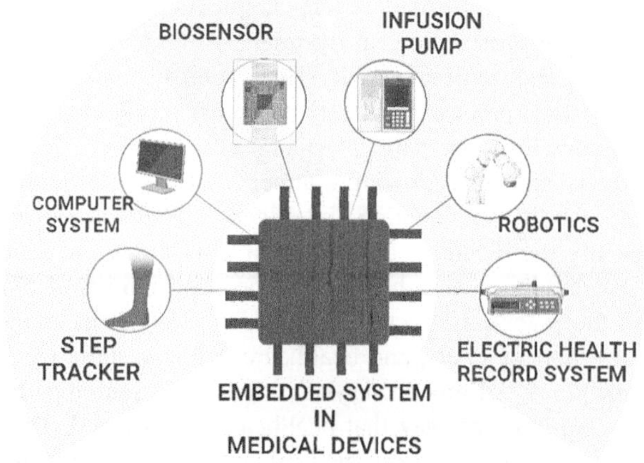

FIGURE 6.1 Various applications of embedded system in medical devices.

the non-invasive monitoring of biomarkers, such as bacteria, hormones, and metabolites, as well as electrochemical and optical biosensors [63, 64]. Due to advances in computing power, new demands for creative healthcare solutions, and technological advancements, embedded systems in biomedical monitoring have made significant headway as shown in Figure 6.1 [65].

Embedded systems are used by ECG monitors to track heart rate and identify anomalies. They are used by blood pressure monitoring systems to deliver precise, real-time readings for patient monitoring. Using embedded systems, CGM devices continuously check blood glucose levels and provide useful information to patients with diabetes [66]. Electrical stimuli are delivered by embedded systems to cardiac pacemakers, which control heart rhythms. Furthermore, implantable cardioverter defibrillators (ICDs) rely on embedded systems to keep an eye on cardiac rhythms and shock the patient when they identify potentially fatal arrhythmias. Wearable technology that tracks various metrics such as activity levels, sleep patterns, and physiological data is powered by embedded systems. This permits ongoing remote patient observation. Wearables with integrated sensors can monitor a patient's vital signs and provide real-time health data [67]. Computer systems called embedded systems are made to carry out a particular job or function inside of a bigger system. Since they enable communication between medical devices and central healthcare systems, enabling telemedicine consultations and remote patient management, they have grown in importance in the medical field. Electronic Health Record (EHR) systems rely heavily on embedded systems for the safe and effective archiving, retrieval, and transfer of patient data [68].

To deliver medicine dosages precisely and programmatically, infusion pumps depend on embedded systems. Systems with integrated inhalers increase drug compliance for respiratory ailments. Healthcare biometric devices employ embedded systems to identify patients via fingerprint or retinal scans, thereby enhancing security. Amputees' quality of life can be improved by prosthetic limbs with embedded systems because they allow for more natural and adaptive movement. In rehabilitation, robotic devices with embedded systems help patients regain their mobility and motor skills. To diagnose neurological disorders, EEG devices use embedded systems to monitor and analyze brain activity. Embedded systems are used in biomedical monitoring to collect precise and timely data, which helps medical professionals make better decisions, improve patient outcomes, and improve healthcare delivery [24]. However, because of the growing number of attacks stemming from security threats and vulnerability exploitation, intelligent embedded device security has become strategically significant. In addition, problems with rapid data delivery, node failures, and connectivity pose a challenge to the development of e-health systems. To fully realize the potential effects of embedded systems in medical devices on treatment efficacy, patient safety, and healthcare delivery, these technical obstacles must be overcome [25, 27]. Embedded systems are now essential parts of the medical device industry, changing the way that healthcare is delivered. These systems are seamlessly integrated into a variety of medical devices to improve their capabilities, efficiency, and precision. They are distinguished by their small size and specialized functionality. Fundamentally, an embedded system in a medical device is a specialized computing platform intended to carry out particular tasks reliably and effectively, frequently in real time [26]. Consequently, embedded sensor systems have become an essential part of medical device advancements due to their remarkable adaptability. They make it possible to develop state-of-the-art diagnostic and patient monitoring tools that can be used in both hospital and home environments. The medical device industry is regulated by several national notification or regulatory bodies. Two of the main regulatory bodies in the world are the European Commission Directorate and the US Food and Drug Administration (FDA) [69].

Embedded systems are now found in all categories of health technology, not just those that monitor medical equipment. They are utilized in prognostic (PET, digital X-ray, and MRI), diagnostic (blood glucose monitors), patient management (self-test devices for remote patient monitoring), and telemedicine applications [70]. Among the cutting-edge embedded devices are defibrillators, which employ embedded technology to check a patient's heart for abnormal rhythms and, in case of need, gently shock the heart back into normal rhythm. Doctors configure the defibrillator to fit each patient using an external device. The external paddle (manual) defibrillators are no longer necessary when a defibrillator is implanted in the patient. Patients may experience no change at all until the machine functions. Using a specialized stethoscope, one can listen to the baby's heartbeat for external monitoring. External monitoring is most frequently carried out with two flat devices (sensors) fastened to the abdomen with elastic belts. One sensor monitors the baby's heart rate by using ultrasonography or reflected sound waves. The length of your contractions is measured by the additional sensor. A device that records the data is connected to the sensors [71, 72]. Additionally, pulse oximetry is a straightforward, reasonably priced, and non-invasive method of oxygenation monitoring. It keeps track of the proportion of oxygen-saturated hemoglobin. Always maintain an oxygen saturation level above 95%; however, in patients with chronic respiratory conditions or cyanotic congenital heart disease, this level may be lower, depending on the severity of the ailment [73–75].

Furthermore, wireless sensor networks and embedded systems have made it possible for real-time patient health monitoring and alarm systems, which have improved patient outcomes, particularly for those who are ill during their regular lives. Moreover, the incorporation of non-medical devices for chronic dyspnea into complex social systems has highlighted how the patient, caregiver, and clinician triads collaborate and impact the processes of integration and implementation. Embedded systems in medical devices have taught us important lessons about the importance of trust and security in intelligent embedded systems, especially when it comes to maintaining user trust and privacy preservation [76–78]. Additionally, the importance of optimized embedded healthcare industry models with lightweight computing has been shown by the integration of e-health data transmission to medical experts for real-time treatments, supported by a digital mobile network. Additionally, the potential drawbacks of asthma patients switching inhaled drugs and devices without consent highlight how important it is to take into account elements like medication, design, and user-friendliness when creating embedded medical devices. Moreover, a significant advancement in real-time patient monitoring has been data analytics. Deep learning and medical technology can now be combined for the best possible patient care due to edge computing's ability to save bandwidth, improve availability, and reduce latency [79–82]. Additionally, the prevention and control of illnesses like COVID-19 have been greatly aided by the use of big data and predictive analytics in the healthcare industry [83].

Additionally, a focus area has been interoperability and connectivity across various devices. Interoperability between medical devices is becoming more common and is thought to be the direction that medical technology will take. Modern medicine is beginning to demand the interconnection of medical devices, and many communication standards have been put forth to make this happen. It is thought that the interoperability reference model put forth will advance the AI medical device sector [84].

6.5 CHALLENGES OF EMBEDDED SYSTEMS IN TREATMENT

Healthcare applications present a unique set of requirements and constraints for embedded systems used in biomedical monitoring [85]. The integration of embedded systems in medical devices is beset with concerns in the USA, mainly related to cybersecurity threats and compatibility standardization. Risks associated with cybersecurity include the possibility of data breaches and remote hacking, which endanger patient privacy. As medical technology advances, healthcare IT systems are becoming more interconnected, making them more susceptible to cyberattacks [86]. This raises questions regarding patient data security and the possibility of remotely manipulating medical equipment. Standardizing interoperability is also essential for guaranteeing smooth device communication and resolving compatibility problems [87]. Since data communication between devices is still being researched and standardized, one of the biggest obstacles to achieving interoperability is the heterogeneity of medical devices from various suppliers. The Medical Device Amendments Act reaffirms the FDA's authority to assess the efficacy and safety of medical devices marketed in the United States.

However, due to their increased connectivity to current computer networks, medical devices are now more vulnerable to cybersecurity threats [88]. Therefore, to determine the effect on patient health and the exploitability of these vulnerabilities, risk assessments and enhanced protection are necessary. Additionally, to facilitate communication between medical information systems across organizational, geographic, and system boundaries, medical device interoperability standards must be developed [89]. It takes a lot of work to ensure data accuracy and to properly secure embedded systems that are meant to gather data from sensors and transmit it to a storage server. Even though the cloud is becoming a fairly developed system, there is still room for improvement in many areas, including security. This is because the cloud is still relatively new compared to other IT systems [90].

Limited memory and processor speed on embedded systems, as illustrated in Figure 6.2, is another problem with machine learning. Memory capacity, processor speed, energy consumption, latency, cost, security, and privacy are all crucial factors to take into account when integrating deep learning or machine learning with embedded systems. High dimensionality from large datasets increases the need for computations and data transfer [91]. Additionally, the requirement for programmability leads to an increase in data movement and computation. When implementing machine learning in an embedded system, a variety of calculation types and quantities must be performed to analyze the data. Since the internet is involved in all of these computations, sending data to the cloud raises security, privacy, and latency concerns. In certain circumstances, a prompt response is required. An application might not be able to withstand the time lag brought on by cloud transmission [92, 93]. Furthermore, the data may be private and restricted from outside sharing or transfer. To overcome these difficulties, all classifications in machine learning methods such as neural

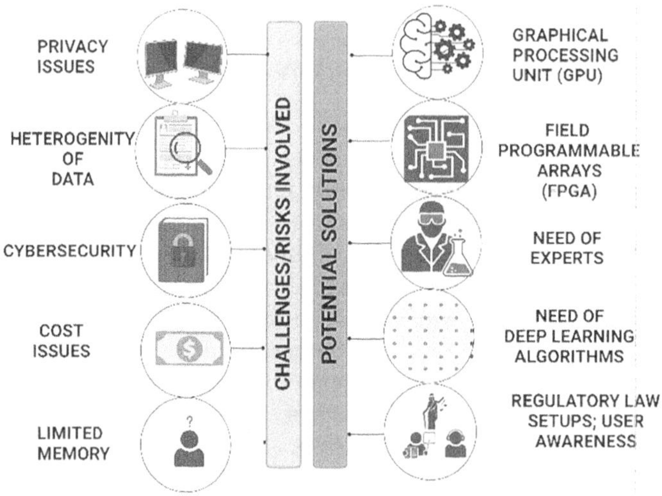

FIGURE 6.2 Pictorial representation of challenges and solution of embedded system in treatment.

networks are represented by matrix multiplications [93]. Multiply and accumulate, the two primary operations in neural network processing, produce partial sums that are accumulated at the output feature maps. The number of these computations increased due to the high dimensionality of the data. Machine learning algorithms such as Decision Tree Classification and Support Vector need to be accelerated because large datasets require a lot of processing power. Therefore, to minimize computation overhead and accelerate computations, GPUs are used in embedded systems [94].

While the most widely utilized solution is the graphical processing unit (GPU), Field Programmable Arrays (FPGA) offer an even better option. FPGA has proven to perform noticeably better than GPU in a variety of applications, including image processing, digital signal processing, pattern recognition, etc. Therefore, one of the most widely used, potent, and parallel processing reprogrammable devices for hardware in machine learning or deep learning algorithms is the FPGA. FPGAs can achieve powerful computing capabilities at low cost and energy consumption, which is crucial for achieving the three main objectives of reduced latency, increased throughput, and lower energy consumption [95–97]. They are even better than GPUs in terms of constraints for computational systems. FPGA's ability to be reprogrammed increases its flexibility and adaptability to changes. Accelerators can also be used to optimize data movement and, by extension, energy consumption, by lowering access from the price level of the memory hierarchy. Pruning is a technique that reduces the amount of multiplication and accumulation operations required by getting rid of weights that don't affect output [98]. Energy models are used to reduce energy costs and consumption by doing away with the weights. The ALU processing elements are designed so that they cannot perform matrix multiplications when the inputs are zero. Consequently, in this manner, the energy consumption can be cut by 45%. It is preferable to perform all calculations locally on the system, rather than utilizing the cloud, to address concerns related to latency, security, and privacy. Completing calculations on-site will also minimize data movement, which will lower energy usage and associated costs [99, 100].

For embedded systems, machine learning models need a lot of room and time to train. Rather, train the model in a deep learning environment first on a laptop. Models like Resnet, Mobilenet, and Squeezenet can be used with embedded systems to reduce storage needs once the network has been trained. However, computations still lead to storage problems; therefore, shallower neural networks can be used for embedded systems [101]. It is preferable to execute all computations locally on the system rather than using the cloud to reduce latency and enhance security and privacy. Minimizing data movement by completing computations on-site will also reduce energy usage and associated costs. For embedded systems, machine learning models need a lot of room and time to train. Rather, first, train the model in a deep learning environment on a laptop [102]. Models like Resnet, Mobilenet, and Squeezenet can be used with embedded systems to reduce storage needs once the network has been trained. However, storage issues arise from computations as well; thus, shallower neural networks can be applied to embedded systems. Embedded systems have the potential to significantly influence the future of healthcare by transforming patient care and medical treatment. Smart processing has the power to change how healthcare is provided and how patients are treated by connecting different physical objects with embedded technology for perception and communication [103]. Furthermore, it is anticipated that the implementation of Industry 4.0 technologies in the pharmaceutical, healthcare, and medical domains will tackle issues related to medical data integrity and aid in surmounting healthcare obstacles such as those presented by the COVID-19 pandemic [104]. To meet one or more of the security requirements, an increasing number of embedded system designers must support a variety of security solutions. The complexity of security protocols and increasing data rates lead to significant obstacles in the embedded system design process. The first is the processing gap, which occurs when embedded system architectures cannot keep up with the computational demands of security processing, requiring a high or large number of transactions in the system. The second issue is the battery gap, which develops as a result of the extremely high energy consumption required to support security on embedded systems with limited battery life. Flexibility is yet another prerequisite for security. Since embedded systems frequently need to implement multiple security standards and protocols to satisfy multiple security objectives and enable interoperability in various environments, it is preferable to have a sufficiently flexible security structure (programmable) to easily adapt to changing requirements. Therefore, the integration of machine learning and predictive analytics, the use of cutting-edge technology, and the revolution in healthcare will shape the future of embedded systems in medical devices in the United States. These advancements could lead to better patient care, medical care, and the resolution of significant healthcare problems [110].

6.6 CONCLUSION

The aging population and new healthcare concerns have caused constant change in the medical device sector. The development of new tools and solutions that facilitate disease prevention, diagnosis, monitoring, treatment, recovery, and care streamlining has been made possible by technological advancements in fields like AI and the IoT. As embedded sensor systems are so versatile, they have become an essential part of medical device innovations. They enable the creation of state-of-the-art patient monitoring and diagnostic systems that are suitable for use in both home and hospital settings. Embedded systems have significantly transformed the healthcare industry by offering cost-effective and secure communication interfaces for healthcare services, as well as by continually monitoring essential indicators such as vital signs and blood sugar levels. AI diagnostic algorithms can be employed for data post-processing to improve the precision of diagnosis. For example, pacemakers equipped with integrated systems can monitor heart rate and detect cardiovascular problems. Currently, embedded systems are utilized in prognostic, diagnostic, patient management, and telemedicine applications, which are all domains within the field of health technology. Due to their high level of controllability and ability to be customized, they play a vital role in the medical device sector. Embedded systems enhance patient outcomes and quality of life by integrating biological and technological processes. Implantable medical devices, such as pacemakers and medication delivery systems, depend on integrated technology to guarantee accurate and constant operation inside the human body. These devices' embedded systems offer critical functions like vital sign monitoring, precise medication administration, and therapeutic capabilities that improve patient outcomes and care quality. These advancements have the potential to address significant healthcare issues, raise the standard of medical care, and improve patient care.

REFERENCES

1. Petretto DR, Pili R. Ageing and COVID-19: What is the role of elderly people? *Geriatrics*. 2020 Apr 26;5(2):25.
2. Rabi FA, Al Zoubi MS, Kasasbeh GA, Salameh DM, Al-Nasser AD. SARS-CoV-2 and coronavirus disease 2019: What we know so far. *Pathogens*. 2020 Mar 20;9(3):231.
3. Bahl S, Singh RP, Javaid M, Khan IH, Vaishya R, Suman R. Telemedicine technologies for confronting COVID-19 pandemic: A review. *Journal of Industrial Integration and Management*. 2020 Dec 31;5(04):547–61.
4. He W, Zhang ZJ, Li W. Information technology solutions, challenges, and suggestions for tackling the COVID-19 pandemic. *International Journal of Information Management*. 2021 Apr 1;57:102287.
5. Ruan K, Wu Z, Xu Q. Smart cleaner: A new autonomous indoor disinfection robot for combating the covid-19 pandemic. *Robotics*. 2021 Jul 12;10(3):87.
6. Moisello E, Malcovati P, Bonizzoni E. Thermal sensors for contactless temperature measurements, occupancy detection, and automatic operation of appliances during the COVID-19 pandemic: A review. *Micromachines*. 2021 Feb 3;12(2):148.
7. Luks AM, Swenson ER. Pulse oximetry for monitoring patients with COVID-19 at home. Potential pitfalls and practical guidance. *Annals of the American Thoracic Society*. 2020 Sep;17(9):1040–6.
8. Alanazi A. IoT and AI in healthcare: A systematic literature review. *PLOMS AI*. 2021 May 22;1(1), 1–6.
9. Wani SU, Khan NA, Thakur G, Gautam SP, Ali M, Alam P, Alshehri S, Ghoneim MM, Shakeel F. Utilization of artificial intelligence in disease prevention: Diagnosis, treatment, and implications for the healthcare workforce. In *Healthcare* 2022 Mar 24 (Vol. 10, No. 4, p. 608). MDPI.
10. Jennings D, Little MM, Johnson-Jennings M. Developing a tribal health sovereignty model for obesity prevention. *Progress in Community Health Partnerships: Research, Education, and Action*. 2018;12(3):353–62.
11. Chui KT, Alhalabi W, Pang SS, Pablos PO, Liu RW, Zhao M. Disease diagnosis in smart healthcare: Innovation, technologies and applications. *Sustainability*. 2017 Dec 18;9(12):2309.
12. Mansour RF, El Amraoui A, Nouaouri I, Díaz VG, Gupta D, Kumar S. Artificial intelligence and internet of things enabled disease diagnosis model for smart healthcare systems. *IEEE Access*. 2021 Mar 17;9:45137–46.
13. Al Banna MH, Ghosh T, Taher KA, Kaiser MS, Mahmud M. A monitoring system for patients of autism spectrum disorder using artificial intelligence. In *International Conference on Brain Informatics*. 2020 Sep 15 (pp. 251–262). Cham: Springer International Publishing.
14. Li X, Zhou HP, Zhou ZJ, Du N, Zhong EH, Zhai K, Liu N, Zhou L. Artificial intelligence-powered remote monitoring of patients with chronic obstructive pulmonary disease. *Chinese Medical Journal*. 2021 Jul 5;134(13):1546–8.
15. Troisi J. Artificial intelligence in medicine: Disease diagnosis, drug development and treatment personalization. *Current Medicinal Chemistry*. 2021 Oct 1;28(32):6509–11.

16. Tahri Sqalli M, Al-Thani D. On how chronic conditions affect the patient-AI interaction: A literature review. In *Healthcare*. 2020 Sep 1 (Vol. 8, No. 3, p. 313). MDPI.
17. Fouad H, Hassanein AS, Soliman AM, Al-Feel H. Analyzing patient health information based on IoT sensor with AI for improving patient assistance in the future direction. *Measurement*. 2020 Jul 15;159:107757.
18. Chow JC. Artificial intelligence in radiotherapy and patient care. In *Artificial Intelligence in Medicine*. 2021 Jul 11 (pp. 1–13). Springer International Publishing.
19. Anliker U, Beutel J, Dyer M, Enzler R, Lukowicz P, Thiele L, Troster G. A systematic approach to the design of distributed wearable systems. *IEEE Transactions on Computers*. 2004 Jun 21;53(8):1017–33.
20. Park S, Jayaraman S. Enhancing the quality of life through wearable technology. *IEEE Engineering in Medicine and Biology Magazine*. 2003 Jul 22;22(3):41–8.
21. DeVaul R, Sung M, Gips J. MIThril 2003: Applications and architecture. In *Seventh IEEE International Symposium on Wearable Computers, 2003. Proceedings*. 2003 Oct 1 (p. 4). IEEE Computer Society.
22. Van Laerhoven K, Schmidt A, Gellersen HW. Multi-sensor context aware clothing. In *Proceedings. Sixth International Symposium on Wearable Computers*. 2002 Oct 10 (pp. 49–56). IEEE.
23. Chiuchisan I, Geman O. Trends in embedded systems for e-Health and biomedical applications. In *2016 International Conference and Exposition on Electrical and Power Engineering (EPE)*. 2016 Oct 20 (pp. 304–308). IEEE.
24. Zavitsanou S, Chakrabarty A, Dassau E, Doyle III FJ. Embedded control in wearable medical devices: Application to the artificial pancreas. *Processes*. 2016 Sep 23;4(4):35.
25. Sonko S, Monebi AM, Etukudoh EA, Osasona F, Atadoga A, Daudu CD. Reviewing the impact of embedded systems in medical devices in the USA. *International Medical Science Research Journal*. 2024 Feb 9;4(2):158–69.
26. Chang R, Jiang L, Xie Y, He H, Chen D, Ren L. Implementing a hardware-assisted memory management mechanism for arm platforms using the b method. *Concurrency and Computation: Practice and Experience*. 2019 Nov 10;31(21):e4659.
27. Haseeb K, Saba T, Rehman A, Ahmed I, Lloret J. Efficient data uncertainty management for health industrial internet of things using machine learning. *International Journal of Communication Systems*. 2021 Nov 10;34(16):e4948.
28. Kurien J, Koutsoukos X, Zhao F. Distributed diagnosis of networked embedded systems. In *Proceedings of the 13th International Workshop on Principles of Diagnosis (DX-2002)*. 2002 May 2 (pp. 179–188). Semmering Austria.
29. Pham MT, Kim JM, Kim CH. Deep learning-based bearing fault diagnosis method for embedded systems. *Sensors*. 2020 Dec 2;20(23):6886.
30. Mhamdi L, Dammak O, Cottin F, Dhaou IB. Artificial intelligence for cardiac diseases diagnosis and prediction using ECG images on embedded systems. *Biomedicines*. 2022 Aug 19;10(8):2013.
31. Ge N, Nakajima S, Pantel M. Online diagnosis of accidental faults for real-time embedded systems using a hidden Markov model. *Simulation*. 2015 Oct;91(10):851–68.
32. Dias D, Paulo Silva Cunha J. Wearable health devices—vital sign monitoring, systems and technologies. *Sensors*. 2018 Jul 25;18(8):2414.
33. Anand S, Nath V. Study and design of smart embedded system for remote health monitoring using internet of things. In *Nanoelectronics, Circuits and Communication Systems: Proceeding of NCCS 2017*. 2019 (pp. 409–414). Springer Singapore.
34. Ottaviano D, Cinque M, Manduchi G, Dubbioso S. Virtualization of accelerators in embedded systems for mixed-criticality: Rpu exploitation for fusion diagnostics and control. *Fusion Engineering and Design*. 2023 May 1;190:113518.

35. Hu X, Ding X, Bai D, Zhang Q. A compressed model-agnostic meta-learning model based on pruning for disease diagnosis. *Journal of Circuits, Systems and Computers*. 2023 Jan 30;32(02):2350022.
36. Abdallah IB, Bouteraa Y. A newly-designed wearable robotic hand exoskeleton controlled by EMG signals and ROS embedded systems. *Robotics*. 2023 Jul 1;12(4):95.
37. Aldaajeh SH, Harous S, Alrabaee S. Fault-detection tactics for optimized embedded systems efficiency. *IEEE Access*. 2021 Jun 22;9:91328–40.
38. Heit J. Impact of methods and mechanisms for improving software dependability on non-functional requirements (Doctoral dissertation, Universitätsbibliothek der Universität Stuttgart).
39. France RB, Kim DK, Ghosh S, Song E. A UML-based pattern specification technique. *IEEE Transactions on Software Engineering*. 2004 Mar 8;30(3):193–206.
40. Bogner J, Wagner S, Zimmermann A. Using Architectural Modifiability Tactics to Examine Evolution Qualities of Service-and Microservice-Based Systems: An Approach Based on Principles and Patterns. *SICS Software-Intensive Cyber-Physical Systems*. 2019 Jun 1;34:141–9.
41. Wojcik R, Bachmann F, Bass L, Clements P, Merson P, Nord R, Wood W. Attribute-driven design (add), version 2.0, Softw. Eng. Inst., Carnegie Mellon Univ., Tech. Rep. CMU/SEI-2006-TR-023, 2006. [Online]. Available: https://resources.sei.cmu.edu/library/asset-view.cfm?AssetID=8147
42. Bachmann F, Bass L, Nord R. Modi ability tactics, Softw. Eng. Inst., Carnegie Mellon Univ., Tech. Rep. CMU/SEI-2007-TR-002, 2007. [Online]. Available: https://resources.sei.cmu.edu/library/asset-view.cfm?AssetID=8299
43. Kim DK. The role-based metamodeling language for specifying design patterns. In *Design Pattern Formalization Techniques*. 2007 (pp. 183–205). IGI Global.
44. Mazzia V, Khaliq A, Salvetti F, Chiaberge M. Real-time apple detection system using embedded systems with hardware accelerators: An edge AI application. *IEEE Access*. 2020 Jan 7;8:9102–14.
45. Oliveira F, Costa DG, Assis F, Silva I. Internet of intelligent things: A convergence of embedded systems, edge computing and machine learning. *Internet of Things*. 2024 Mar 4:26:101153.
46. Zhang X. RETRACTED: Energy-saving design of civil engineering buildings based on FPGA and embedded system. 2021 June: 103970.
47. Liu Y, Yu W, Rahayu W, Dillon T. An evaluative study on IoT ecosystem for smart predictive maintenance (iot-spm) in manufacturing: Multi-view requirements and data quality. *IEEE Internet of Things Journal*. 2023 Feb 22; 10: 11160–11184.
48. Babaei A, Khedmati M, Akbari Jokar MR, Tirkolaee EB. Designing an integrated blockchain-enabled supply chain network under uncertainty. *Scientific Reports*. 2023 Mar 9;13(1):3928.
49. Mazumdar H, Kaushik A, Gohel HA. To mitigate primary user emulation attack trajectory using cognitive single carrier frequency division multiple access approaches: Towards next generation green IoT. *Engineering Reports*. 2023 Dec;5(12):e12672.
50. Mishra N, Pandya S. Internet of things applications, security challenges, attacks, intrusion detection, and future visions: A systematic review. *IEEE Access*. 2021 Apr 15;9:59353–77.
51. Xue X, Marappan R, Raju SK, Raghavan R, Rajan R, Khalaf OI, Abdulsahib GM. Modelling and analysis of hybrid transformation for lossless big medical image compression. *Bioengineering*. 2023 Mar 6;10(3):333.
52. Potočnik J, Foley S, Thomas E. Current and potential applications of artificial intelligence in medical imaging practice: A narrative review. *Journal of Medical Imaging and Radiation Sciences*. 2023 Apr 14;26:101153.

53. El-Shafai W, Hemdan EE. Robust and efficient multi-level security framework for color medical images in telehealthcare services. *Journal of Ambient Intelligence and Humanized Computing*. 2023 Apr;14(4):3675–90.
54. El-Shafai W, Khallaf F, El-Rabaie ES, El-Samie FE. Proposed 3D chaos-based medical image cryptosystem for secure cloud-IoMT eHealth communication services. *Journal of Ambient Intelligence and Humanized Computing*. 2024 Jan;15(1):1–28.
55. Ansari Z, Mateenuddin Q, Abdullah A. Performance research on medical data classification using traditional and soft computing techniques. *International Journal of Recent Technology and Engineering*. 2019;8:990–5.
56. Kermany DS, Goldbaum M, Cai W, Valentim CC, Liang H, Baxter SL, McKeown A, Yang G, Wu X, Yan F, Dong J. Identifying medical diagnoses and treatable diseases by image-based deep learning. *Cell*. 2018 Feb 22;172(5):1122–31.
57. Sudheer Kumar E, Shoba Bindu C. Medical image analysis using deep learning: A systematic literature review. In *Emerging Technologies in Computer Engineering: Microservices in Big Data Analytics: Second International Conference, ICETCE 2019, Jaipur, India, February 1–2, 2019, Revised Selected Papers 2* 2019 (pp. 81–97). Springer Singapore.
58. Perumal S, Velmurugan T. Preprocessing by contrast enhancement techniques for medical images. *International Journal of Pure and Applied Mathematics*. 2018;118(18):3681–8.
59. Zhang J, Zhang X, Wei X, Xue Y, Wan H, Wang P. Recent advances in acoustic wave biosensors for the detection of disease-related biomarkers: A review. *Analytica Chimica Acta*. 2021 Jun 15;1164:338321.
60. Brazaca LC, Sampaio I, Zucolotto V, Janegitz BC. Applications of biosensors in Alzheimer's disease diagnosis. *Talanta*. 2020 Apr 1;210:120644.
61. Rodrigues Ribeiro Teles FS, Pires de Tavora Tavira LA, Pina da Fonseca LJ. Biosensors as rapid diagnostic tests for tropical diseases. *Critical Reviews in Clinical Laboratory Sciences*. 2010 Jun 1;47(3):139–69.
62. Threm D, Nazirizadeh Y, Gerken M. Photonic crystal biosensors towards on-chip integration. *Journal of Biophotonics*. 2012 Aug;5(8–9):601–16.
63. Parker RN, Grove TZ. Designing repeat proteins for biosensors and medical imaging. *Biochemical Society Transactions*. 2015 Oct 1;43(5), 856–860.
64. Pourasl AH, Ahmadi MT, Rahmani M, Chin HC, Lim CS, Ismail R, Tan ML. Analytical modeling of glucose biosensors based on carbon nanotubes. *Nanoscale Research Letters*. 2014 Dec;9:1–7.
65. Bandodkar AJ, Jeerapan I, Wang J. Wearable chemical sensors: Present challenges and future prospects. *Acs Sensors*. 2016 May 27;1(5):464–82.
66. Heikenfeld J, Jajack A, Rogers J, Gutruf P, Tian L, Pan T, Li R, Khine M, Kim J, Wang J. Wearable sensors: Modalities, challenges, and prospects. *Lab on a Chip*. 2018;18(2):217–48.
67. Matzeu G, Florea L, Diamond D. Advances in wearable chemical sensor design for monitoring biological fluids. *Sensors and Actuators B: Chemical*. 2015 May 1;211:403–18.
68. Liu Y, Pharr M, Salvatore GA. Lab-on-skin: A review of flexible and stretchable electronics for wearable health monitoring. *ACS Nano*. 2017 Oct 24;11(10):9614–35.
69. Gao W, Emaminejad S, Nyein HY, Challa S, Chen K, Peck A, Fahad HM, Ota H, Shiraki H, Kiriya D, Lien DH. Fully integrated wearable sensor arrays for multiplexed in situ perspiration analysis. *Nature*. 2016 Jan 28;529(7587):509–14.
70. Pohl K, Hönninger H, Achatz R, Broy M, editors. *Model-based Engineering of Embedded Systems: The SPES 2020 Methodology*. 2012 Nov 8. Springer.
71. Kulkarni S, Kulkarni SG. Remote health monitoring using embedded systems. *International Journal of Emerging Research in Management & Technology*. 2015;4(6): 295–300.

72. Kim D, Jeong D, Kim J, Kim H, Kim J, Park SM, Ahn S. Design and implementation of a wireless charging-based cardiac monitoring system focused on temperature reduction and robust power transfer efficiency. *Energies*. 2020 Feb 24;13(4):1008.
73. Niu H, Tian H, Chang C, Li D, Fan Y. Development of a device for negative pressure wound therapy based on arm9 embedded system. In *2011 5th International Conference on Bioinformatics and Biomedical Engineering* 2011 May 10 (pp. 1–4). IEEE.
74. Gibson LL, Fahey NM, Hafer N, Buchholz B, Dunlap DR, Murphy RL, Achenbach C, Stone C, Cleeton R, O'Neal J, Frediani JK. The RADx Tech Clinical Studies Core: A model for academic based clinical studies. *IEEE Open Journal of Engineering in Medicine and Biology*. 2021 Apr 28;2:152–7.
75. Ohenhen PE, Chidolue O, Umoh AA, Ngozichukwu B, Fafure AV, Ilojianya VI, Ibekwe KI. Sustainable cooling solutions for electronics: A comprehensive review: Investigating the latest techniques and materials, their effectiveness in mechanical applications, and associated environmental benefits. *World Journal of Advanced Research and Reviews*. 2024;21(1):957–972.
76. Leidy NK, Beusterien K, Sullivan E, Richner R, Muni NI. Integrating the patient's perspective into device evaluation trials. *Value in Health*. 2006 Nov 1;9(6):394–401.
77. Lesén E, Björholt I, Ingelgård A, Olson FJ. Exploration and preferential ranking of patient benefits of medical devices: A new and generic instrument for health economic assessments. *International Journal of Technology Assessment in Health Care*. 2017;33(4):463–71.
78. Orieno OH, Ndubuisi NL, Ilojianya VI, Biu PW, Odonkor B. The future of autonomous vehicles in the US urban landscape: A review: Analyzing implications for traffic, urban planning, and the environment. *Engineering Science & Technology Journal*. 2024 Jan 15;5(1):43–64.
79. Prihartadi AS, Licastro GI, Pearson M, Johnson MJ, Luckett T, Swan F. Non-medical devices for chronic breathlessness: Use, barriers and facilitators for patients, carers and clinicians-a scoping review. *BMJ Supportive & Palliative Care*. 2023 Nov 1;13(e2):e244–53.
80. Tan L, Yu K, Bashir A, Cheng X, Ming F, Zhao L, … Zhou X. Toward real time and efficient cardiovascular monitoring for covid-19 patients by 5g-enabled wearable medical devices: A deep learning approach. *Neural Computing and Applications*. 2021;35(19):13921–13934.
81. Taylor CR, Venkatasubramanian K, Shue CA. Understanding the security of interoperable medical devices using attack graphs. In *Proceedings of the 3rd International Conference on High Confidence Networked Systems* 2014 Apr 15 (pp. 31–40).
82. Venkatasubramanian KK, Vasserman EY, Sokolsky O, Lee I. Functional alarms for systems of interoperable medical devices. In *2014 IEEE 15th International Symposium on High-Assurance Systems Engineering* 2014 Jan 9 (pp. 247–248). IEEE.
83. Al-Aubidy KM, Derbas AM, Al-Mutairi AW. Real-time patient health monitoring and alarming using wireless-sensor-network. In *2016 13th International Multi-Conference on Systems, Signals & Devices (SSD)* 2016 Mar 21 (pp. 416–423). IEEE.
84. Kramer DB, Fu K. Cybersecurity concerns and medical devices: Lessons from a pacemaker advisory. *Jama*. 2017 Dec 5;318(21):2077–8.
85. Kruse CS, Frederick B, Jacobson T, Monticone DK. Cybersecurity in healthcare: A systematic review of modern threats and trends. *Technology and Health Care*. 2017 Jan 1;25(1):1.
86. Gowda V, Schulzrinne H, Miller BJ. The case for medical device interoperability. In *JAMA Health Forum* 2022 Jan 4 (Vol. 3, No. 1, p. e214313). American Medical Association.

87. Touahria IE, Khababa A. A component based framework to enable medical devices communication. *Ingénierie des Systèmes d Inf.* 2021 Jun;26(3):295–302.
88. Williams PA, Woodward AJ. Cybersecurity vulnerabilities in medical devices: A complex environment and multifaceted problem. *Medical Devices: Evidence and Research.* 2015 Jul 20;21:305–16.
89. Dobrin A, Stamatescu G, Dragana C, Sgarciu V. Cloud challenges for networked embedded systems: A review. In *2016 20th International Conference on System Theory, Control and Computing (ICSTCC)* 2016 Oct 13 (pp. 866–871). IEEE.
90. Nadeski M. Bringing machine learning to embedded systems. *Texas Instruments.* 2019 Mar;11:1–5.
91. Horowitz M. 1.1 computing's energy problem (and what we can do about it). In *2014 IEEE International Solid-State Circuits Conference Digest of Technical Papers (ISSCC)* 2014 Feb 9 (pp. 10–14). IEEE.
92. Chen YH, Emer J, Sze V. Using dataflow to optimize energy efficiency of deep neural network accelerators. *IEEE Micro.* 2017 Jun 14;37(3):12–21.
93. Mathieu M, Henaff M, LeCun Y. Fast training of convolutional networks through ffts. 2013 Dec 20. arXiv preprint arXiv:1312.5851.
94. Dubout C, Fleuret F. Exact acceleration of linear object detectors. In *Computer Vision–ECCV 2012: 12th European Conference on Computer Vision, Florence, Italy, October 7–13, 2012, Proceedings, Part III 12* 2012 (pp. 301–311). Springer.
95. Cong J, Xiao B. Minimizing computation in convolutional neural networks. In *International Conference on Artificial Neural Networks* 2014 Sep 15 (pp. 281–290). Springer International Publishing.
96. Lavin A, Gray S. Fast algorithms for convolutional neural networks. In *Proceedings of the IEEE Conference on Computer Vision and Pattern Recognition 2016* (pp. 4013–4021).
97. Afifi SM, GholamHosseini H, Poopak S. Hardware implementations of SVM on FPGA: A state-of-the-art review of current practice. 2015 Nov 2, (11):733–752.
98. Chen Y, Luo T, Liu S, Zhang S, He L, Wang J, Li L, Chen T, Xu Z, Sun N, Temam O. Dadiannao: A machine-learning supercomputer. In *2014 47th Annual IEEE/ACM International Symposium on Microarchitecture* 2014 Dec 13 (pp. 609–22). IEEE.
99. Kim D, Kung J, Chai S, Yalamanchili S, Mukhopadhyay S. Neurocube: A programmable digital neuromorphic architecture with high-density 3D memory. *ACM SIGARCH Computer Architecture News.* 2016 Jun 18;44(3):380–92.
100. Chen YH, Krishna T, Emer JS, Sze V. Eyeriss: An energy-efficient reconfigurable accelerator for deep convolutional neural networks. *IEEE Journal of Solid-State Circuits.* 2016 Nov 8;52(1):127–38.
101. Dinh TM, Mesnilgrente F, Conédéra V, Kyeremateng NA, Pech D. Realization of an asymmetric interdigitated electrochemical micro-capacitor based on carbon nanotubes and manganese oxide. *Journal of the Electrochemical Society.* 2015 Jul 28;162(10):A2016.
102. Lee S, Lee T, Jin G, Hong J. An implementation of wireless medical image transmission system on mobile devices. *Journal of Medical Systems.* 2008 Dec;32:471–80.
103. Raskovic D, Martin T, Jovanov E. Medical monitoring applications for wearable computing. *The Computer Journal.* 2004 Jan;47(4):495–504.
104. Ow J. The future of healthcare in Singapore. The challenges and benefits of integrated use of Industry 4.0 technologies and how likely the general public and institutions are to adopt the integration of Industry 4.0 technologies. 2021 Nov 4. Available at SSRN 3957676.

7 Enhancing Remote Healthcare

Integration of ATOM ECG with eSanjeevani

R. Ananthakrishnan, Nitish Naik, Raghav Bansal, Abhinav Cardea, Mukesh Roy, Avval Gupta, Rohit Kumar Kushwaha, Vivek Shahi, and Manish Jawa

7.1 INTRODUCTION

Cardiovascular Disease (CVD) is the leading cause of mortality worldwide, accounting for approximately 17.9 million deaths each year, which is about 32% of all global deaths [1]. A 12-lead ECG, preferably recorded simultaneously, is a critical component for evaluating patients with cardiac ischemia. While the ECG tracings offered by conventional paper-based ECG machines are reliable, these devices are often bulky and difficult to transport. Moreover, even though such ECG machines are available in rural settings, such as Primary Health Centers (PHCs), the unavailability of cardiologists or even general physicians to interpret the ECG becomes a major concern. Consequently, patients physically carry the ECG reports to a central or district hospital for consultation with an expert. In urban settings, ECG machines are typically available in hospitals or laboratories, which can be challenging to access at the time of urgency at home.

The development and adoption of portable 12-lead ECG devices has revolutionized cardiac monitoring, offering greater accessibility and convenience for both patients and healthcare providers. Recent advancements have significantly improved the accuracy and usability of these devices, making them indispensable tools in modern cardiology. Studies have demonstrated that portable ECG devices, such as the CardioSecur Active, have achieved an accuracy comparable to traditional 12-lead ECG systems, enabling their use in both emergency and routine clinical settings [2]. The use of portable ECG devices in ambulances has been shown to improve the early management of acute coronary syndromes by providing immediate ECG data to hospital teams [3]. Furthermore, the global Holter ECG monitoring market is expected to grow significantly, with advancements in wireless technology and extended monitoring capabilities [4].

DOI: 10.1201/9781003508199-7

Integration with mobile technology has made ECG monitoring more accessible, allowing for real-time data transmission and remote diagnostics [5]. Portable ECG devices have been instrumental in the early detection of atrial fibrillation, which is crucial for the management and prevention of ischemic strokes. Additionally, wearable ECG devices have evolved to include multi-lead capabilities, offering comprehensive cardiac monitoring without the need for bulky equipment [6]. Point-of-care testing using portable ECG devices has improved patient outcomes by enabling rapid decision-making in critical care environments [7]. The cost-effectiveness and portability of these devices have made them widely accessible, particularly in low-resource settings [8]. Moreover, the integration of artificial intelligence in portable ECG devices has enhanced diagnostic accuracy and predictive analytics, leading to more personalized patient care [9]. Future developments in sensor technology and data analytics are expected to further improve the functionality and diagnostic capabilities of portable ECG devices [10]. These advancements underline the transformative impact of portable ECG technology on cardiac care, highlighting their growing importance in both clinical and remote settings.

Several devices and mobile applications catering to m-health have recently emerged. For instance, it has been reported that the AliveCor KardiaMobile device has shown 94% sensitivity and 97% specificity for detecting atrial fibrillation. Devices such as the 6-lead ECG of AliveCor or the single-lead Apple Watch Series 4 allow users to monitor arrhythmias [11, 12]. However, a portable, medical-grade ECG device that can plot all 12-channel signals simultaneously on a smartphone and send the recording in a standard ECG format to a cardiologist instantly via mobile application services such as WhatsApp or email would be highly beneficial for Indian scenarios. This would be applicable in both rural and urban hospital areas, as well as for at-home monitoring.

Despite some attempts in this direction, many wearable devices capture fewer leads and do not provide complete 12-lead information. Additionally, these devices often require expensive phones to function. Addressing these limitations, Cardea Labs, Bangalore, has designed and manufactured a promising device called "ATOM ECG". ATOM allows users to view all 12-channel ECG signals simultaneously on smartphones in real time and generates a standard 12-lead ECG report in PDF format. As a promising screening device, independent study and clinical validation are necessary before recommending it for field usage.

The first part of this paper presents the findings of a comparative analysis of the ECG tracings from ATOM—a novel 12-lead simultaneous ECG on a mobile phone device—against the reports generated by traditional paper-based ECG machines serving as the gold standard for clinical validation. The study was conducted at the Department of Medicine and Cardiology, INHS Asvini, Mumbai, over a 30-day period. Electrode arrangements were made to ensure both devices recorded the ECG signals simultaneously from the same patient. The signals generated by the ATOM device on the smartphone were compared with the paper-based recordings of the BPL Lifeline 150 to assess its accuracy, sensitivity, and specificity for all major time-based parameters.

The second part of this paper presents the findings of a blinded study of the ECG tracings from the ATOM ECG device compared to the recordings of the Philips MS-150. This study aimed to determine if the ATOM ECG could accurately capture different arrhythmias in 34 patients at the Department of Cardiology, AIIMS New Delhi. Conducted over one month, the ECGs were simultaneously recorded from both machines. The recordings were blinded and sent to two different cardiologists to establish if the ECG tracings resulted in the same arrhythmia findings.

The third part of this paper presents an overview of the field trial conducted on 5103 subjects at 10 primary health centers in the state of Rajasthan by the WISH Foundation supported by BIRAC, Dept of Biotechnology, Government of India.

The fourth part of this paper presents an integrated cloud architecture deployed to seamlessly transmit ECGs generated by the ATOM ECG device to eSanjeevani. This cloud integration aims to broaden the reach of the ATOM ECG device through telemedicine facilities, significantly enhancing the accessibility and effectiveness of cardiac care.

7.2 ABOUT ATOM—ACCURATE TELEECG ON MOBILE

ATOM, an innovation by Cardea Labs located in Bangalore, India provides a clinical quality trace of simultaneously recorded 12-lead ECG signals over an Android phone. This device allows real-time data viewing, and with the press of a button, the tracing gets saved in a PDF file in the form of a standard 12-lead ECG record. In addition to the standard tracing, a 10-second rhythm tracing of all 12 leads forms an annexure to the PDF file. Additionally, a vector cardiogram (VCG) to show the QRS axis is also generated on the third page of the three-page PDF file. ATOM has been designed with technical know-how from BARC, Bombay, and with clinical inputs from AIIMS, New Delhi. The device utilizes several proprietary algorithms, making it highly useful in clinical settings.

The ATOM mobile application is designed to be compatible with nearly all variants of Android devices. The mobile application ensures that all 12 ECG channels are easily viewable on any screen size of Android phones. Data from the ATOM device is transmitted wirelessly to the mobile application via Bluetooth.

The mobile application displays up to all 12 ECG channels in real time and generates a three-page PDF file saved locally on the phone. The first page contains a standard ECG report with all 12 channels recorded for 2.5 seconds each, along with a 10-second ECG of lead II at the bottom. To minimize the need for repeat ECGs, the second page provides a 10-second ECG of all 12 leads. Additionally, the third page includes a vector cardiogram to help quickly identify any axis deviations.

Recent research and advancements in portable ECG technology support the efficacy and utility of such devices. For instance, studies have demonstrated that modern portable ECG devices can provide accurate diagnostics comparable to conventional ECG systems [2–4]. The use of mobile applications to visualize ECG data in real time and generate comprehensive reports has been shown to enhance clinical workflows and patient management [5].

Integration of Bluetooth technology in medical devices like ATOM allows for seamless data transfer and real-time monitoring, which is crucial in emergency and remote settings [6–8]. The implementation of vector cardiography for detecting axis deviations in ECG reports further enhances diagnostic capabilities, ensuring a comprehensive analysis of cardiac health [9, 10] (Figures 7.1–7.3).

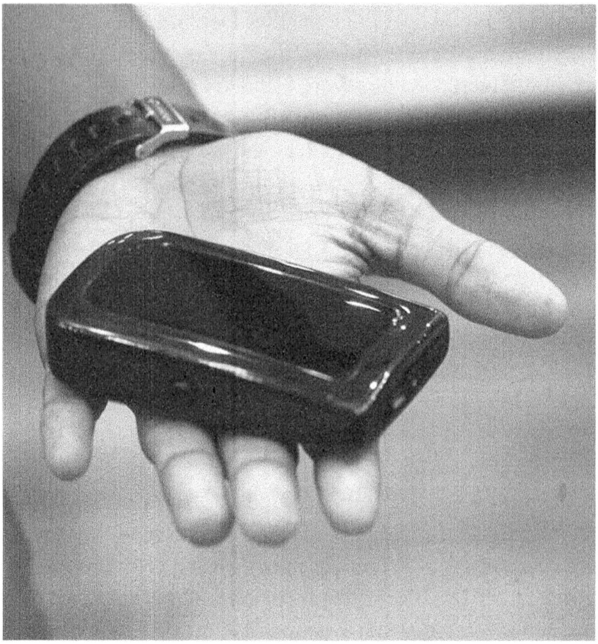

FIGURE 7.1 Image showcasing the hand-held size of ATOM.

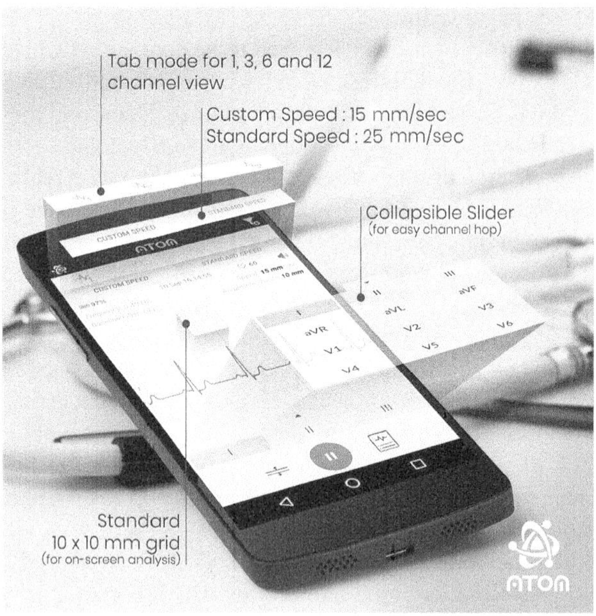

FIGURE 7.2 Image showcasing the features of single channel view of ATOM Android application.

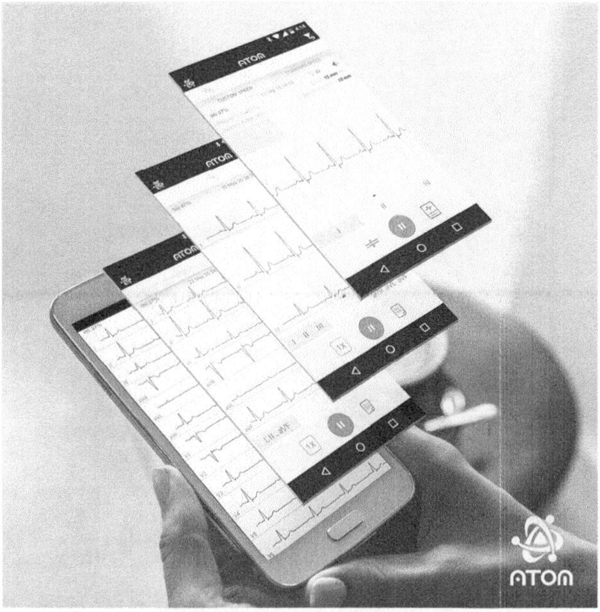

FIGURE 7.3 Image showcasing single, 3, 6 and all 12 simultaneous channel views of ATOM Android application.

7.3 MATERIALS AND METHODS/STUDY DESIGN

A study was conducted to validate the performance of the ATOM ECG device by comparing its ECG signals against the tracings of paper-based ECG machines, serving as the gold standard. Ethics committee clearance and written informed consent were obtained prior to the study. ECGs generated by the ATOM device and traditional paper-based machines were simultaneously recorded on 105 referred patients, comprising 90 males and 15 females, within the age group of 18–70. These patients were recommended to obtain their ECGs by their consulting physicians or cardiologists.

The study was conducted over the course of one month at a tertiary care hospital in Mumbai, specifically at the Department of Medicine and Cardiology, INHS Colaba. Electrodes were arranged to ensure both devices recorded the ECG signals simultaneously from the same positions on the patient. A qualified ECG technician was assigned to perform the simultaneous recording of ECGs using both the ATOM device and conventional machines.

ATOM ECG reports were recorded on an affordable Android smartphone with OS version 8.1.1, with each ECG record size being approximately 500 KBs. The conventional ECG reports were provided in the form of graphical paper printouts. Recordings were conducted in nearly equal numbers at four locations: the Ward, the Outpatient Department (OPD), the Emergency department, and the Intensive Care Unit (ICU).

Subsequently, the recorded ECGs from both the conventional machines and ATOM were presented to a cardiologist for interpretation. The cardiologist's interpretations were used to assess the performance and accuracy of the ATOM ECG

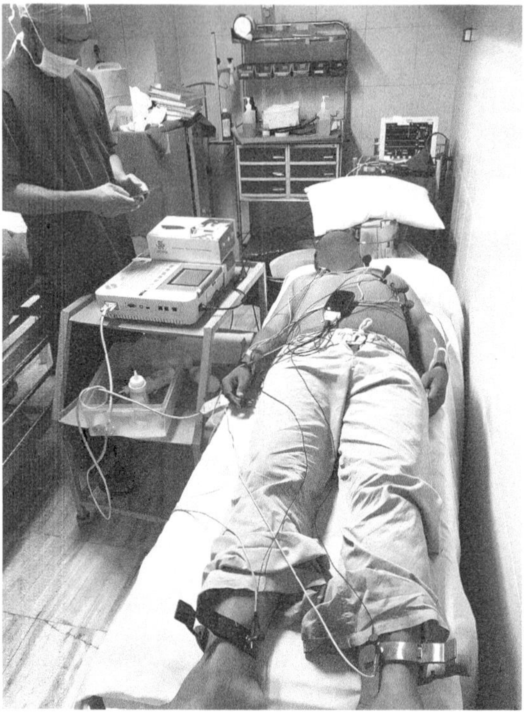

FIGURE 7.4 Image of patient with both devices connected simultaneously.

device compared to traditional paper-based ECG machines. Features such as heart rate, ST-T changes, PR interval, QT interval, and arrhythmia detection were tabulated for comparison. Accuracy, sensitivity, and specificity were calculated based on these features.

Additionally, a questionnaire was given to the ECG technician to gather feedback, which was then tabulated for further analysis (Figure 7.4).

7.4 STATISTICAL ANALYSIS

The ECG reports generated from the two devices were blinded and tabulated in an Excel sheet. A statistical analysis of the data was then performed to compare the performance of the two devices.

7.4.1 Boxplot

A boxplot was utilized to summarize the duration and axis variables as measured by ATOM in comparison with the standard of care (SoC). The boxplot indicates a strong correlation between the measurements of the two devices, which is confirmed by linear correlation and Bland–Altman Plot analysis [13, 14] (Figure 7.5).

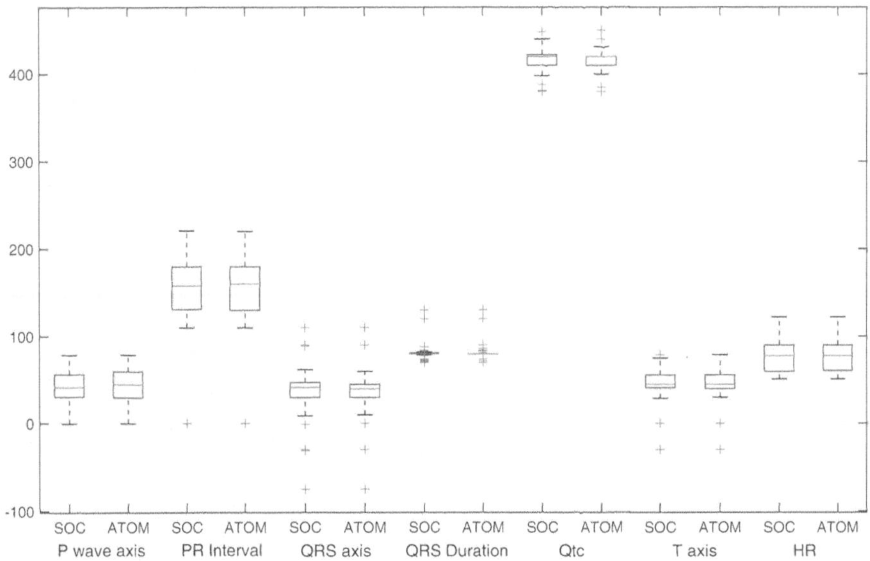

FIGURE 7.5 Boxplot of ATOM and SoC.

7.4.2 Pearson Coefficient and Linear Correlation Analysis

Linear Correlation Analysis was employed to evaluate the relationship between the measurements by ATOM and the SoC. The correlation, denoted by r, measures the amount of linear association between two variables. The R-squared value, denoted by R^2, is the square of the correlation and measures the proportion of variation in the dependent variable that can be attributed to the independent variable [15, 16]. The Pearson's correlation coefficients of the duration variables and heart rate were also measured and tabulated as shown in Table 7.1.

The linear correlation graphs indicate a strong correlation between the measurements of two devices.

TABLE 7.1
Data for Pearson Coefficient and Linear Correlation Analysis

Parameters	Pearson's Correlation	R square
QRS Duration	0.9901319 (p-value < 0.01)	0.9803611
PR Interval	0.9982711 (p-value < 0.01)	0.9965453
QTc	0.9960291(p-value < 0.01)	0.992074
Heart Rate	0.9994245(p-value < 0.01)	0.9988493

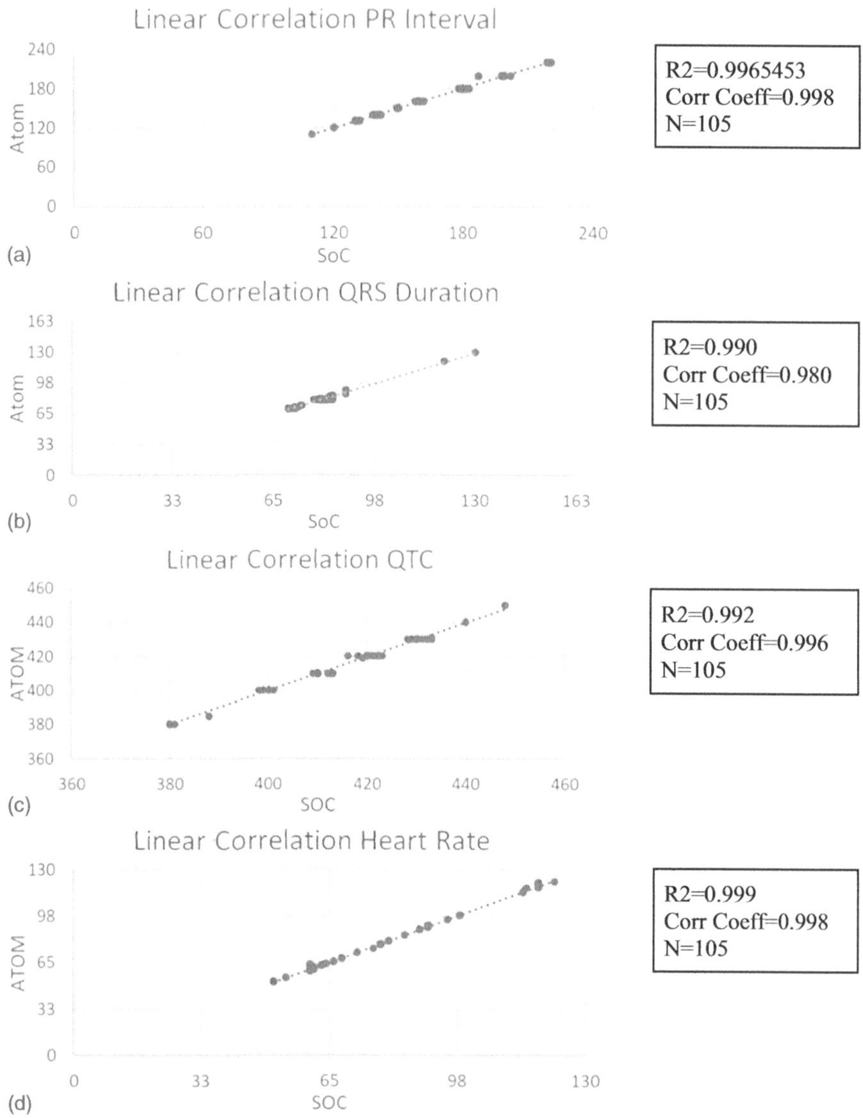

FIGURE 7.6 Linear correlation graphs indicate a strong correlation between the measurements (a) PR interval, (b) QRS Interval, (c) QTc, and (d) Heart Rate of the two devices. Figures 7.6 (a)-(d) Shows the linear correlation between SoC and ATOM of PR interval, QRS Interval, QTc, and Heart Rate, respectively.

7.4.3 Mean Absolute Error

Absolute Error, which is the difference between the measured value and the "true" value, was calculated. The Mean Absolute Error (MAE), which is the average of all absolute errors, was also calculated and tabulated. Mean absolute percentage

TABLE 7.2
Various Parameters and Errors

Parameter	Mean Absolute Error	Mean Absolute Percentage Error (%)
QRS Duration	0.6326531	0.78
PR Interval	0.75	0.44
QTc	0.65625	0.15
Heart Rate	0.1666667	0.21

error—the average absolute percent error for each time period minus actual values divided by actual values—was also calculated (Table 7.2) [17, 18].

7.4.4 Bland–Altman Plot

The Bland–Altman method calculates the mean difference between two methods of measurement and 95% limits of agreement as the mean difference ± 2 SD (or more precisely ± 1.96 SD). It is expected that the 95% limits include 95% of differences between the two measurement methods [19, 20] (Figure 7.7).

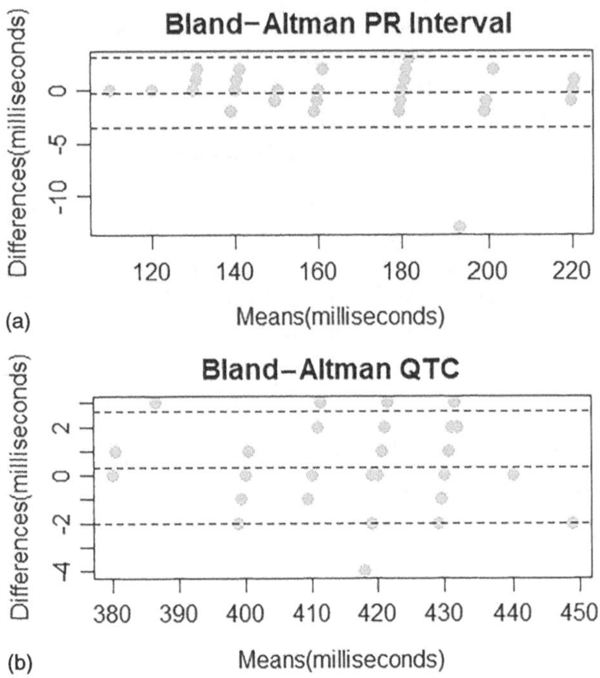

FIGURE 7.7 Shows comparison of differences vs means using Bland Altman Plot. Figures 7.7(a)–(b). show Bland–Altman Plot of PR interval, QTc Interval, QRS interval, and Heart Rate, respectively.

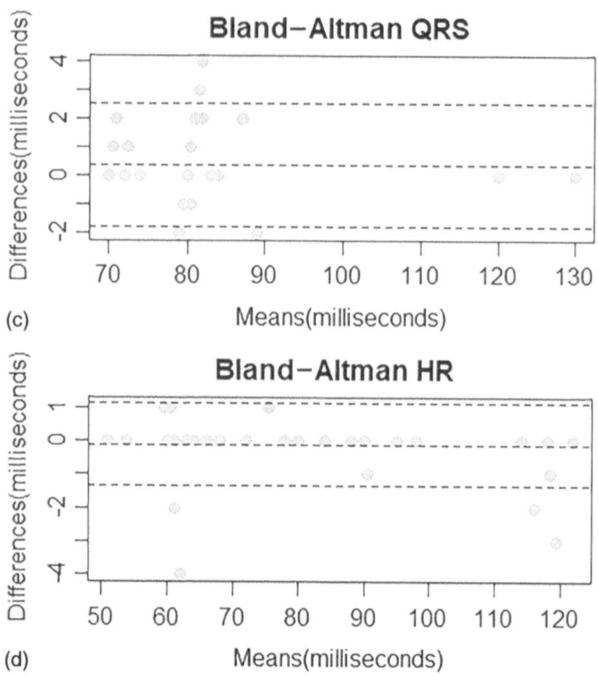

FIGURE 7.7 (*CONTINUED*) Shows comparison of differences vs means using Bland Altman Plot. Figures 7.7(c)–(d). show Bland–Altman Plot of PR interval, QTc Interval, QRS interval, and Heart Rate, respectively.

7.4.5 Questionnaire-Based Competitive Benchmarking

A questionnaire was prepared asking the experienced ECG technician to provide an experiential score for ATOM and the traditional paper-based ECG device (Table 7.3). A rating score of 1–4 was prepared for six parameters: Cost, Ease of Use, File Storage/Transfer, Maintenance, Portability, and Battery Life. The scores were then used to create a radar plot for comparison, which is depicted in Table 7.3.

TABLE 7.3
Experiential Score for ATOM and the Traditional Paper-based ECG Device

Parameter	ATOM Score	BPL Cardiart 9108
Cost	4	1
Ease of Use	4	3
File Storage/Transfer	4	2
Maintenance	4	3
Portability	4	1
Battery Life	3	4

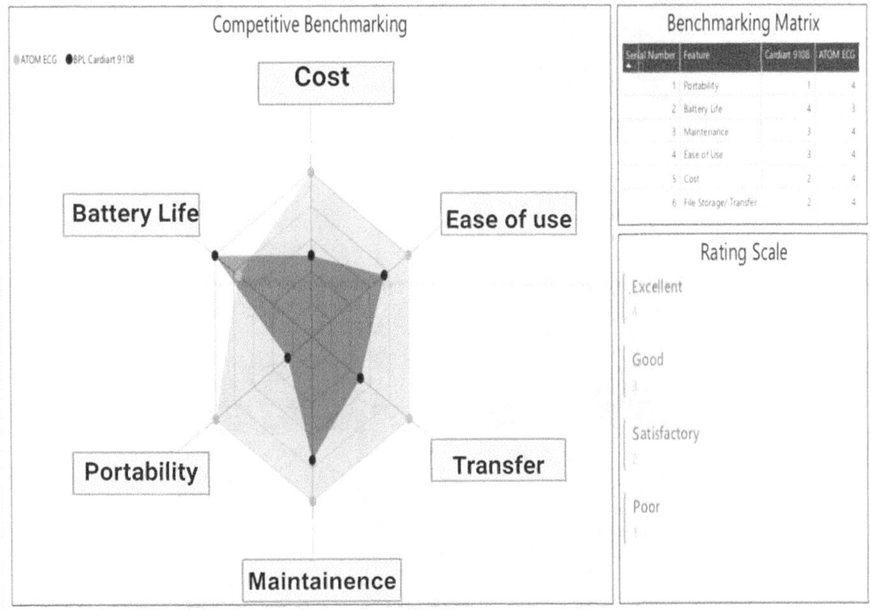

FIGURE 7.8 Radar plot of ATOM ECG with Cardiart9108.

The radar plot summarizes these scores, highlighting the comparative advantages of the ATOM ECG device over traditional paper-based ECG devices [21, 22] (Figure 7.8).

7.5 CLINICAL VALIDATION OF ATOM AT AIIMS NEW DELHI

The validation of the ATOM ECG device to assess its efficacy in identifying patients with arrhythmia was conducted at the Department of Cardiology, AIIMS New Delhi. The study included 34 patients with known diagnoses of cardiac anomalies, carefully selected for their high risk of arrhythmias. After obtaining ethical clearance, the study was performed by simultaneously acquiring ECG signals using an ATOM ECG device and a Philips ECG page writer TC70 machine.

The reports generated from both devices were recorded and subsequently blinded. These blinded reports were then independently evaluated by two cardiologists to ensure an unbiased assessment. The goal was to compare the accuracy of arrhythmia detection between the ATOM ECG device and the conventional Philips ECG machine.

The study aimed to determine if the ATOM ECG device could reliably identify various arrhythmias and provide comparable results to the standard Philips ECG machine. This validation is crucial as accurate arrhythmia detection is vital for appropriate patient management and treatment [13–15]. The comparative analysis included measuring heart rate, PR interval, QRS duration, and QT interval, and detecting specific arrhythmias such as atrial fibrillation, ventricular tachycardia,

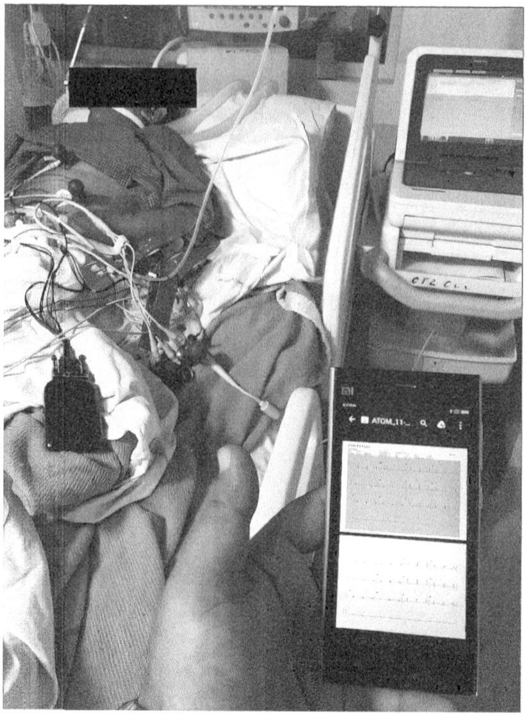

FIGURE 7.9 Image of patient with both the devices connected simultaneously at AIIMS New Delhi.

and others. The results showed a high degree of correlation between the two devices, supporting the efficacy of the ATOM ECG in clinical settings [6, 7, 16] (Figure 7.9).

7.6 FIELD TRIAL AT THE STATE OF RAJASTHAN

WISH Foundation, in partnership with the Department of Biotechnology, Government of India, organized a six-month field trial for further validation of the ATOM ECG device under the aegis of BIRAC. A total of 5103 candidates participated in the field trials across ten primary health centers in Rajasthan. WISH Foundation runs these PHCs under a public–private partnership model with the Government of Rajasthan. The CARDEA project was supported with funds from the Biotechnology Industry Research Assistance Council (BIRAC), Department of Biotechnology (DBT), Government of India. The protocol remained the same, where the ECG tracings were recorded simultaneously from a paper-based ECG machine (GE MAC 600) along with an ATOM ECG device. Subsequently, those ECGs were sent remotely to a cardiologist, and his findings were recorded. The reports from both machines were then compared to validate the efficacy of ATOM ECG (Figure 7.10).

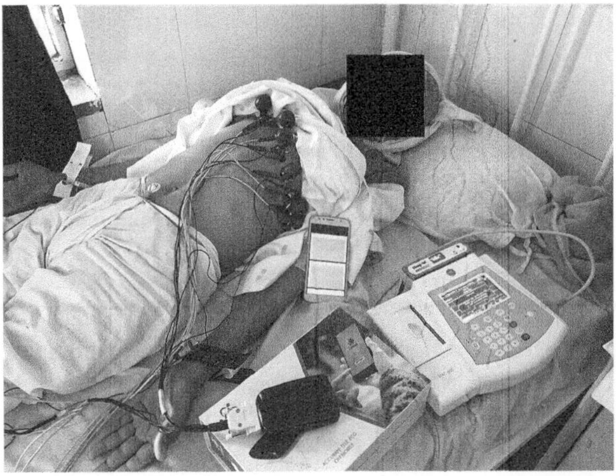

FIGURE 7.10 Image of patient with both devices connected simultaneously at a PHC in Rajasthan.

7.7 RESULTS OF CLINICAL TRIALS AND FIELD TRIALS

The clinical studies and the field study concluded that the ATOM ECG device consistently produces reliable ECG tracings. The MAE during the analysis of all measured parameters showed below 1%. Parameters such as heart rate, QRS duration, QTc interval, and PR interval showed good precision and reliability. Additional statistical analysis such as linear correlation and Bland–Altman plots of QRS duration, QTc interval, PR interval, and heart rate also showed good agreement between the ATOM ECG device and the conventional ECG machines. Pearson correlation coefficients were well above 0.90 in value, showing a strong linear correlation between the tracings of the two devices. The clinical trial at Colaba demonstrated that ATOM ECG achieved an overall sensitivity of 99.96% and a specificity of 99.41% in generating the ECG tracings of cardiac abnormalities including arrhythmias, thereby confirming its reliability and accuracy.

The Mean Absolute Error (MAE) and Mean Absolute Percentage Error (MAPE) confirmed that the ATOM device performs within globally recommended limits for clinical operation. Further, the agreement between the devices is strengthened by Bland–Altman plots, demonstrating that the differences between devices are within the 95% limits of agreement, another standard statistical measure used in clinical validation studies [9, 10, 19]. The results of these clinical trials confirm that the ATOM ECG device is a robust, precise, and feasible tool for cardiac monitoring. Its portability and small hand-held size make it useful in various settings, including its usage at home.

Clinical studies at AIIMS New Delhi confirmed that the recordings from ATOM ECG device produced identical arrhythmia tracings when compared to the gold-standard ECG machines. Clinical trials conducted at AIIMS New Delhi concluded that the ECG tracings obtained from ATOM ECG device showed comparable arrhythmia findings when compared with the gold standard. This included the detection of various arrhythmias such as atrial fibrillation, ventricular tachycardia, and other significant cardiac anomalies. The clinical trials also reported numerous practical benefits of the ATOM ECG device over a traditional ECG machine.

The field trials conducted in the state of Rajasthan on 5103 patients demonstrated a high correlation of ST-T findings, heart rate, PR interval, and QT interval between ATOM ECG and the traditional paper-based ECG machine. A paper demonstrating a few case studies highlighting how ATOM device effectively identified high-risk cardiac patients at the last mile in India has already been published [23]. It was also concluded that because ATOM generates a PDF format of ECG reports, the user can also take a printout on a normal A4 sheet, thereby removing the dependency on ECG paper rolls which is the case in paper-based ECG devices. The digital report on the smartphone in PDF format can also be transmitted instantly through various mobile application platforms like WhatsApp for quick medical consultations and timely interventions and could be life-saving in times of emergency.

7.8 OVERVIEW OF ATOM CLOUD ARCHITECTURE

The architecture of ATOM cloud system has been designed to be user-friendly, easily scalable, highly secured, low maintenance, and a robust system. Additionally, the cloud system can be easily integrated with external cloud systems such as eSanjeevani to expand the usability and reliability of the interconnected systems.

7.8.1 Distributed Cloud Infrastructure

The ATOM cloud architecture is a distributed cloud infrastructure that applies different cloud services to implement the functions of data processing, storage, and transmission. The core of this infrastructure is the serverless infrastructure that mainly applies to Vercel to deploy serverless functions [24]. This guarantees dynamism, given that the infrastructure will scale up or down depending on demands at that specific time. Furthermore, the use of serverless functions is a smart approach to cut down the operational overhead as there is no direct management of actual servers, and the servers are provisioned on demand.

7.8.2 Data Management and Storage

The architecture of ATOM cloud embeds data handling. The system harbors Neon PostgreSQL, a cloud-native RDBMS that is used for storage and management of ECG data. It is meant to be highly performant, reliable, and scalable for the management of vast volumes of health data [25]. The developed database is built in such a way that it withstands the occurrence of complex queries and provides on-demand data mining. This is highly useful especially when real-time medical diagnostics and analyses are needed.

Cloudinary is a multimedia file and storage management application with ECG reports in PDF. The service avails storage solutions that are scalable in nature and contains advanced media-processing features for efficient management of large files yet making them highly accessible. Integrating Cloudinary into the architecture provides smooth handling of file uploads and retrievals, which are necessary for both healthcare providers and patients to access time-critical data [26].

7.8.3 Secure Data Transmission

Security is of utmost importance while designing the ATOM cloud architecture, especially given its role as a health data system. The system uses HTTPS for data communication to ensure the safety of data flow between the mobile application, API [27] server, cloud storage, and external systems. The SSL certificates establish secure connections, which securing data from being accessed by any unauthorized person during the transmission.

This architecture includes a two-factor authentication as an extra security protocol for system access [28]. This provides another layer of safety to ensure that sensitive patient data cannot be accessed by anyone without permission.

7.8.4 Event-Driven Architecture

The event-driven nature of the system makes the ATOM cloud architecture quick and responsive and fail-safe which makes the system react to various events such as file upload, upload failures, retries failed jobs, etc. This along-the-line processing pattern is also facilitated by message queues and serverless functions, allowing event-based scheduling and processing of tasks [29]. For instance, when the mobile application captures as ECG, the data is further transmitted and stored in the cloudinary storage service, which triggers an event to upload the file to vendor's servers as well, such as eSanjeevani's server and also notify the user about the status and retry file upload in case of upload failure.

7.8.5 Interoperability and API Integration

ATOM cloud architecture is self-sufficient in terms of its compatibility features. The system is necessarily compatible with nearly all telemedicine platforms, including eSanjeevani, through its RESTful APIs. This API facility ensures secure data exchange across different systems and provides comprehensive patient care. RESTful API design follows industry best practices and is reliable and efficient in integrating data between different platforms.

7.8.6 Automated Task Management

The automated task management system supports cloud-based architecture to run without manual intervention. This includes functions such as file uploads, real-time notifications, and automated health checks. ATOM uses Qstash, a message queuing service, which schedules and tracks tasks perfectly well, further reducing the latency of the system and improving the operational efficiency of the system.

7.8.7 Mobile Application Interface

An integral part of ATOM cloud architecture is ATOM mobile application. It first communicates with the ECG hardware via Bluetooth to gather the ECG data which is then sent to the cloud. The mobile application provides real-time notifications and system-event alerts, through which the user is notified about the important event that happens within the system.

The API server, developed in JavaScript and TypeScript using Next.js, deals with all the requests made from the mobile application and outside systems. The server is hosted at the Vercel platform, which allows the API server to scale dynamically, which further provides system agility and handles data management safely and effectively.

7.9 METHODOLOGY

The architecture integrates scalability and reliability with secure data transport using standard protocols, such as HTTP, and this responsiveness is further enhanced with event-driven processing. Scheduling mechanisms embedded within the architecture automate the management of tasks and provide for real-time execution. Security is further enhanced by the use of two-factor authentication and encryption. Additionally, the architecture supports interoperability through the use of RESTful APIs. SSL certification [30] encrypts HTTP communication [31], thereby ensuring that the data is secure from unauthorized users [32]. The designed system is efficient, scalable, safe, and interoperable, and hence this architecture serves as a paradigm for accomplishing a reliable ECG data management solution. Figure 7.11 showcases the overview of the ATOM cloud architecture.

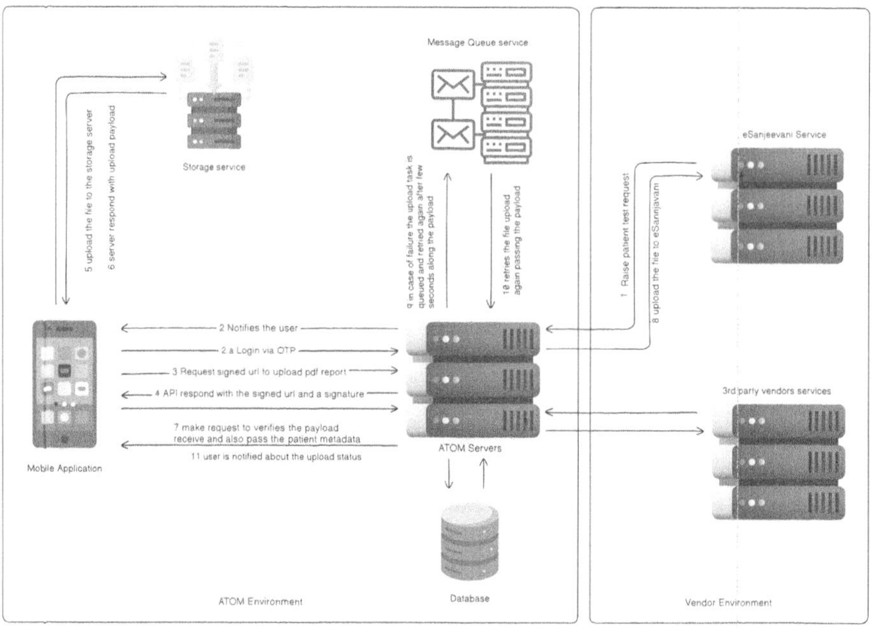

FIGURE 7.11 ATOM cloud architecture.

7.10 COMPONENTS OF THE SYSTEM

The key components enabling the entire process are:

- ATOM Mobile Application: It captures ECG data, generates PDF reports, and interacts with the ATOM API server.
- ATOM API Server: Manages ECG data, handles requests from the mobile application, and integrates with external services such as eSanjeevani.
- Storage Server: Provides centralized storage for ECG reports, with seamless integration via REST API and Node.js SDK [26].
- Message Queue Service: Acts as a message queue system for task scheduling [33], progress tracking, and notifications.
- Database: A serverless database with fast retrieval and sub-millisecond response time, accessed through a specialized Node.js SDK utilizing REST API [25].
- Rest API interface for vendors: External systems collaborating with ATOM, benefiting from data exchange and collaboration.

7.10.1 ATOM Mobile Application

The ATOM mobile application works as an interface for ECG data capture and transmission. It communicates with the ATOM hardware via Bluetooth, generates PDF reports, and interacts with cloud system functionalities. Figure 7.12 illustrates this at a high level. The mobile application also serves as a primary interface for important notifications on events within the system; consequently, the user can take relevant actions. It provides notifications and alerts that are sent on time through the API server and the message queue provides updates about the data and system activities to its users.

7.10.2 ATOM API Server

The heart of the ATOM cloud system is the REST API server, processing requests coming from the mobile application and other vendors, including eSanjeevani. It processes the ECG data and coordinates with the other components and scales dynamically based on the traffic [24]. Developed using JavaScript [34], TypeScript [35], and Next.js [36], it runs on top of Node.js and is hosted on Vercel. Running on Vercel's serverless functions, the API server brings cost efficiency, dynamic scalability, and security, all in rapid development. Next.js code-splits vastly improve the efficiency of API calls and enable serverless functions to scale at a granular level, which in other words, support any magnitude of load seamlessly. The Next.js powered REST API server on the Vercel platform provides a strong, responsive, and a reliable foundation for handling diverse requests and for processing ECG data.

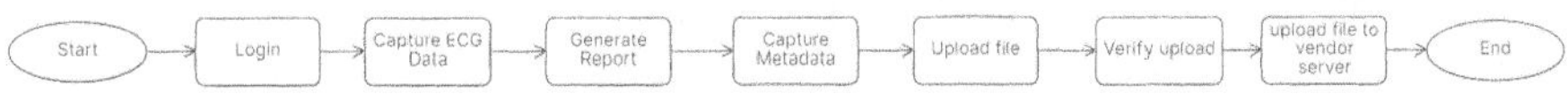
Start
Login
Capture ECG Data
Generate Report
Capture Metadata
Upload file
Verify upload
upload file to vendor server
End

FIGURE 7.12 High-level overview of the entire process.

7.10.3 Storage Server

A good industry practice dictates that a system that supports a stateless API server should have a different system for storage which ensures that the data is persistent. Cloudinary fills this gap by offering high delivery throughput, cost-effectiveness, low maintenance, and secure transmission [26]. Driven by a REST API, it allows Node.js SDK for user custom functions. Cloudinary's REST API enables the system to be compatible, while with the Node.js SDK, one can provide a particular extent of customization. This helps to achieve a system that is very cost-effective in a manner where the PDF reports are securely stored and require less maintenance with high delivery throughput.

7.10.4 Message Queue Service

Qstash [33] is a vital messaging queue service that allows the cloud systems to move with a fail-safe approach. It can handle long asynchronous functional tasks reliably—e.g., upload of files. It works like a sort of buffer for producers and workers queuing for tasks to be executed after the restoration of the system. For example, a network problem failure to upload is retained in the queue for retry immediately after the system is restored. The other form of services that this system performs ensures that the data integrity is not lost, a must for healthcare data. The system also monitors the progress of tasks; therefore, it maintains a transparency in the system to efficiently respond to any problems. Failed tasks are flagged and alerted to administrators for proactive management. This component ensures persistence, resilience, and continuous fail-safe performance.

7.10.5 Database

Serverless PostgreSQL by Neon.tech is used in this architecture, which decouples computational resources from storage for the best use of resources and scalability in the best way possible [25]. It operates with multi-region clusters using REST API interfaces, which reduce network latency and, at the same time, provide near real-time responses (10 ms to 100 ms) [25]. It, therefore, practices frictionless user experience delivery and effective real-time data processing. By also integrating a solution from Neon.tech, this system is flexible, scalable, and cost-effective to be able to handle varying workloads with maximum performance and reliability trade-offs [37]. This system can scale and remain cost-effective under workloads, all while offering high performance and reliability. A typical architecture of a neon serverless database is shown in Figure 7.13.

7.10.6 REST API Interface for Vendors

The ATOM API server is a secure and private endpoint for vendors such as eSanjeevani [30]; this gives the platform the capability of being both extensible and interoperable across boundaries [38]. Secured access would ensure that it is available exclusively for legitimate stakeholders, which again would generate partnerships for improved capabilities and reach. Patient services are enhanced with access to increased resources and expertise, eventually improving patient care and outcomes.

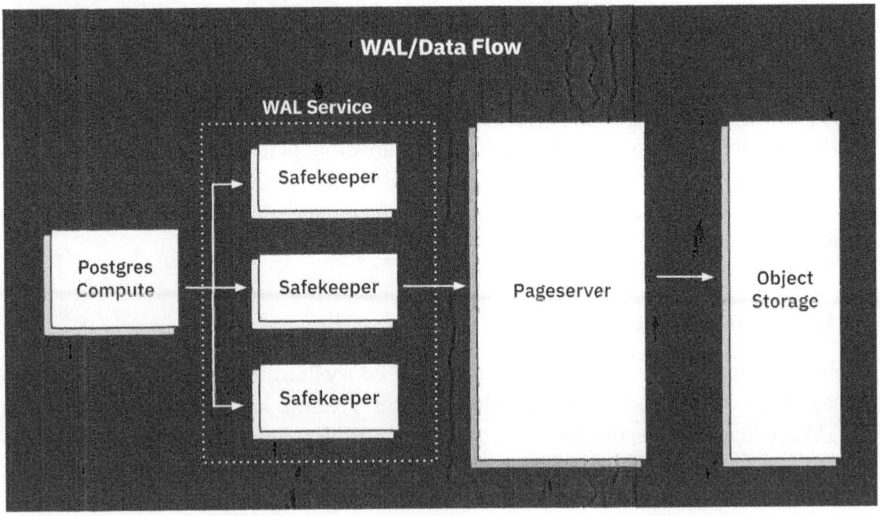

FIGURE 7.13 Neon database architecture split compute engine and storage engine.

7.11 IMPLEMENTATION

The ATOM ecosystem interconnects and manages data from ECG in real time. The ATOM mobile application is developed in Java using the Android SDK and communicates with the ATOM API Server for managing data and vendor integration such as eSanjeevani. ECG reports are handled by Cloudinary, and Qstash from Upstash.com manages task scheduling and notifications. Neon is backed by serverless PostgreSQL, which lets it fetch any data under a millisecond, provided by the Node.js SDK for optimization. SSL certifications also encrypt transmissions, and their misuse by unauthorized users is prevented and reported.

7.11.1 ATOM Mobile Application

ATOM mobile application is written in Java [39] based on the Android SDK [40] and supports all Android devices with Android 7 OS and above. To exchange data, the mobile application communicates with the API server by making HTTP requests [31]. The application processes the data to create a detailed PDF report that displays the ECG tracings along with the rate and rhythm of the heart. These reports are then uploaded by users onto the ATOM server, which forwards it further for analysis to a cardiologist using eSanjeevani.

7.11.2 ATOM API Server

Next.js with Vercel is a powerful platform for developing and deploying RESTful APIs. Next.js has automated code splitting, server-side rendering, and built-in routing so that it can be used to make both frontend and backend components. Using its API Routes, one can easily create RESTful APIs right within the same codebase, enhancing maintenance [36]. Vercel simplifies deployment with instant scaling, global distribution, and seamless Git integration [41]. Serverless functions and edge caching boosts performance and reliability [38]. Deploying a Next.js application on Vercel is easy and optimized for efficiency, meaning fewer steps to complete. With the ever-evolving nature of web development, developers in such a setup can quickly build modern web APIs and deploy them with ease, all coupled with the simplicity of Next.js and Vercel, which enhances performance and provides cost-effective solutions.

7.11.3 Storage Server

Implementation of Cloudinary in the ATOM ecosystem provides a cohesive data management system between ATOM and other vendors such as eSanjeevani. The ATOM application uses the REST API to upload PDF reports to Cloudinary for storage. The ECG PDF reports can be frequently viewed and easily shared or downloaded by users. Cloudinary handles operational overheads for developers and administrators in a reliable manner even when it scales. Vendors benefit from efficient data exchange, increased collaboration, and improved patient care. Figure 7.14 Storage server architecture.

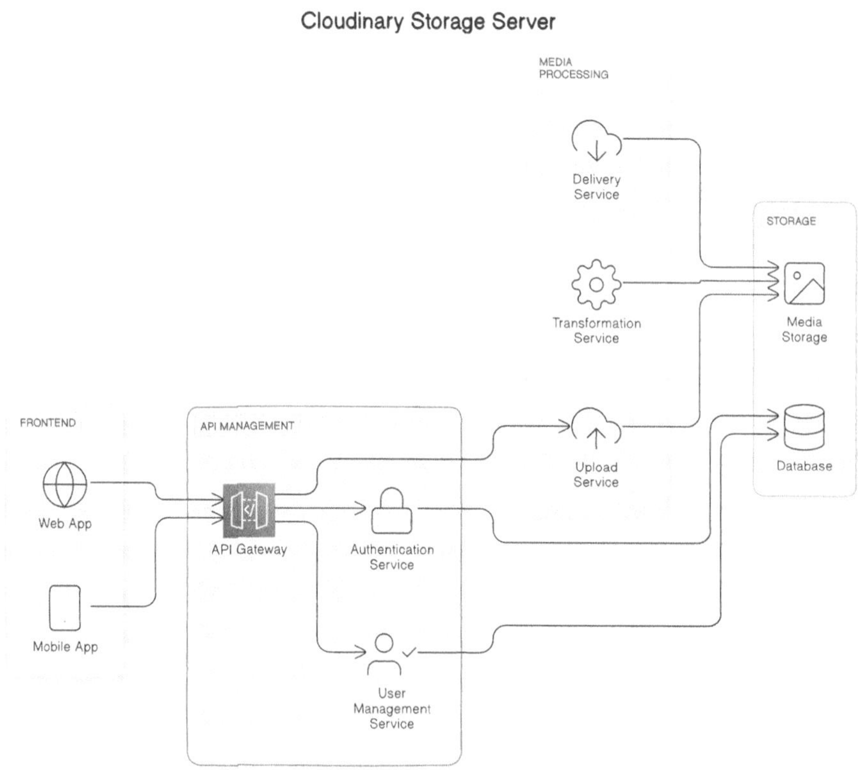

FIGURE 7.14 Cloudinary system architecture.

7.11.4 Message Queue Service

Qstash from Upstash.com is integrated in ATOM cloud which improves the scheduling of tasks, monitors the task progress, and manages task notifications [33]. Qstash also manages file upload tasks through its REST API and the Node.js SDK [42]. Qstash executes the uploaded task and informs the ATOM API about the failure or success. Following the task of uploading, Qstash sends a signal to ATOM API, which in turn reports to the Android application through application notification via Google Firebase Cloud Messaging platform, where the user is also notified. This incorporation provides better task management, system communication, and user engagement to ensure real-time updates and responsiveness within the ATOM ecosystem. Figure 7.15 represents the stash message queue architecture.

7.11.5 Database

The Neon Serverless Postgres database is a suitable match for the serverless architecture of the ATOM cloud. This database allows quick data access, with response

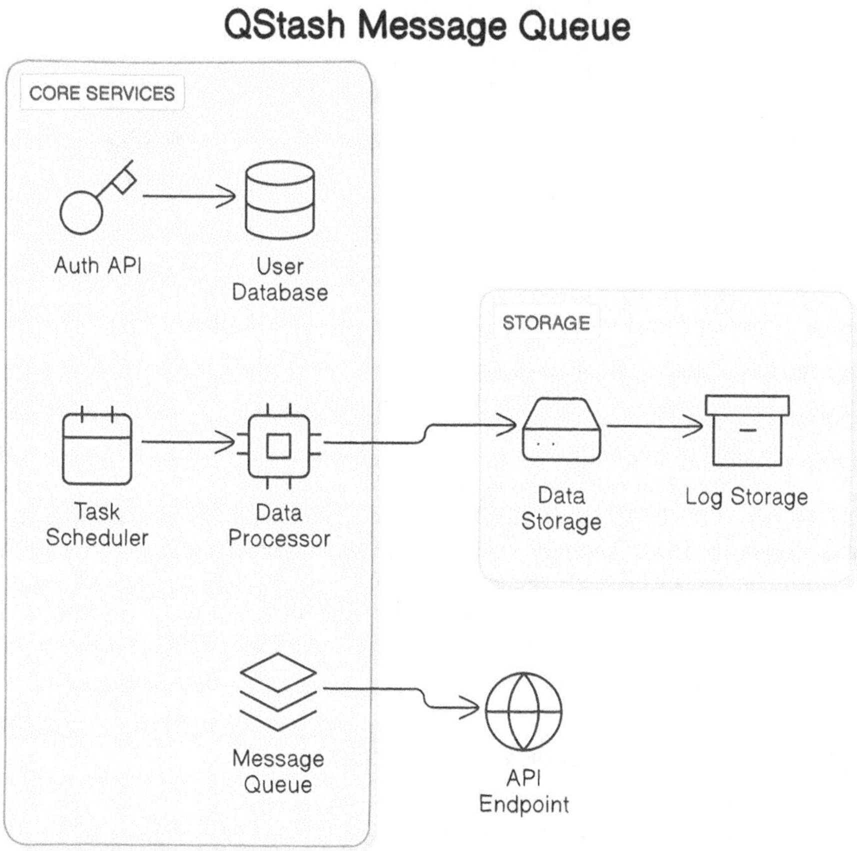

FIGURE 7.15 System design of Qstash service acting as a message queue.

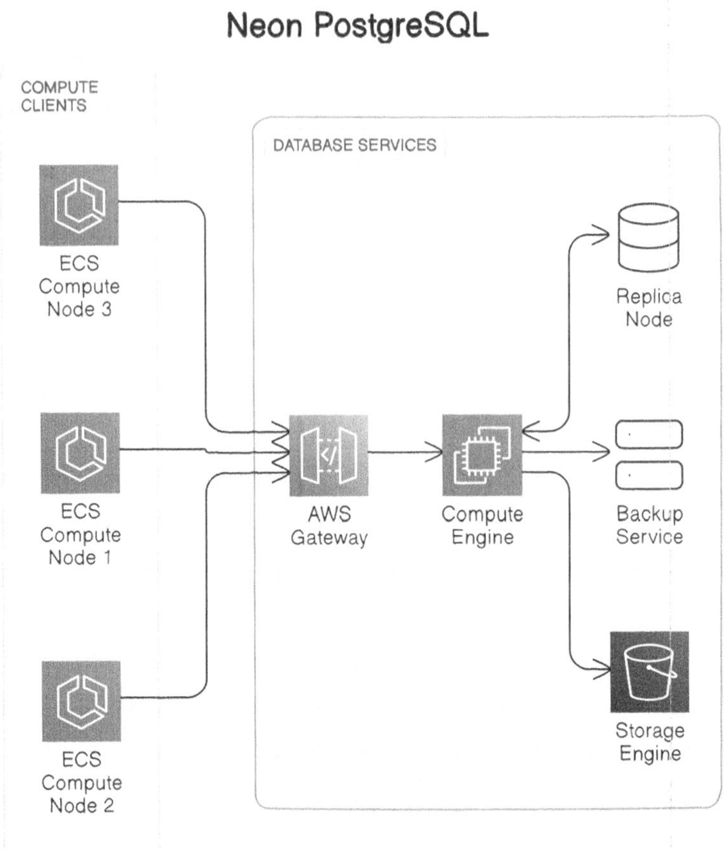

FIGURE 7.16 Neon database architecture.

times measured in sub-milliseconds, averaging between 10 and 100 milliseconds. It abstracts the details of such interactions with databases in the best possible manner, enabling the ATOM API to effectively carry out data operations for enhanced real-time data accessibility and user experiences. The non-blocking property of Node.js ideally interacts with the SDK, thus promoting very efficient database operations and lightweight development. This consequently optimizes the sharp responsiveness of the ATOM ecosystem. The architecture of the Neon PostgreSQL is illustrated in Figure 7.16 [25].

7.11.6 Overall Interaction Flow of the System

User authentication is the first step of the system. On entering the phone number and OTP verification, the user lands on the home screen. Clicking on the patient screen enlists the list of patients and the option for selecting the patient. After selecting the patient, the application scans for ATOM ECG device through Bluetooth [43], and after successful pairing the ECG is recorded and the patient information screen is displayed to enter the details of the patient such as his height, weight, and complaints (if any). A PDF containing all these information along with the ECG tracings is generated. The generated report is uploaded automatically to the ATOM server and the status of upload is shown. If the upload fails because of some reason, the application reattempts for five times till the file is uploaded. If the file is not uploaded even after five attempts, the application informs the user, and the user can retry later. Figure 7.17 provides an overall description of the system's flow.

7.11.6.1 ECG Test Initiation from Vendor

The system begins when eSanjeevani (vendor) initiates a test from their server. The vendor server obtains an access token [44] by calling predefined endpoints. Once the access token is acquired, it submits the ECG request to the ATOM server. Figure 7.18 shows how the request is received from the vendor.

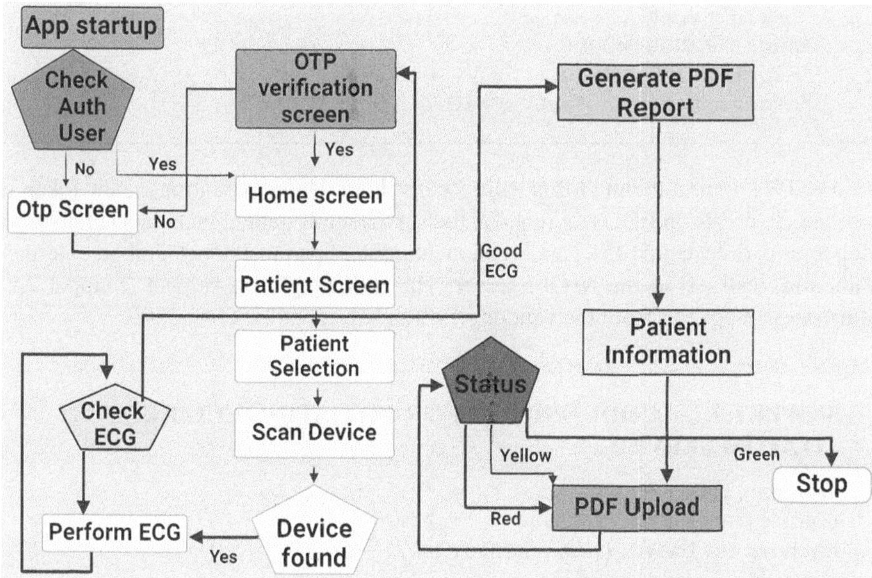

FIGURE 7.17 Detailed system flow diagram.

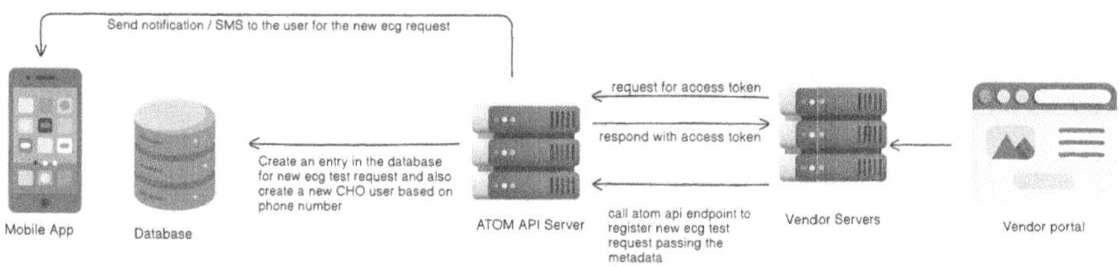

FIGURE 7.18 Request flow from eSanjeevani.

The access token, a JWT Bearer token [44], is valid for one hour. Upon expiration, a new token is needed. To create an ECG test request, the eSanjeevani or vendor server sends patient metadata (firstName, dob, gender, phoneNumber, operatorPhoneNumber, externalPatientId, and testList) to the ATOM server. The following code snippet (Snippet 7.1) illustrates the api call by the vendor servers to get access tokens.

SNIPPET 7.1 CODE SNIPPET FOR OBTAINING ACCESS TOKEN

```
Request Sample
POST {{url}}/auth/token
{
    "client_id": "{{clientId}}",
    "client_secret": "{{clientSecret}}",
    "grant_type": "{{grantType}}"
}
Response sample
{
  "token_type": "Bearer",
  "sub": "ANONYMOUS",
  "expires_in": 3600,
  "access_token": "eyJhbGciOiJ. . . .0EDc"
```

The JWT Bearer token [44] is valid for one hour. Upon expiration, a new token is needed. To create an ECG test request, the server sends patient metadata (firstName, dob as unix timestamp [45], gender, phoneNumber, operatorPhoneNumber, externalPatientId, testList) to the ATOM server. The following code snippet (Snippet 7.2) illustrates an api call from the vendor server to submit an ECG request.

SNIPPET 7.2 CODE SNIPPET FOR INITIATING ECG REQUEST TO ATOM SERVER

```
Request Sample
POST {{url}}/patient
Authorization: {{accessToken}}
{
    "firstName": "Patient First Name",
    "dob": 1674950400,
    "gender": "MALE",
    "phoneNumber": "+911231231",
    "operatorPhoneNumber": "+91 1231231",
    "externalPatientId":
  "911231231-89631360000_1695149129037",
    "testList": [
        "ECG"
    ]
}
Response Sample
```

```
{
  "success": true,
  "message": "Patient registered successfully",
  "status": "200"
}
```

The 'externalPatientId' is globally unique, combining patient ID, vendor ID, and Unix Timestamp to prevent duplicates. `operatorPhoneNumber` identifies the user in ATOM. When a new ECG request is received, ATOM adds the `operatorPhoneNumber` to its database and notifies the mobile application if the number already exists.

7.11.6.2 Login Process

Only individuals whose phone numbers are listed in the ECG test request can log into ATOM. A third-party service sends an OTP via SMS [46] to the user's phone number specified in the ECG test request [28]. Users enter their number in the mobile application, which calls ATOM's API, prompting the third-party server to send an OTP. Figure 7.19 illustrates the OTP Login flow.

The following code snippet (Snippet 7.3) illustrates the API call made by the mobile application to get the OTP.

SNIPPET 7.3 CODE SNIPPET FOR USER TO LOGIN VIA PHONE

```
Request Sample
POST {{url}}/auth/cdac_login
{
    "phone": "+91 1231231231"
}
Response Sample
OK
```

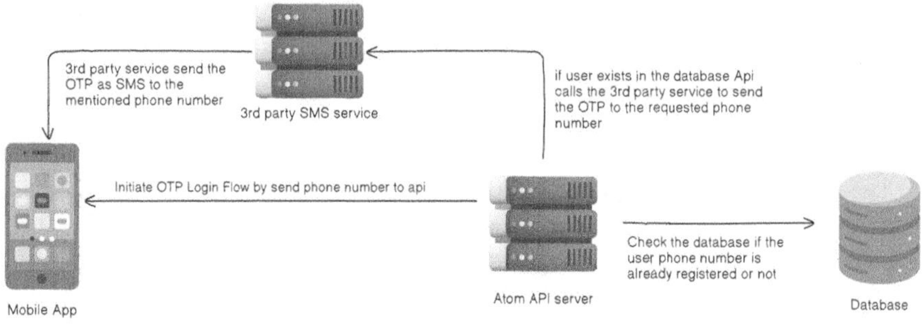

FIGURE 7.19 OTP login flow.

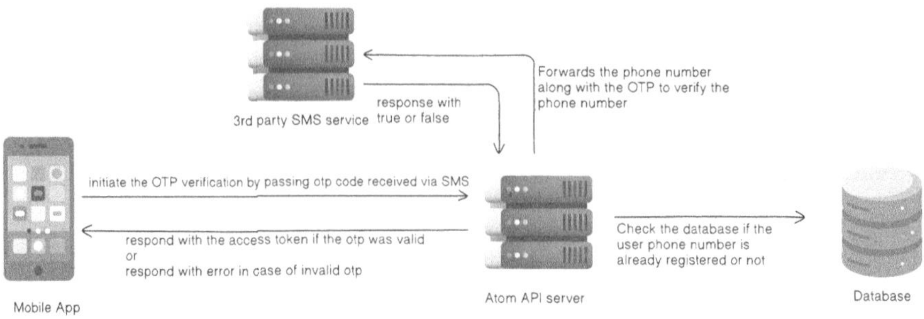

FIGURE 7.20 OTP verification flow.

7.11.6.3 OTP Verification

After receiving the OTP via SMS [28], users enter it in the mobile application for verification. If valid, the ATOM server provides access and refreshes JWT tokens [44]. These tokens are stored temporarily on the device, enabling API requests. Upon expiration, the application uses the refresh token to obtain a new access token. The process includes using the Google Firebase Cloud Messaging package [47] for notifications. Figure 7.20 shows the interaction of 3rd party SMS service.

The following code snippet (Snippet 7.4) illustrates the api call from mobile application to verify OTP.

SNIPPET 7.4 CODE SNIPPET FOR VERIFYING OTP

```
Sample Request
POST {{url}}/auth/cdac_login_verify
{
    "phone": "+91 1231231231",
    "code": "132132",
    "deviceToken": "lkajsdasldj.........asdjasido"
}
Sample Response
{
  "accessToken": "eyJhbGciOiJIUzI1N......iOJ5Gua7hl3wz7Y",
  "refreshToken": "eyJhbGciOiJI......OOeTU"
}
```

The following code snippet updates the device token of the user's mobile device, as it can change over time. Regular updates ensure that the user receives notifications for any associated events. This process maintains notification integrity, ensuring users are alerted for relevant events. The following code snippet (Snippet 7.5) is an example of registering device tokens into an ATOM server for sending notifications later.

Figure 7.21 depicts the login flow within the application.

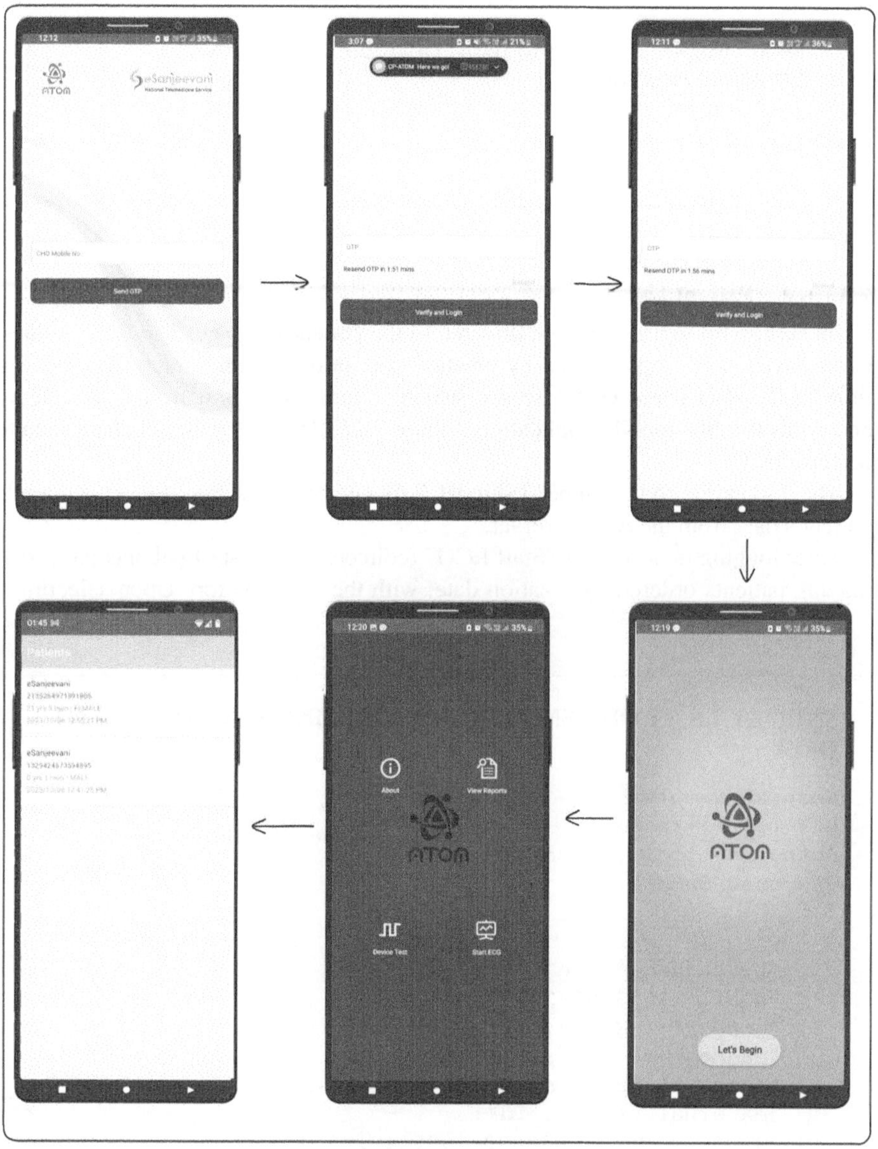

FIGURE 7.21 Login flow within the application.

SNIPPET 7.5 CODE SNIPPET FOR UPDATING DEVICE TOKEN

```
Sample Request
POST {{url}}/device/token
Authorization: {{accessToken}}
```

```
{
 "deviceToken": "eGsc1g3BCAI:APACbHQJy. . .fkS-
   QXRECKniv98KTUhCl"
}
Sample Response
OK
```

7.11.6.4 Patient List

Upon successful login, users are directed to the patient list page. The latest request is displayed at the top, ordered by creation date in descending order. The application fetches data from ATOM server, which in turn retrieves it from the database and sends it to the mobile application. Figure 7.22 illustrates getting patient data to perform ECG.

The following code snippet (Snippet 7.6) demonstrates how to get a sample patient's data from the ATOM server.

After logging in, selecting "Start ECG" redirects to the list of patients page, displaying patients ordered by creation date, with the latest on top. Upon selecting a

SNIPPET 7.6 CODE SNIPPET FOR GETTING LATEST PATIENT DATA

```
Request Sample
GET {{url}}/patient
Authorization: {{accessToken}}
Response Sample
[
  {
    "first_name": "eSanjeevani",
    "dob": "2023-01-29T00:00:00.000Z",
    "gender": "MALE",
    "phone_number": "+911231231",
    "operator_phone_number": "+91 1231231",
    "external_patient_id":
  "911231231-896313600000_1695149129037",
    "test_list": [
      "ECG"
    ],
    "created_at": "2024-05-07T16:12:08.452Z"
  }
  .
  .
  .
  ]
```

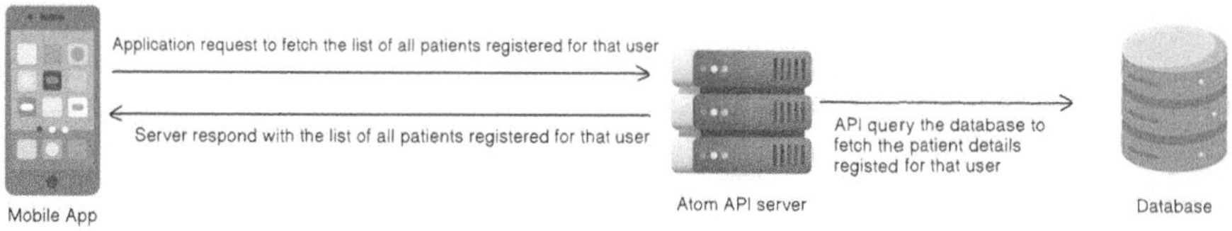

FIGURE 7.22 Flow of fetching latest patient data.

patient, users proceed to scan for the ATOM ECG device via Bluetooth. Upon successful pairing, users conduct the ECG and record it.

Subsequently, users generate the PDF after filling in the patient's details such as weight, height, blood pressure, activity, smoking/drinking habits, and any additional operator comments such as chest pain, palpitations, etc. A few necessary information such as external patient ID, gender, and age is fetched and automatically filled from the metadata provided by eSanjeevani when initiating a test request.

Finally, the generated PDF is uploaded to the ATOM servers in a three-step process: (1) obtaining a signed URL, (2) direct upload to the ATOM storage server using the signed URL, and (3) verification of the uploaded file by transmitting metadata and patient information to the ATOM server.

Each step involves precise technical operations, including data transmission protocols, authentication mechanisms, and server interactions to ensure seamless functioning within the system architecture.

7.11.6.5 Signed URL

Before uploading, the mobile application requests for a secured and signed URL from the ATOM server. This URL is used to upload the file directly to the ATOM storage server along with the file itself. Figure 7.23 shows an application request for a signed URL for uploading an ECG report to a storage server.

The following code snippet (Snippet 7.7) illustrates an api call from the mobile application to the ATOM server.

SNIPPET 7.7 CODE SNIPPET FOR GENERATING SIGNED URL FOR UPLOADING ECG REPORT

```
Request Sample
POST {{url}}/report/signed_url
Authorization: {{accessToken}}
Response Sample
{
  "timestamp": 1715099632,
  "signature": "1368a10e63836234645e483300eb9effcc74a807",
  "uploadPreset": "m362s32fdfsd1346defa3346ult"
}
```

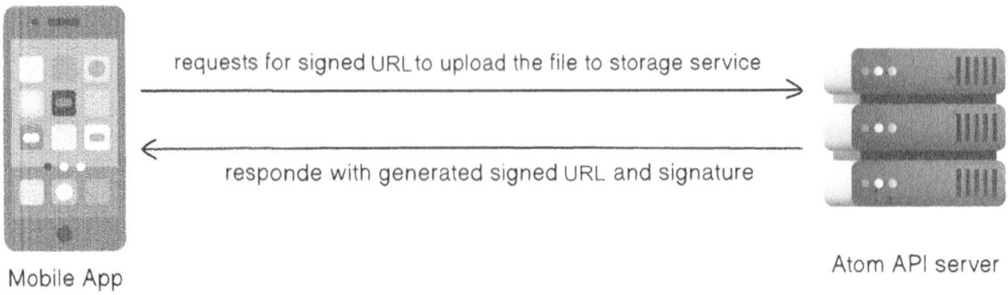
requests for signed URL to upload the file to storage service
responde with generated signed URL and signature
Mobile App
Atom API server

FIGURE 7.23 Signed URL flow.

The application uploads a file to the storage server by passing the signature, timestamp, upload preset, and the file itself. The following code snippet (Snippet 7.8) shows how the file is uploaded to the storage server.

SNIPPET 7.8 CODE SNIPPET FOR FILE UPLOAD

```
Request Sample
curl -X POST \
{{secureUrl}} \
--form 'api_key="XXXXXXXXXXXXXX"' \
--form 'uploadPreset="XXXXXXXXXXXXX"' \
--form 'timestamp="XXXXXXXXXX"' \
--form 'signature="XXXXXXXXXXXXXXXXXXXXXXXXXXXXXXXXXX"' \
--form 'file=@file_location'
Response Sample
{
    "asset_id": "asset123",
    "public_id": "public123",
    "version": 1,
    "version_id": "version123",
    "signature": "signature123",
    "width": 800,
    "height": 600,
    "format": "jpg",
    "resource_type": "image",
    "created_at": "2024-05-07T12:00:00Z",
    "tags": ["tag1", "tag2"],
    "bytes": 1024,
    "type": "upload",
    "etag": "etag123",
    "placeholder": false,
    "url": "https://example.com/image.jpg",
    "secure_url": "https://example.com/image.jpg",
    "folder": "uploads",
    "original_filename": "example.jpg"
}
```

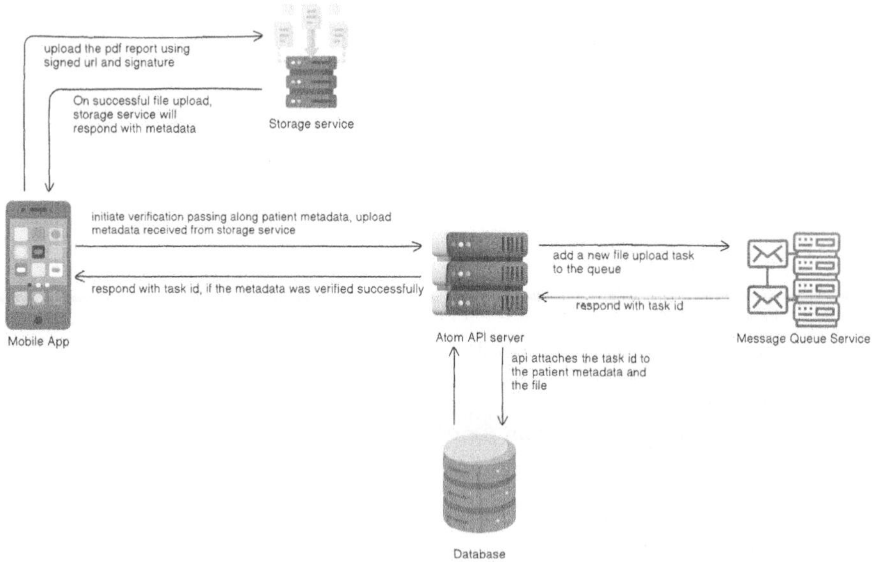

FIGURE 7.24 File upload flow chart.

After successful file upload, the mobile application sends the upload response and patient information to the ATOM server endpoint for verification, thereby reducing network I/O. Figure 7.24 illustrates the file upload verification process.

The code snippet makes an API call to the server for file verification, schedules the upload process via Message Queue service to eSanjeevani or vendors, updates the database, and tracks upload progress and retries. The ATOM server responds with a message and a tracking ID for status monitoring. The following code snippet (Snippet 7.9) demonstrates the payload which is sent to ATOM server for upload verification.

SNIPPET 7.9 CODE SNIPPET FOR VERIFYING UPLOADED ECG REPORT

```
Request Sample
POST {{url}}/report/verify-upload
Authorization: {{accessToken}}
{
  "file_upload_response": {
    "asset_id": "asset123",
    "public_id": "public123",
    "version": 1,
    "version_id": "version123",
    "signature": "signature123",
    "width": 800,
    "height": 600,
    "format": "jpg",
```

```
        "resource_type": "image",
        "created_at": "2024-05-07T12:00:00Z",
        "tags": ["tag1", "tag2"],
        "bytes": 1024,
        "type": "upload",
        "etag": "etag123",
        "placeholder": false,
        "url": "https://example.com/image.jpg",
        "secure_url": "https://example.com/image.jpg",
        "folder": "uploads",
        "original_filename": "example.jpg",
        "api_key": "api_key123"
    },
    "patientData": {
        "patientName": "John Doe",
        "age": "35",
        "sex": "Male",
        "weight": "75 kg",
        "height": "180 cm",
        "BP": "120/80 mmHg",
        "lifestyle": {
            "activity": "Moderate",
            "smoking": "No",
            "drinking": "Occasional"
        },
        "external_patient_id": "pat123",
        "comments": "Patient appears to be in good health.",
        "recorded_at": "2024-05-07T10:30:00Z"
    }
}
Response Sample
{
    "message": "File uploaded successfully",
    "trackingId": 123456
}
```

7.11.6.6 HTTP Polling

To manage the time-consuming file upload process asynchronously, a message queue system is implemented, necessitating the introduction of tracking IDs within the ATOM system. After file verification, the server response includes the tracking ID. The mobile application then polls the ATOM server every 5 seconds [48] for up to 5 minutes using this ID. Upon success or failure, the server updates the database, halting the polling. This method efficiently tracks and manages the upload process, with HTTP polling typically completing within 1 minute due to rapid server-to-server communication. To conserve battery, polling ceases after 5 minutes if the process hasn't concluded. The following code snippet retrieves the latest status of the upload process. Figure 7.25 illustrates the asynchronous file upload process and its tracking.

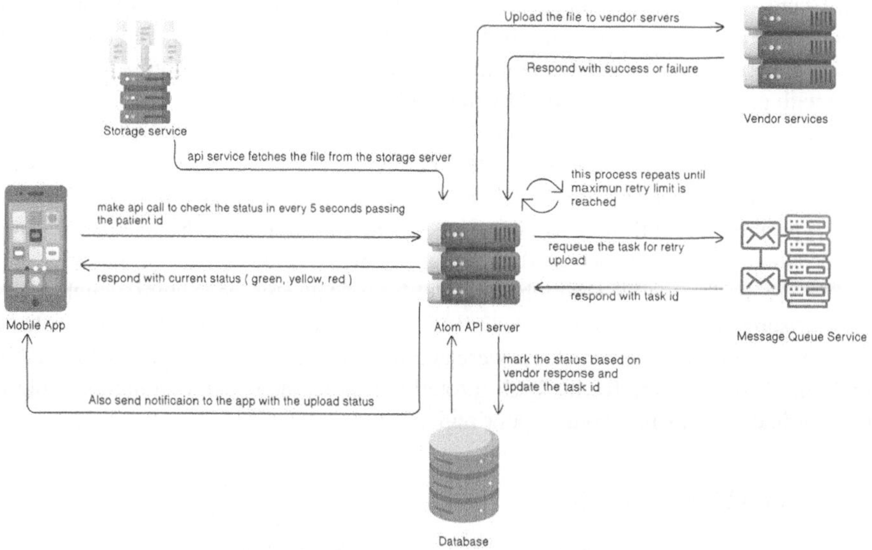

FIGURE 7.25 HTTP polling flow.

The following code snippet (Snippet 7.10) demonstrates how to get the status of the ongoing file upload process.

SNIPPET 7.10 CODE SNIPPET TO GET THE STATUS OF ONGOING FILE UPLOAD TO VENDOR'S SERVER

```
Request Sample
POST {{url}}/report/status
Authorization: {{accessToken}}
{
  "trackingId": 987654
}
Response Sample
{
  "status": "pending"
}
```

7.12 RESULTS

The clinical and field trials of the device demonstrated the reliability and accuracy of the 12 lead simultaneously acquired ECG tracings generated from the ATOM ECG when compared with the heavy, paper-based traditional ECG machines. The clinical trial at INHS Colaba showcased that the mean absolute error for all measurable parameters such as heart rate, QRS duration, QTc interval, and PR interval, was below 1%, indicating high precision. Strong agreement was observed in linear correlation and Bland–Altman plots. The calculated Pearson coefficient values showcased high precision. At the clinical trial at AIIMS New Delhi, the cardiologists interpreting the ECGs generated by ATOM were able to detect all different arrhythmias as was the case with paper tracings provided by the gold standard.

The field trials in Rajasthan validated the efficacy of the ATOM ECG device for mass screening. The field trials reported that the ATOM ECG device correlates well with the gold-standard devices.

All possible capabilities have been integrated within the ATOM ECG ecosystem by the cloud technology. Secure data management and scalable patient-data management were made possible through the cloud-based data storage system, which, similarly, ensures instant access to historical ECG records for remote consultations. Data from the cloud-embedded systems were automatically synchronized and analyzed in real time, thus allowing for the high-throughput screening of large numbers of high-risk cardiac patients in resource-poor regions.

7.13 FUTURE WORKS

While the device is already well received by the stakeholders, future work will be focused in advancing the functionalities and capabilities of ATOM ECG device. Efforts are being made to make the device support Bluetooth Low Energy (BLE) protocol. This protocol will help the system work for longer hours on a single charge.

ATOM trials extending the validation dataset to a more heterogeneous patient cohort for testing the device's accuracy across different demographic and clinical conditions are also planned. This will also include test subjects from the pediatric populations of patients. The second priority is additional integration with telemedicine platforms beyond eSanjeevani. Develop APIs and software plugins for the ATOM ECG device to make it compatible with other global telehealth services by ATOM ECG for broader use. Besides, the machine learning algorithms of the device for automated detection and prediction of arrhythmias are also planned to enhance diagnostic capabilities and reduce dependency on cardiologist interpretation. For instance, it will ensure that blockchain technology is operational in tamper-proof data logging and advanced encryption standards in protecting patient data. It would be critical to enhance the cloud infrastructure further to support real-time analytics and machine learning model updates to preserve the system's robustness and efficiency. Improvements in the user interface for the mobile application are on the way to make the device even more user-friendly for health providers and patients. Additional studies will guide evidence-based best practices for implementation and provide valuable data to be used as part of the regulatory submission for market expansion of the technology.

7.14 CONCLUSION

Integrating ATOM ECG with eSanjeevani is a giant leap in remote cardiac care, which could potentially revolutionize cardiac care through smartphones for the underserved. This device has been shown to have reliable sensitivity in tracing all types of cardiac arrhythmias. It is able to emanate ECG tracings that can be relied upon in a similar way to traditional machines. Portable, easy to use, and the capability to send data instantaneously to improve service in a telemedicine center are a few of the advantages of such systems. Making the system cloud enabled has readily permitted a secure, scalable, and real-time patient data management in ways that facilitate rapid consultations and improve efficiency in delivering quality cardiac care. Clinical and field trials have confirmed that ATOM ECG analysis is a robust and a practical solution for cardiac monitoring. The device meets clinical standards of accuracy and operation, efficiency, and availability. Future works will include making the system compatible with BLE to reduce battery consumption and will be toward the development of superior algorithms, data security, machine learning for automated analysis, and new vistas toward advanced cloud solutions. All this is needed to ensure easy use for at-home tests and for patients at the last mile who are usually left behind in healthcare.

ACKNOWLEDGMENTS

The authors express their deep gratitude to the officials of the Directorate General Medical Services and the Indian Navy, who extended complete cooperation in conducting the validation study at Colaba, without which this would have never been possible for induction into the armed forces. We owe a special salutation to the late Dr. Rajnish Juneja, Professor of the Department of Cardiology, All India Institute of Medical Sciences, New Delhi, whose clinical acumen and zeal made ATOM a reality. A special thanks to Dr. Dinkar Bhasin from AIIMS, New Delhi for facilitating the data collection and efficient management of the validation study during the clinical trials. Finally, we would like to thank the officials of CDAC Mohali and Jhpiego who supported us at every stage of the integration with eSanjeevani and were always available for any questions. We gratefully acknowledge valuable support from BIRAC, the Department of Biotechnology, Government of India and to WISH Foundation for the field trials. Lastly, the authors appreciate Mr. Aditya Deshpande from INHS Kochi and the health workers from the PHCs Rajasthan for the efficient and timely collection of ECGs.

REFERENCES

1. World Health Organization. (2021). "Cardiovascular Diseases (CVDs)." Retrieved from https://www.who.int/news-room/fact-sheets/detail/cardiovascular-diseases-(cvds).
2. Spaich S, Kern H, Zelniker TA, Stiepak J, Gabel M, Popp E, Katus HA, Preusch MR. Feasibility of CardioSecur®, a Mobile 4-Electrode/22-Lead ECG Device, in the Prehospital Emergency Setting. *Front Cardiovasc Med.* 2020 Oct 9;7:551796. doi: 10.3389/fcvm.2020.551796. PMID: 33195450; PMCID: PMC7581708
3. Behar J, Oster J, Clifford G. "ECG Monitoring in Ambulances: Benefits and Limitations." Int. J. Cardiol. 2020; 304:72–78.
4. Allied Market Research. "Holter ECG Monitoring Market: Forecast 2023–2028." 2021.
5. Stein PK, Watanabe MA. "Integration of Mobile Technology in Cardiac Monitoring." *IEEE Trans. Biomed. Eng*.2021; 68(10):2930–2941.
6. Shin SR, Park SY, Kang Y. "Wearable ECG Devices: Multi-Lead Capabilities and Clinical Applications." *Sensors* 2019; 19(10):2337.

7. Patel SI, Souter MJ. "Point-of-Care Testing with Portable ECG Devices in Emergency Medicine." *Am. J. Emerg. Med.* 2019; 37(8):1576–1582.
8. Glikson M, Friedman PA. "Cost-Effectiveness of Portable ECG Devices in Low-Resource Settings." *Europace* 2020; 22(5):744–752.
9. Raghunath S, Pfeifer JM, Beaulieu-Jones BK. "Artificial Intelligence in Portable ECG Devices." *JAMA Cardiol.*2021; 6(4):456–463.
10. Chung HU, Kim BH, Lee JY. "Future Directions in Portable ECG Technology." *Nat. Biomed. Eng.* 2020; 4:983–995.
11. Turakhia MP, Desai M, Hedlin H, et al. "Rationale and Design of a Large-Scale, App-Based Study to Identify Cardiac Arrhythmias Using a Smartwatch: The Apple Heart Study." *Am Heart J.* 2019; 207:66–75.
12. Tison GH, Sanchez JM, Ballinger B, et al. "Passive Detection of Atrial Fibrillation Using a Commercially Available Smartwatch." *JAMA Cardiol.* 2018; 3(5):409–416.
13. Cohen J. *Statistical Power Analysis for the Behavioral Sciences.* Routledge 2018.
14. Altman DG, Bland JM. "Measurement in Medicine: The Analysis of Method Comparison Studies." *Statistician* 2019; 32(3):307–317.
15. Schober P, Boer C, Schwarte LA. "Correlation Coefficients: Appropriate Use and Interpretation." *Anesth. Analg.*2018; 126(5):1763–1768.
16. Mukaka MM. "Statistics Corner: A Guide to Appropriate Use of Correlation Coefficient in Medical Research." *Malawi Med. J.* 2018; 24(3):69–71.
17. Willmott CJ, Matsuura K. "Advantages of the Mean Absolute Error (MAE) over the Root Mean Square Error (RMSE) in Assessing Average Model Performance." *Clim. Res.* 2018; 30(1):79–82.
18. Armstrong RA. "When to Use the Bonferroni Correction." *Ophthal. Physiol. Opt.* 2019; 34(5):502–508.
19. Bland JM, Altman DG. "Statistical Methods for Assessing Agreement between Two Methods of Clinical Measurement." *Lancet* 1986; 327(8476):307–310.
20. Giavarina D. "Understanding Bland Altman Analysis." *Biochem. Med.* 2019; 25(2): 141–151.
21. Ng, YC, Alexander, S, Frith, KH. (2018). "Integration of mobile health applications in health information technology initiatives: expanding opportunities for nurse participation in population health. *CIN.*" *Computers, Inf. Nurs.* 36(5), 209–213.
22. Krueger RA, Casey MA. *Focus Groups: A Practical Guide for Applied Research.* SAGE Publications 2019.
23. Dipankar S R, Arvind R, Anand Kumar P et al. "From Screening to Triaging, Timely Referral and Specialist Treatment: Striving for a Paradigm Shift in Cardiac Care for the Last-mile Population in Rajasthan, India." *Quality in Primary Care* 2019; 27(1): 9–12.
24. Vercel. "Vercel Documentation." *Vercel*, https://vercel.com/docs. Accessed 9 May 2024.
25. Neon tech. *Neon – Serverless, Fault-Tolerant, Branchable Postgres*, https://neon.tech/. Accessed 9 May 2024.
26. Cloudinary. "Cloudinary Image & Video Management – Documentation Home." *Cloudinary*, https://cloudinary.com/documentation. Accessed 9 May 2024.
27. Google. "API Design Guide | Cloud APIs." *Google Cloud*, https://cloud.google.com/apis/design. Accessed 9 May 2024.
28. Richards G. "RFC 6560: One-Time Password (OTP) Pre-Authentication." *RFC Editor*, https://www.rfc-editor.org/rfc/rfc6560.html. Accessed 9 May 2024.
29. Bogner Justus, et al. *2019 IEEE International Conference on Software Architecture Companion: ICSA-C 2019: Proceedings: 25-29 March 2019, Hamburg, Germany.* IEEE, 2019. Accessed 9 May 2024.

30. Cloudflare. "What is an SSL Certificate?" *Cloudflare*, https://www.cloudflare.com/learning/ssl/what-is-an-ssl-certificate/. Accessed 9 May 2024.
31. Fielding R, et al. "RFC 2616 – Hypertext Transfer Protocol – HTTP/1.1." *IETF Datatracker*, https://datatracker.ietf.org/doc/html/rfc2616. Accessed 9 May 2024.
32. Freier, Alan O, et al. "RFC 6101 – The Secure Sockets Layer (SSL) Protocol Version 3.0." *IETF Datatracker*, August 2011, https://datatracker.ietf.org/doc/html/rfc6101. Accessed 9 May 2024.
33. Upstash. "Documentation." *Upstash*, https://upstash.com/docs/qstash/overall/getstarted. Accessed 9 May 2024.
34. MDN. "JavaScript | MDN." *MDN Web Docs*, 5 March 2024, https://developer.mozilla.org/en-US/docs/Web/JavaScript. Accessed 9 May 2024.
35. Typescript. "The Starting Point for Learning TypeScript." *TypeScript*, https://www.typescriptlang.org/docs/. Accessed 9 May 2024.
36. Vercel Next.js. "Docs." *Next.js*, https://nextjs.org/docs. Accessed 9 May 2024.
37. PostgreSQL. "Documentation: 16: PostgreSQL 16.2 Documentation." *PostgreSQL*, https://www.postgresql.org/docs/16/index.html. Accessed 9 May 2024.
38. AWS Lambda. "AWS Lambda – Getting Started." *Amazon AWS*, https://aws.amazon.com/lambda/getting-started/. Accessed 9 May 2024.
39. Oracle. "Java Documentation – Get Started." *Oracle Help Center*, https://docs.oracle.com/en/java/. Accessed 9 May 2024.
40. Google Android. "Develop for Android." *Android Developers*, https://developer.android.com/docs. Accessed 9 May 2024.
41. GitHub. "GitHub Docs." *GitHub Docs*, https://docs.github.com/en. Accessed 9 May 2024.
42. Node.js. "Node.js API Documentation." *Node.js*, https://nodejs.org/en/docs/. Accessed 9 May 2024.
43. Bluetooth. "Specifications." *Bluetooth*, https://www.bluetooth.com/specifications/specs/. Accessed 9 May 2024.
44. "RFC 7519: JSON Web Token (JWT)." *RFC Editor*, https://www.rfc-editor.org/rfc/rfc7519.html. Accessed 9 May 2024.
45. IEEE. "IEEE Standard for Information Technology – Portable Operating System Interface (POSIX(TM)) Base Specifications." *Wikipedia*, https://ieeexplore.ieee.org/stamp/stamp.jsp?tp=&arnumber=8277153&isnumber=8277152. Accessed 9 May 2024.
46. Wilde E. "RFC 5724: URI Scheme for Global System for Mobile Communications (GSM) Short Message Service (SMS)." *RFC Editor*, https://www.rfc-editor.org/rfc/rfc5724. Accessed 9 May 2024.
47. Google Firebase. "Introducing Firebase Cloud Messaging." *Firebase*, https://firebase.google.com/docs/cloud-messaging. Accessed 9 May 2024.
48. Backman Annabelle. "RFC 8936 – Poll-Based Security Event Token (SET) Delivery Using HTTP." *IETF Datatracker*, 30 November 2020, https://datatracker.ietf.org/doc/rfc8936/. Accessed 9 May 2024.

8 Artificial Intelligence in Embedded Systems for Biomedical Applications

Sena Nur Karabekiroglu, Meral Usta, Deniz Uygunoz, and Mert Akın Insel

8.1 INTRODUCTION

With today's technology, detecting diseases early offers a better lifestyle for people and increases their comfort. High hospital costs and increasing working hours and pace prevent people from applying to hospitals for health problems. Therefore, automatic detection using signal treatment and pattern recognition techniques poses a potential for providing diagnostic information. Thanks to technological developments in the field of medicine, the development of diagnosis and treatment methods and a better estimation of particular pathologies create the expectation of more efficient and better healthcare services [1].

The high reliability levels of versatile embedded systems that enable the evolution of new diagnostic and modern monitoring machines for patients in home and hospital conditions and the provision of effective solutions in health have accelerated the applications of data processing and storage in the biomedical field in recent years [2, 3]. In addition, positive developments in battery and wireless technologies, decreasing the size of electronic circuits day by day, have enabled the production of portable biomedical devices for monitoring and diagnosis. Working on the embedded system principle, these biomedical devices scan vital functions and develop the concept of wireless systems with embedded biosensors. It can assess stress factors by monitoring physical and psychological stress by evaluating the person's monitored variables. It also allows monitoring the perceiver's response to changes in the environment. Embedded systems must instantly respond to essential function changes to detect health issues or avoid life-threatening changes. Medical devices in an embedded system can also track a patient's activity, sleep, and medication use. These qualities make embedded systems essential for biomedical diagnosis and monitoring [4].

The most basic embedded system medical applications are imaging equipment. Ultrasound (US), computed tomography (CT), positron emission tomography (PET), and magnetic resonance (MR) are examples of embedded systems that function according to different concepts. These embedded systems facilitate the exact diagnosis and treatment planning by enabling the processing, acquisition,

 DOI: 10.1201/9781003508199-8

and display of medical imaging data [5]. Biomedical applications of embedded systems include defibrillators that monitor the heartbeat irregularly and restore it to normal when anything is wrong. Electrocardiograms, private health care systems, portable diagnostic systems, biomedical power units, glucose monitors, clinical and biotechnological analyzers, mobile patient monitoring systems, pacemakers, and reliable wearable electronic devices use the embedded system principle [2, 4]. Rehabilitation also makes substantial use of embedded systems. Treatment and rehabilitation systems necessitate the utilization of a diverse array of technologies, such as electric stimulators, rehabilitation robots, prostheses, and other similar tools. All these devices work with embedded systems to monitor their function. These devices can be made more precise and effective in therapy and rehabilitation tasks by means of embedded systems. For example, with rehabilitation robots, the possibility of recovery can be increased by providing a more stable and effective treatment by enabling the robot to move according to the specified trajectory, the embedded system can enable the patient to move their lower or upper limbs continuously and passively, thus increasing the efficiency of rehabilitation [6].

The requirement for more effective medical systems with fast and personalized support is increasing day by day. An attempt is made to respond to this demand by integrating artificial intelligence (AI) into the field of medicine by capitalizing of its capacity to acquire from a compact and complex database, process great amounts of information, give accurate results, and control processes to create the optimum outcome [1, 7]. AI technologies, whose core is embedded technology, are mostly implemented through image processing, speech recognition, and smart robots [8]. This technology is beneficial in assisting physicians in decision-making processes in both diagnosis and treatment, such as monitoring patients and examining drug efficacy tests, promoting, and caring for the patient recovery process, prevention, treatment, and overcoming diseases [1, 3]. AI which covers computer vision (CV), neural networks (NN), machine learning (ML), and natural language processing (NLP) is playing a critical role in the development and data observation of the healthcare industry and robotics with the help of the Internet of Things (IoT) [9, 10]. With more detailed results obtained, AI increases treatment accuracy and allows for minimizing test errors and misdiagnoses. AI technology plays a major role in reducing the cost of treatment and increasing the survival rate in acute diseases such as cancer, tumors, and some viruses. In addition, AI has vital importance such as robot-assisted surgeries, obtaining faster laboratory results through better and higher success rate review of records, high surgical success rate, early prediction, and a better understanding of the disease [10]. Besides, to preserve cardiovascular patients' health, it is of extreme significance that their diseases are recognized immediately. Sensors produce great amounts of data in the IoT environment, and this data has priceless healthcare knowledge. Thus, analysis of these data is important for enhancement in medical technologies. Herein, AI and ML technology would be extraordinarily beneficial for accomplishing classification, data analytics, and predicting healthcare specifications based on this data [11]. AI-integrated systems update real-time health monitoring, efficiency in therapeutic pharmaceutical production, and predictive forecasting [7]. In addition, in terms of making a significant contribution to daily life, it is possible to examine many health parameters such as calories burned during sports, step calculation, stress measurement, oxygen saturation, and blood pressure measurement by using technologies combined with AI [10].

8.2 FUNDAMENTALS OF EMBEDDED SYSTEMS IN BIOMEDICAL APPLICATIONS

An embedded system is an association of various electronic devices, sensors, and processors that form part of a larger system, including hardware and software components, designed to accomplish a function or control a range of functions [2, 12, 13]. These systems are based on microprocessors and are not designed for independent programming by the user. They are systems that are expected to operate with minimal or no human interaction [12, 13]. Embedded systems typically engage in direct interaction with processes or the surrounding environment, generating inputs and making instant decisions based on the inputs. It is essential for embedded systems to respond in real time and be reactive to process inputs for the proper functioning of the system [12]. Embedded systems and real-time systems operate reactively and in constrained environments where processing power and computer memory are limited [12, 14].

The inputs to an embedded system consist of parameters and process variables that are received through input/output (I/O) ports and sensors. For users or other application subsystems, the system generates control actions on system actuators or processed data. A user interface, which can contain various display devices such as LEDs, LCDs, keys, buttons, sensors, and similar components, can facilitate user input-output communication. A set of instructions that are programmed into a system's central processing unit (CPU) to perform specific functions or activities is referred to as software. It includes software applications that control how physical components operate [3]. Hardware, consisting of electronic and physical elements, enables the embedded system to fulfill its functionality [3]. While the layout of different systems may vary greatly depending on their intended use, there are three essential hardware components that are necessary for an embedded system: the Central Processing Unit (CPU), a collection of input-output ports, and system memory. The CPU is responsible for executing software instructions that determine the system's functionality and process system inputs. Necessary data and programs for system operation are stored by memory. Signal transmission between the external environment and the CPU is provided by I/O ports [12]. To get the most effective benefit from embedded systems, the system should use minimum program memory and run faster than the system requires. Embedded software must be highly readable and easy to intervene in the system [15].

Microprocessor-based embedded systems, microcontrollers, board-based embedded systems, and extended microcontrollers are classified as embedded systems [13]. Embedded systems are mostly used in mass-produced electrical and electronic devices (cameras, toys, televisions, microwave ovens, dishwashers, washing machines, dryers, sound systems, media players, and mobile phones), medical equipment, transportation (avionics, aerospace, automotive), anti-lock brakes and airbag deployment mechanisms, trains, power distribution, and factory automation systems [12, 14].

Nowadays, the importance of new technology for health products that detect diseases faster and more reliably is increasing. By using new data analysis techniques developed on the basis of ML, it becomes possible to detect increasing risks and increase the chance of recovery. In addition to diagnosis, treatments can also be supported with personalized medicines supported by AI. Examples of these technologies include new devices to assist disabled patients, new devices to support surgery [16]. In medical devices, embedded systems consist of computing elements and medical equipment which aim to achieve some specific functions such as data processing, monitoring, and control [5]. Embedded system technologies provide much better tools to control the positive or negative effects of the applied treatment, with the possibility of improved monitoring of test results [16]. The accelerating number of smart devices operating based on embedded systems allows continuous monitoring of vital marks, leading to significant developments in the healthcare sector. For healthcare monitoring, sensors are usually utilized for measuring vital signs such as body temperature, heart rate, blood pressure, and respiratory rate [3].

The design of an embedded system encompasses several key elements, including the architecture of digital hardware and software, the formal design process, development and optimization, security, safety, and reliability considerations. It also involves the design of digital hardware and software (or firmware), the interface with analog and digital signals from the physical world, as well as the debugging, troubleshooting, and testing of the design. The embedded system design process involves the completion of tasks such as defining requirements, creating system specifications, developing functional and architectural designs, and creating prototypes [17]. Embedded system should have the least power consumption and be designed to be size- and cost-efficient. Also, they usually must be fully predictable and highly dependable [18].

Embedded systems are designed to respond to events in real time and operate autonomously without human intervention [14]. AI-integration of embedded systems improves the quality of healthcare field, such as monitoring cardiac arrhythmia, surgery assisting, and diabetes control. To further analyze and improve decision-making abilities, ML enhances the processing of large and complex sensor data efficiently. The use of AI/ML in the separation of analytical data from lower resolution or noise information sets is also functional. Moreover, the AI methods provide better sensitivity, measurement time, signal strength, and specificity [7]. NLP, which is a method of AI, may be utilized to automatically separate data from unstructured clinical files, such as physician notes or discharge summaries. NLP and ML techniques can be able to automatize assignment process suitable medical codes to patient diagnoses, treatments, and procedures. They also help the evolution of virtual assistants and chatbots for e-healthcare. Another vital advantage of these techniques is clinical decision-making by evaluating patient info, medical literature, and curing guidelines [19].

The main factors that affect and shape the life cycle of embedded system design are design constraints [12]. Unfortunately, the design of such autonomously embedded systems is a hard and costly process, since they are generally integrated into different medical devices and used for the vast majority of biomedical applications, but lacking an overarching architecture that includes hardware and software components. In addition, every prototype requires testing and validation to consider the

TABLE 8.1
Pros and Cons of AI-integrated Systems in Healthcare [19]

Opportunities	Challenges
Improved healthcare and lifetime	Power consumption
Real-time disease management and prevention	Data management
Cheaper and simple healthcare	Cost efficacy
Medication and automatic alerts on time	Scalability

architecture's effectiveness as well as its advantages for developing integrated biomedical embedded systems [20].

Embedded systems require high stability and reliability in the operation process, due to their wide application area, as well as having advantages of small size and low power consumption. It is able to complete design and installation within a limited space [8]. The most fundamental constraints in the design and implementation of embedded systems are memory and power consumption, high real-time requirements, cost and processing power, limited hardware resources, and strong environmental adaptability [8]. Constraints such as memory, timing, and speed affect the use of real-time operating systems in embedded software [14]. The high volume of production of devices operating on the embedded system principle increases the cost and creates a limiting factor in design [12]. Because most operate as wireless sensor networks and are small in physical size, biomedical embedded systems have a very limited number of options for providing a constant power supply. A battery can be used to produce integrated power; however, it provides only a limited amount of energy. If the device is implanted in the body, it will be more complicated to replace the batteries as required. Instead, vibration and solar are not feasible and maintain a deficient power for continuous operation. The available power supply limits embedded systems computation which makes it difficult for them to be used continuously in all biomedical devices integrated into the body [20]. Another critical challenge with AI-integrated embedded systems is the management of comprehensive data, also described as big data. The risk of the system crashing is high due to this problem that occurs when there are too many inputs. To prevent this problem, a smart ML algorithm is needed to process very large data [7]. Even though AI may perform healthcare duties in many cases equally or better than humans and have so many advantages, challenges will inhibit the work of health experts from being considerably computerized for a noticeable period (Table 8.1) [21].

8.3 INTRODUCTION TO ARTIFICIAL INTELLIGENCE IN BIOMEDICAL APPLICATIONS

The healthcare sector has frequently utilized information technologies in recent years to develop modern applications, as well as to improve diagnostic and treatment processes. In this context, AI has been in the limelight for researchers and biomedicine applications because of its ability to process large amounts of data, produce accurate results, and control processes for optimal results [22].

AI is generally defined as the development of algorithms and programs to make devices efficient and intelligent for use in tasks that require human intelligence [23].

In the healthcare sector, AI has the potential to completely transform a number of processes, including patient care, diagnosis, and treatment. However, this technology includes a number of subcategories, such as speech recognition, deep learning (DL), fuzzy logic, ML, and traditional neural networks, each with unique features and capabilities. These features have the potential to enhance the effectiveness of contemporary medical sciences. Such intelligent systems can simplify human intervention in decision-making skills such as diagnosing diseases, recommending treatment options, medical imaging, and extracting meaningful information from large data sets [7, 24].

According to some researchers, the use of AI in biomedical applications falls into two directions: virtual applications (more commonly DL) where ML is used, and physical applications where AI is performed by robots. Also, it is anticipated that AI technologies will soon have an impact on other aspects of emergency medicine and healthcare delivery [25].

8.3.1 Overview of Artificial Intelligence and Machine Learning Techniques

AI is the ability of computer systems to perform human-like intelligence functions, or an attempt to simulate this ability. Its main goal is to provide computer systems with capabilities like human intelligence, such as thinking, learning, problem-solving, language understanding, perception, and decision-making [26]. The concept of AI was introduced for the first time in 1956 at the Dartmouth workshop led by Minsky and McCarthy [27].

There have been periods in the past when the potential of AI could not be realized due to limitations in data, computing power, and funding. However, the current era of improved communication power and access to data volumes, coupled with increased funding, presents a more optimistic picture for the implementation of AI [28].

AI encompasses a variety of subfields, including computer vision, NLP, robotics, DL, and ML [29]. However, many researchers consider ML as a special part of AI [23] In general, learning is an important aspect of human cognition, where humans process large amounts of information using abstract knowledge that helps them better understand incoming inputs. ML models can mimic human cognitive abilities thanks to their adaptive nature [30]. In other words, MLs are a collection of techniques that are employed to address a variety of real-world issues by utilizing computer systems that have the ability to learn how to solve them [31].

8.3.2 Importance of AI-Driven Approaches in Analyzing Biomedical Data

Over the past 50 years, there has been a profound transformation in the field of information technology (IT), resulting in the generation and storage of exponentially increasing amounts of data. This data has enabled researchers to develop a wide range of products and services, not only in the technology sector but also in other industries. Currently, big data possesses unparalleled potential to enhance medical results and the health of the population [32, 33].

The data sets obtained in biomedical research are often large and complex. Coming from a variety of sources such as genomic data, hospital records, imaging data, and biological signals, these data can be difficult and time-consuming to analyze manually. In order to convert the data into actionable analytical knowledge, the implementation of analytical techniques, such as AI algorithms, is necessary, as the data in question is not particularly informative on its own [34]. Additionally, AI algorithms that necessitate a diverse array of data to prevent overfitting particularly benefit from such large and lengthy data. [29].

In this context, the use of AI algorithms in the analysis of biomedical data brings a new perspective to biomedical research in many areas such as disease diagnosis, treatment planning, drug development, and disease risk prediction (Figure 8.1). With the proper application of this technology, faster progress can be made in biomedical research and innovative solutions can be produced for human health. [25].

8.3.3 Challenges and Considerations Specific to AI in Biomedical Applications

AI has benefits for biological research but also challenges. Data integrity, security, scalability, and ethics may limit AI use. However, well-designed approaches and algorithms can overcome these constraints [35]. Limited data sets are the biggest challenge for ML systems. When dealing with a small data set, overfitting arises

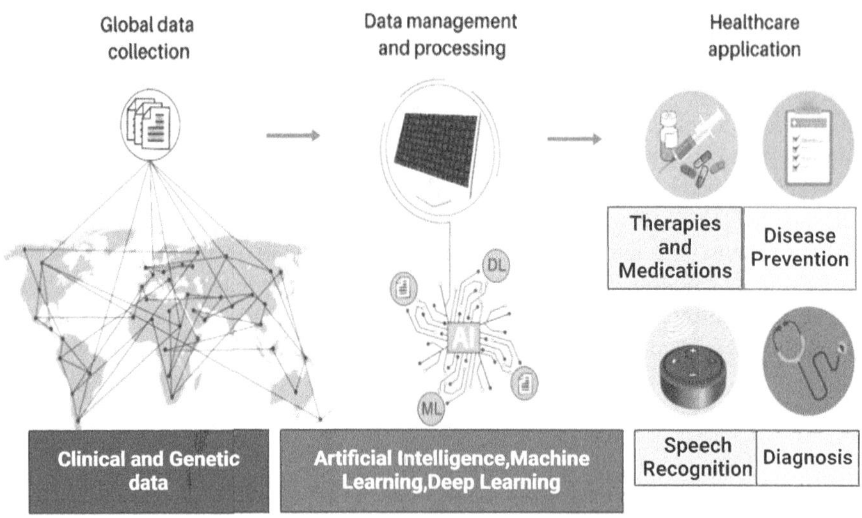

FIGURE 8.1 Integration of globally collected data into healthcare services after processing with artificial intelligence algorithms.

(Reproduced with permission from [25].)

because ML algorithms' precision and applicability depend on data quality and quantity. An algorithm memorizes its statistical variances in a specific data set, which performs well, but fails on a bigger data set [36]. Low-quality training data might potentially hurt algorithm prediction. Working with huge data sets and methodically preparing them before training is essential [37]. DL and ML face major hurdles, including the "black box problem". The black box problem is the inability to view an algorithm's decision-making process, comprehend how many neural connections achieve a certain conclusion, and discern which input data properties affect the output. 2020 [38]. DL methods are opaque, making it difficult to gather more data, identify flaws, and improve models. This limits the use of DL algorithms in clinical AI [22]. Other subfields, such as robotics, face restrictions such as the lack of high-quality, diverse data sets, the necessity for sufficient technological and computational infrastructure, and the high costs of implementation and maintenance [39]. Finally, AI incorporation into biological applications raises ethical and legal issues in addition to technological ones. AI replacing humans raises ethical issues such as prejudice, inequity, patient confidentiality, and privacy [40]. Due to the "black box" nature of AI in medical responsibility and accountability, comprehensive validation and regulatory approval are needed to ensure AI methods' safety, efficiency, transparency, and equity [36].

8.4 INTEGRATION OF ARTIFICIAL INTELLIGENCE WITH EMBEDDED SYSTEMS

Embedded systems are hardware systems that are specifically designed to perform a particular task. They consist of mechanical and electronic components, along with an operating system and processor. Typically, they function responsively and in real-time with restricted resources, without direct engagement with the end user [5].

Imaging devices like MRI, PET, CT, and US are widely recognized as the most prevalent medical applications of embedded systems, despite their distinct operational principles. Embedded systems encompass a variety of devices, such as defibrillators, digital flow sensors, blood pressure devices, glucose test sets, fetal heart monitoring machines, and device designs that enable users to monitor values like heart rate, blood pressure, and glucose levels [41].

These examples show how versatile and effective embedded systems can be used to meet a variety of needs in the healthcare sector. However, these devices enable the collection of continuous and large amounts of data. This large and complex data is not very informative on its own, so innovative approaches are needed to draw meaningful conclusions from it [41].

The integration of embedded systems with AI is a technology that has the potential to provide better service to patients by providing significant innovations in the healthcare sector. In addition, the data collected through embedded systems can be analyzed by AI algorithms to optimize hospital resources and improve patient care by providing benefits in many areas such as disease diagnosis, treatment planning, drug development, and disease risk prediction [2].

8.4.1 Rationale for Combining AI with Embedded Systems in Biomedical Applications

Global economic, environmental, and social progress, along with resulting shifts in lifestyle, have caused a significant surge in chronic illnesses such as cardiovascular disease, diabetes, and cancer. Presently, this poses the most significant peril to human well-being. Healthcare professionals and researchers are seeking a contemporary system that can monitor a patient's vital signs and offer accurate diagnoses and recommendations regarding their health, considering their complete medical history. Due to the recent pandemic, remote health monitoring has emerged as a significant concern [35].

IoT is a developing bioanalytical tool that integrates interconnected biomedical devices with a software application to enhance human health. These systems enable healthcare providers to monitor remotely their patients and supervise their treatment. The advent of IoT technology has effectively eradicated the geographical barriers and limitations that once separated doctors and patients. Furthermore, it has facilitated the provision of cutting-edge medical services to patients residing in remote regions, who frequently lack access to such amenities [2].

The integration of IoT devices, such as wearable monitors, smart pills, and sensors, enables healthcare practitioners to collect data in real time, thereby facilitating continuous data collection. Nevertheless, AI algorithms are necessary to analyze and handle this vast and intricate data. By incorporating AI-powered embedded systems, it is possible to analyze this data to identify variations in a patient's condition, suggest treatment alternatives, and recognize patterns. This facilitates the early detection of diseases, enhances patient outcomes, and expedites the discovery and availability of new treatments [24].

8.4.2 Synergies between AI Techniques and Embedded Systems Design Principles

Embedded systems are computer systems that require a comprehensive understanding of their intricacies and functionalities in order to effectively manipulate and manage them. An embedded system is a combination of hardware and software elements, consisting of a microprocessor, memory for storing data and programs, transducers such as microcontrollers or digital signal processors (DSP), actuators, sensors, and different interfaces [15]. Since embedded systems fulfill critical tasks in various fields, the occurrence of a fault can cause serious material losses and even loss of life [15]. Therefore, making embedded systems reliable and fault-tolerant is a priority in design and development processes [11].

The processes involved in designing and implementing embedded systems are divided into two parts. The hardware component, utilizing the Internet of Medical Things (IoMT), also referred to as health IoT, oversees the physiological variables that impact a patient's well-being. Meanwhile, the software design component is employed to forecast the patient's health condition using the collected data [15]. The novel aspect of IoT-based remote monitoring is that contemporary technologies such as AI and ML can be employed to analyze patient data, thereby facilitating more informed decision-making [2].

Tremendous technological innovations such as IoT and AI offer improvements to address the need in the current scenario of transforming the traditional healthcare system into a smart healthcare system. IoT and AI are technologies that have different purposes and capabilities but when used together create powerful and efficient systems [42].

8.4.3 Examples of AI Algorithms and Methods Suitable for Integration with Embedded Systems

Globally, cardiovascular diseases (CVD) cause the most deaths. Genetics, lifestyle, and stress are the biggest cardiovascular disease risk factors [7]. Heart function anomalies can be diagnosed via cardiac CT scans, ECGs, stress tests, Holter monitoring devices, and blood biomarker profiles [43]. Modern electrocardiograms (ECGs) measure cardiovascular activity in real time [44]. However, ECG data is large and time-consuming to get manually. Therefore, an automated tool to evaluate measurement precision and manage these large data sets is necessary. The researchers used ML methods to diagnose arrhythmic heartbeats and forecast problems [7]. Cloud computing and data analysis allow AI to monitor cardiac electrophysiology and imaging. AI systems have been examined for ECG noise categorization, arrhythmia detection, atrial fibrillation prediction, and genomic sequence analysis [7]. Kachuee et al. suggested a DL ECG analysis technique. The algorithm can describe ECG signals for pulse irregularity detection and signal recognition [45]. Due to rising diabetes rates in healthcare, blood glucose monitoring is important. Hypo or hyperglycemia patients should test their blood glucose periodically. Unlike glucose meters, which provide a brief summary of glucose patterns, a CGM gives patients and caregivers real-time glucose updates. Estimating glucose levels is difficult and time-consuming due to blood dynamics [46]. AI can predict diabetes patterns and identify at-risk individuals to improve diabetes management. In this case, glucose monitoring devices use AI to improve clinical precision [7]. Khanam et al. created an AI-powered glucose sensor. Age, pregnancy status, BMI, glucose, and insulin levels were used to train the system in this study. The dataset was evaluated using NN, random forest (RF), decision tree (DT), and k-nearest neighbor (KNN) approaches. All models measured glucose with over 70% accuracy [47]. AI can also improve cancer research in areas like early detection, large-scale screening, tailored treatment, and clinical trials of novel [48]. AI algorithms can be used to forecast disease outcomes, cancer cell spread to lymph nodes, and therapeutic efficacy [49]. Clinical, pathologic, and genetic polymorphism data were used to create an artificial neural network model that predicted stomach cancer preoperative stage with 82% accuracy. Researchers used AI algorithms to create cancer prediction models [7].

ML combined with AI is known to be effective in the detection, diagnosis, and classification of cancer subtypes. ML algorithms are an alternative tool of choice for pattern identification in cases such as breast cancer. Decision-prediction algorithms such as decision trees, support vector machines, and nearest neighbor algorithms use crowded datasets to extract clinical features [7]. For example, Fan et al. developed an AI-powered method for detecting multiple tumors and diagnosed breast cancer with high selectivity (100%) and sensitivity (95%) [50].

8.5 APPLICATIONS OF ARTIFICIAL INTELLIGENCE IN EMBEDDED SYSTEMS FOR BIOMEDICAL APPLICATIONS

With the increase in studies on the genome, biomedical applications, on which studies are concentrated, have revealed many difficulties along with their development. First, parsing information obtained from the entire genome, gene transcription and phenotype outputs has introduced nonlinear modeling requirements. Secondly, the difficulty in understanding the interconnection of high-dimensional data types has made the work in this field difficult. Insufficient data labels have further increased the difficulty of analyzing missing or mismatched data. Along with all this, the continuation of new discoveries has increased the burden of the list of things to be solved. However, the increase in variant-specific diagnoses and treatments being tested in the clinical setting has caused implementation complexity for healthcare professionals, and ML has emerged as an indispensable tool to overcome these challenges. It has enabled the processing of large-scale genomic data, analysis, modeling and analysis, modeling and construction of these data. AI algorithms have been and continue to be used at various stages of healthcare to answer a variety of questions, from biomolecular exploration studies to the annotation of genomic sequence elements [9].

The AI techniques and mind map depicted in Figure 8.2 exemplify the application of AI techniques in several significant activities, including the analysis of extensive genetic data, pattern recognition, disease risk assessment, and prediction of prospective treatments. These techniques encompass a range of AI technologies, including DL, ML, NLP, and data mining. [9, 51].

8.5.1 The Role of Artificial Intelligence in the Diagnosis and Treatment of Diseases

In clinical diagnostics, AI can accurately explain health facts in their natural condition. These AI frameworks are trained on health data (e.g., clinical images,

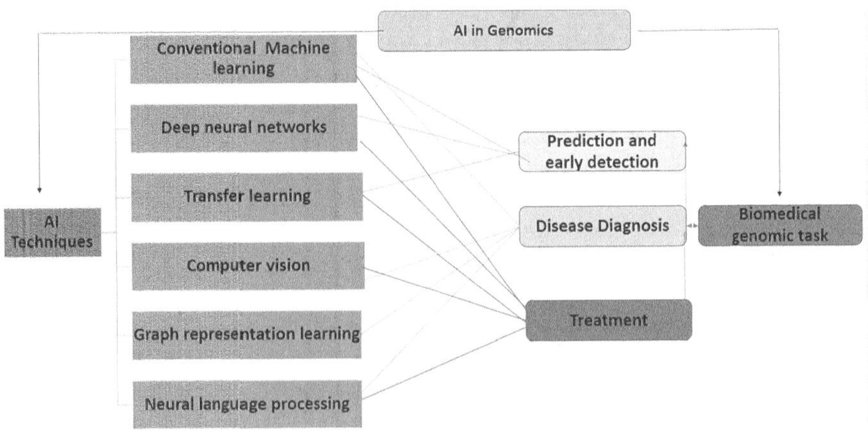

FIGURE 8.2 The AI techniques and mind map of biomedical topics.

(Reproduced with permission from [9].)

examinations, and results) interpreted by healthcare professionals and minimally processed before exposure to the AI system to efficiently interpret large complex data sets. The trained AI system then interprets similar health data. Clinical diagnosis can predict disease states. Healthcare workers can better identify and treat patients by understanding the disease's genetics.

The functions of AI can be divided into classes such as image processing, data analysis, identity recognition, and NLP. All of these abilities are important qualities for solving problems [51, 52].

8.5.1.1 Genetic Diseases and Detection

The human genome includes 20,000 protein-coding genes as well as 25,000 non-coding genes. While some genes are vital for life, some are important for a healthy life. Some of the genes can be deleted completely without causing any visible damage [53].

An essential feature of the gene is the existence of alternative segments known as introns and exons. The demarcation between these regions is established by the sequence patterns of the nucleotide, and numerous disease-causing mutations function by interrupting these patterns. Spinal muscular atrophy (SMA) is a genetic disorder that leads to insufficient production of the survival motor neuron (SMN) protein. This is caused by the absence or mutation of the SMN1 gene in an infant's genome. SMA is particularly severe in infants and can result in death. Genomic medicine is currently of crucial significance. One of its primary objectives is to forecast the potential hazards of these diseases based on a genotype. Developing models that predict the impact of genotype on "cell variables" like protein concentrations simplifies the ML problem and allows for the exploration of targeted therapies (Dias & Torkamani, 2019; Leung et al., 2016).

Doctors have a tremendous issue in evaluating the medical significance of novel variations in a patient's genome, which involves forecasting the harmfulness of mutations. DL approaches have the capacity to analyze and combine many forms of data, enabling them to provide more precise predictions of pathogenicity compared to current methods [51].

Moreover, the fact that ML also contributes a role in phenotype prediction cannot be ignored. It is clear that genetic data, incorporating complex traits such as height and disease risk, play an active role in predicting disease risk. DL also contributes to the development of such models. DL can further improve such models by using its ability to integrate (medical images, clinical history, etc.).

8.5.1.2 Cancer Prognosis and Detection

Cancer diagnosis is one of the important applications of AI-assisted genomic analysis. There are various studies conducted on the early diagnosis of many cancer diagnoses.

A study was conducted with the objective of developing an efficient diagnostic method for the early detection of liver disorders. The study concludes that the ML methods given can effectively address several restrictions in healthcare, including misdiagnosis, missing data, cost, and time constraints [54]. Another study came to a conclusion supporting this and derived an ensemble ML model for early diagnosis of liver cancer.

Several investigations have led to the creation of a generalized linear model, which has been enhanced by the addition of group models. This model has been effectively used as a diagnostic tool in the treatment of various types of cancer, including leukemia, breast cancer, lung cancer, endometrial carcinoma, and other combinations of cancer types [9].

One of the important studies showing that cancer treatments can be greatly improved with AI applications investigates the relationship between genetic mutations in breast cancer tissue and changes in metabolic products [55]. It identifies different subtypes of breast cancer with the combined application of LASSO (Least Absolute Shrinkage and Selection Operator) and SVM (Support Vector Machine) algorithms. Another study is a gene signature study conducted in stage I lung adenocarcinoma patients to optimize risk classification and create an integrated decision tree and nomogram to measure risk assessment [56].

8.5.1.3 Anatomy and Physiology Investigations

The role of AI in biomedical applications in embedded systems provides great contributions to anatomical and physiological research. Some of these applications are Medical Imaging Analysis, Patient Monitoring, processing and analysis of biological signals such as Electrocardiogram (ECG), electroencephalography (EEG), Patient Customized Treatment Planning, Anatomy Education and Simulation.

In a study by [57], they performed AI-based anatomy definition of ultrasound results. According to recorded ultrasound images evaluated by two experts, it was concluded that AI technology can effectively explain anatomical structures in real-time sonography and that the accuracy of color overlays is reliable and consistent. It was concluded that this study would be valuable in helping anesthesiologists.

In the study conducted by 19 experts on ultrasound in 6 anatomical regions, 100 structures were annotated with 30 ultrasound images and expert explanations were compared with AI color overlay, the automatic identification and coloring of objects or structures in digital images using AI. As a result, it was concluded that experts and AI showed the same adaptation model in the sono-anatomical structure. This was considered a promising study [58].

8.5.1.4 Drug Development and Clinical Trials

AI is widely believed to have the potential to greatly transform the pharmaceutical industry by expediting the process of creating novel medications. AI models provide the capability to detect drug targets, repurpose pharmaceuticals, enhance clinical trial results, forecast pharmacokinetics and toxicity, and include natural products into the process of drug development. These models facilitate the identification of potential drug candidates, evaluation of drug-target interactions, and analysis of clinical trials, academic literature, and biological research. It enhances the process of medicine design by analyzing extensive data from databases. AI has the potential to revolutionize the process of designing and manufacturing medications. Examples include optimizing industrial processes, assuring high product quality, and enhancing the design of medicinal formulations [59].

The most commonly used algorithms in AI applications (Figure 8.3), which shows the AI procedures used in the drug discovery process, are Random Forest, Multiple

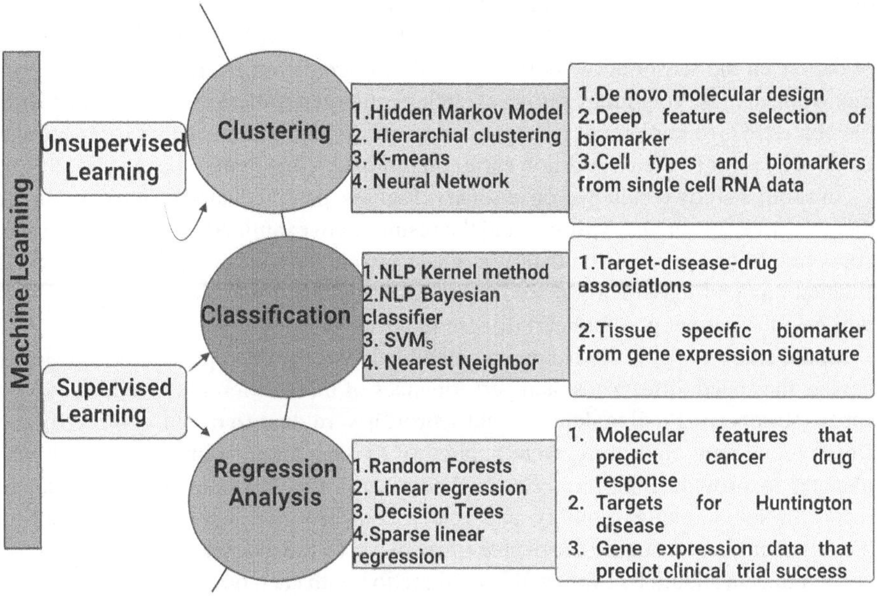

FIGURE 8.3 The artificial intelligence procedures used in the drug discovery process. **(Reproduced with permission from [60].)**

Linear Regression (MLR), Logistic Regression (LR), and Layered Perceptron (MLP). By utilizing these applications, it benefits from the advances of AI in adding or removing features to drugs, the most common of which is drug design [60].

8.5.2 Artificial Intelligence-Supported Embedded Systems in Hospital and Healthcare Systems Integration

8.5.2.1 Biomedical Data Acquisition and Monitoring

In recent years, the integration of AI into embedded systems has gained popularity in many industries. One of these sectors is the health sector. One notable application is the collection, processing, and analysis of biomedical data. It is envisaged that thanks to this established system, the monitoring, diagnosis, and treatment optimization of diseases will be improved and it will be possible to develop health systems. The inclusion of AI algorithms in embedded systems has enabled them to process multi-data studies with high speed and accuracy and to provide valuable information about patient health.

An investigation was carried out on a distant patient monitoring system that makes use of the IoMT, AI, and edge computing. The study focused on creating wearable sensors that are integrated into a prototype device. These sensors enable the remote monitoring of individuals with cardiovascular disorders. This system facilitates the surveillance of physiological indicators, including body temperature, heart rate, and blood oxygen saturation, while also allowing for the transmission of the gathered data to designated locations. The system is coupled with an ML model that utilizes up-to-date data to forecast health issues. Furthermore, it facilitates the transmission of data from the sensor network to the cloud through the utilization of edge computing, while also serving many purposes such as emergency alert messages. Therefore, the objective is to implement preventive measures for individuals with cardiovascular conditions prior to their condition escalating into a medical emergency [11].

In another study conducted on coronary diseases, patient data were recorded using the pulse rate sensor and Arduino, and the results were examined on the Google page, converted to csv go, and the data was made visible. It was then processed with AI calculations and classification studies. It was concluded that the proposed system will help the patient predict heart disease in the early stages [61].

In the study of [62] to develop an embedded system-based portable ECG Holter device, the speed differences, and performances of three different embedded system cards (Raspberry Pi, Beaglebone, and Odroid) were analyzed and compared, and signal processing algorithms were applied (C++ language). With this study, it was planned to provide long-term EKG (Electrocardiography) data recording and to record these data daily, monthly, and yearly, compare them with each other during the treatment, and examine the degree of recovery of the disease [62].

Health data should be evaluated in conjunction with each other. Data sources need to be combined and these bodies of information evaluated with the clinical knowledge of a healthcare professional. In order to diagnose a disease, it is important to consider the data regarding physical examination, laboratory test results, and patient history as a whole. The data collected can form the basis for modeling based on the prediction of results [63].

8.5.2.2 Applications of Embedded AI Systems in Hospital Settings

Data quality and accurate use of clinical information are particularly important in the effort to provide quality healthcare. The final decisions taken for patients in hospitals are obtained by blending the clinical process and the cognitive skills of healthcare professionals. Healthcare organizations (hospitals, clinics, emergency services, etc.) have realized that AI will enable personalized disease diagnoses, verify the consequences of diseases, detect early diagnosis, increase clinician capabilities, contribute to operational efficiency, and improve medical service accessibility [64].

In order for the clinical process to proceed successfully, a modeling that includes data interactions and mimics the cognitive skills of clinicians is required. CDSSs (Clinical Decision Support Systems) are important systems developed using AI techniques and methods that analyze clinical data and access medical knowledge bases, thus providing support in making clinical decisions [63].

Clinical Decision Support Systems (CDSS), commonly referred to as CDSS, provide doctors with intelligently filtered or timely information to enhance health and healthcare. This approach effectively reduces clinical practice errors while also improving patient safety. In order to effectively fulfill their intended function, the output of CDS systems should precisely capture the cognitive load and real-world decision-making process of clinicians.

From major academic medical institutions to small hospitals or clinics, applying AI in healthcare environments is important for the quality and efficiency of service.

In addition to the services offered in the hospital, remote health monitoring is one of today's main concerns. Healthcare professionals, clinicians, and researchers have sought systems that would not only track vitals but also consider medical diagnoses and treatments based on the patient's history. Bluetooth-enabled glucometers, manometers, and spirometers are the most frequently employed and essential remote patient monitoring devices in use today. These devices facilitate the transfer of data to the cloud through a mobile application. The integration of embedded systems in trackable devices with AI in healthcare organizations enables healthcare professionals to establish more reliable and effective relationships with their patients. In addition, it has the opportunity to create a dataset by transferring data from the devices used [11]. Such systems are important in providing quality and safe service to patients and providing evidence-based recommendations to clinicians in making accurate diagnoses.

8.6 CONCLUSION

As discussed so far, the application of AI in embedded systems for biomedical applications implies the beginning of a revolution in healthcare. This is especially the case for patient monitoring, diagnosis, and treatment strategies. These systems will enable the detection of diseases at an early stage and provide personalized diagnostic information by incorporating the data obtained from wearable devices, smart sensors, or IoT technologies. This actuality can indicate a change in healthcare management where the interventions are customized to meet the individual needs of each patient utilizing real-time data analytics.

Moreover, there are significant opportunities for advancements in precision medicine and personalized treatment methods with the integration of AI with embedded systems. By utilizing AI methods in analyzing the comprehensive patient datasets the healthcare providers will be able to enhance the effectiveness of treatments, which implies individualized, and effective interventions that prioritize the unique characteristics and requirements of each individual patient.

It should also be mentioned that the embedded systems that are enhanced with AI have attracted great attention in drug discovery and development. Both unsupervised and supervised learning are utilized to design molecules, identify cell types by feature selection and reduction, classify target-disease-drug associations, and predict clinical trial successes. These methodologies will likely enhance the identification, validation, and utilization of new drugs significantly, yielding more agile development timelines and lower costs.

It is also important to note that in the aftermath of the COVID-19 pandemic, there has been a significant increase in applications of telemedicine and remote patient monitoring. The AI-powered embedded systems have been shown to enable remote diagnostics, teleconsultations, and remote patient management. Thus, it is demonstrated that these systems possess the capacity to enhance the accessibility and equity of healthcare.

In conclusion, it is evident that AI is becoming more and more integrated into healthcare systems. Hence, it is of utmost importance to prioritize the resolution of ethical and regulatory concerns. The issues of data privacy, algorithm bias, transparency, and accountability necessitate thorough deliberation to guarantee the responsible implementation of AI-driven embedded systems. Regulatory frameworks must adapt to technological advancements while ensuring the protection of patient rights and safety. This phenomenon highlights the significance of ethical governance and regulatory supervision in fostering trust, transparency, and accountability in AI-driven advancements in healthcare.

ACKNOWLEDGMENT

This study was conducted by the members of the KMA-338 study group of the Chemical Engineering Department, YTU.

REFERENCES

1. Mhamdi L, Dammak O, Cottin F, Dhaou I Ben. Artificial intelligence for cardiac diseases diagnosis and prediction using ECG images on embedded systems. *Biomedicines* 2022;10. https://doi.org/10.3390/biomedicines10082013
2. Nandini KP, Seshikala G. Role of embedded computing systems in biomedical applications-opportunities and challenges. *2021 IEEE International Conference on Distributed Computing, VLSI, Electrical Circuits and Robotics, DISCOVER 2021 – Proceedings*, Institute of Electrical and Electronics Engineers Inc.; 2021, p. 332–5. https://doi.org/10.1109/DISCOVER52564.2021.9663646
3. Arandia N, Garate JI, Mabe J. Embedded sensor systems in medical devices: Requisites and challenges ahead. *Sensors* 2022;22. https://doi.org/10.3390/s22249917
4. Arandia N, Garate JI, Mabe J. Medical devices with embedded sensor systems: Design and development methodology for start-ups. *Sensors* 2023;23. https://doi.org/10.3390/s23052578
5. Sonko Sedat, Monebi Ayodeji Matthew, Etukudoh Emmanuel Augustine, Osasona Femi, Atadoga Akoh, Daudu Cosmas Dominic. Reviewing the impact of embedded systems in medical devices in the USA. *Int Med Sci Res J* 2024;4:158–69. https://doi.org/10.51594/imsrj.v4i2.767
6. Zhao H. *Applications of Embedded Systems in Medicine: Challenges and Future Trends. Highlights in Science, Engineering and Technology*, 2023; 62, 31–35. 2023. https://doi.org/10.54097/hset.v62i.10416
7. Manickam P, Mariappan SA, Murugesan SM, Hansda S, Kaushik A, Shinde R, et al. Artificial intelligence (AI) and internet of medical things (IoMT) assisted biomedical systems for intelligent healthcare. *Biosensors (Basel)* 2022;12. https://doi.org/10.3390/bios12080562
8. Yang L. Evaluation on the design of embedded platform vision system under the background of artificial intelligence. *Measurement: Sensors* 2024;33:101120. https://doi.org/10.1016/j.measen.2024.101120
9. Guo K, Wu M, Soo Z, Yang Y, Zhang Y, Zhang Q, et al. Artificial intelligence-driven biomedical genomics. *Knowl Based Syst* 2023;279. https://doi.org/10.1016/j.knosys.2023.110937
10. Nagrath P, Alzubi JA, Singla B, Rodrigues JJPC, Verma AK. *Smart Distributed Embedded Systems for Healthcare Applications*. Boca Raton: CRC Press; 2023. https://doi.org/10.1201/9781003254119

11. Ashfaq Z, Mumtaz R, Rafay A, Zaidi SMH, Saleem H, Mumtaz S, et al. Embedded AI-based digi-healthcare. *Appl Sci (Switzerland)* 2022;12. https://doi.org/10.3390/app12010519
12. Jiménez M, Palomera R, Couvertier I. Introduction to embedded systems. 2014. https://doi.org/10.1007/978-1-4614-3143-5
13. Heath S. *Embedded Systems Design.* 2nd edition. Newnes, Oxford. 2003.
14. Srovnal V. Using of embedded systems in biomedical applications. *The 3rd European Medical and Biological Engineering Conference, EMBEC'05, Prague* 2005.
15. Dere G. Biomedical Applications with Using Embedded Systems. *Data Acquisition – Recent Advances and Applications in Biomedical Engineering* 2021. https://doi.org/10.5772/INTECHOPEN.96070
16. Marwedel P. *Embedded System Design Embedded Systems Foundations offCyber-Physical Systems, and the Internet of Things* 4th edition. Embedded Systems. Springer. 2018.
17. Peckol JK. *Embedded Systems: A Contemporary Design Tool.* John Wiley & Sons, Inc; 2019.
18. Nicolescu G, Mosterman PJ. *Model-based Design for Embedded Systems.* CRC Press, Boca Raton. 2018.
19. Mathkor DM, Mathkor N, Bassfar Z, Bantun F, Slama P, Ahmad F, et al. Multirole of the internet of medical things (IoMT) in biomedical systems for managing smart healthcare systems: An overview of current and future innovative trends. *J Infect Public Health* 2024;17:559–72. https://doi.org/10.1016/j.jiph.2024.01.013
20. Panneerselvam P. Application of embedded system for a genetic disease, sickle cell anemia. *2014 International Conference on Advances in Electrical Engineering, ICAEE 2014, IEEE Computer Society*; 2014. https://doi.org/10.1109/ICAEE.2014.6838446
21. Parasar D, Ali A, Pillai NM, Shahi A, Alfurhood BS, Pant K. Detailed review on integrated healthcare prediction system using artificial intelligence and machine learning 2023. *3rd International Conference on Advance Computing and Innovative Technologies in Engineering, ICACITE 2023*, Institute of Electrical and Electronics Engineers Inc.; 2023, p. 682–5. https://doi.org/10.1109/ICACITE57410.2023.10182709
22. Jiang F, Jiang Y, Zhi H, Dong Y, Li H, Ma S, et al. Artificial intelligence in healthcare: Past, present and future. *Stroke Vasc Neurol* 2017;2:230–43. https://doi.org/10.1136/SVN-2017-000101
23. Collins C, Dennehy D, Conboy K, Mikalef P. Artificial intelligence in information systems research: A systematic literature review and research agenda. *Int J Inf Manage* 2021;60:102383. https://doi.org/10.1016/J.IJINFOMGT.2021.102383
24. Mansour RF, Amraoui A El, Nouaouri I, Diaz VG, Gupta D, Kumar S. Artificial intelligence and internet of things enabled disease diagnosis model for smart healthcare systems. *IEEE Access* 2021;9:45137–46. https://doi.org/10.1109/ACCESS.2021.3066365
25. Leite ML, de Loiola Costa LS, Cunha VA, Kreniski V, de Oliveira Braga Filho M, da Cunha NB, et al. Artificial intelligence and the future of life sciences. *Drug Discov Today* 2021;26:2515–26. https://doi.org/10.1016/J.DRUDIS.2021.07.002
26. Rai A, Constantinides P, Sarker S. *Next-Generation Digital Platforms: Toward Human-AI Hybrids, MIS Quarterly, MIS Research Center, 43-1*, 2019.
27. McCarthy J, Minsky ML, Rochester N, Shannon CE. A proposal for the Dartmouth summer research project on artificial intelligence, August 31, 1955. *AI Mag* 2006;27:12–12. https://doi.org/10.1609/AIMAG.V27I4.1904
28. Reddy S, Fox J, Purohit MP. Artificial intelligence-enabled healthcare delivery. *J R Soc Med* 2019;112:22–8. https://doi.org/10.1177/0141076818815510/ASSET/IMAGES/LARGE/10.1177_0141076818815510-FIG 1.JPEG

29. Hulsen T. Literature analysis of artificial intelligence in biomedicine. *Ann Transl Med* 2022;10:1284–1284. https://doi.org/10.21037/ATM-2022-50
30. Janiesch C, Zschech P, Heinrich K. Machine learning and deep learning. *Electr Markets* 2021;31:685–95. https://doi.org/10.1007/S12525-021-00475-2/TABLES/2
31. Kühl N, Schemmer M, Goutier M, Satzger G. Artificial intelligence and machine learning. *Electr Markets* 2022;32:2235–44. https://doi.org/10.1007/S12525-022-00598-0/TABLES/2
32. Oliveira AL. Biotechnology, big data and artificial intelligence. *Biotechnol J* 2019;14. https://doi.org/10.1002/BIOT.201800613
33. Car J, Sheikh A, Wicks P, Williams MS. Beyond the hype of big data and artificial intelligence: Building foundations for knowledge and wisdom. *BMC Med* 2019;17. https://doi.org/10.1186/S12916-019-1382-X/METRICS
34. Williams AM, Liu Y, Regner KR, Jotterand F, Liu P, Liang M. Artificial intelligence, physiological genomics, and precision medicine. *Phys Genom* 2018;50:237–43. https://doi.org/10.1152/PHYSIOLGENOMICS.00119.2017
35. Athanasopoulou K, Daneva GN, Adamopoulos PG, Scorilas A. Artificial intelligence: The milestone in modern biomedical research. *BioMed Inform* 2022;2:727–44. https://doi.org/10.3390/BIOMEDINFORMATICS2040049
36. Kulkarni S, Seneviratne N, Baig MS, Khan AHA. Artificial intelligence in medicine: Where are we now? *Acad Radiol* 2020;27:62–70. https://doi.org/10.1016/J.ACRA.2019.10.001
37. Handelman GS, Kok HK, Chandra R V, Razavi AH, Lee MJ, Asadi H. eDoctor: Machine learning and the future of medicine. *J Intern Med* 2018;284:603–19. https://doi.org/10.1111/JOIM.12822
38. Choi RY, Coyner AS, Kalpathy-Cramer J, Chiang MF, Peter Campbell J. Introduction to machine learning, neural networks, and deep learning. *Transl Vis Sci Technol* 2020;9. https://doi.org/10.1167/TVST.9.2.14
39. Ward TM, Mascagni P, Ban Y, Rosman G, Padoy N, Meireles O, et al. Computer vision in surgery. *Surgery* 2021;169:1253–6. https://doi.org/10.1016/J.SURG.2020.10.039
40. Hassoun S, Jefferson F, Shi X, Stucky B, Wang J, Rosa E. Artificial intelligence for biology. *Integr Comp Biol* 2022;61:2267–75. https://doi.org/10.1093/ICB/ICAB188
41. Zhao H. Applications of embedded systems in medicine: Challenges and future trends. *Highlights Sci Eng Technol* 2023;62:31–5. https://doi.org/10.54097/HSET.V62I.10416
42. Shah R, Chircu A. IoT and AI in healthcare: A systematic literature review. *Issues Inf Syst* 2018. https://doi.org/10.48009/3_iis_2018_33-41
43. Karuppaiah G, Velayutham J, Hansda S, Narayana N, Bhansali S, Manickam P. Towards the development of reagent-free and reusable electrochemical aptamer-based cortisol sensor. *Bioelectrochemistry* 2022;145:108098. https://doi.org/10.1016/J.BIOELECHEM.2022.108098
44. Tseng PY, Chen YT, Wang CH, Chiu KM, Peng Y Sen, Hsu SP, et al. Prediction of the development of acute kidney injury following cardiac surgery by machine learning. *Crit Care* 2020;24:1–13. https://doi.org/10.1186/S13054-020-03179-9/FIGURES/6
45. Kachuee M, Fazeli S, Sarrafzadeh M. ECG heartbeat classification: A deep transferable representation. *Proceedings – 2018 IEEE International Conference on Healthcare Informatics, ICHI 2018* 2018:443–4. https://doi.org/10.1109ICHI.2018.00092
46. Hasanzad M, Aghaei Meybodi HR, Sarhangi N, Larijani B. Artificial intelligence perspective in the future of endocrine diseases. *J Diabetes Metab Disord* 2022;21:971–8. https://doi.org/10.1007/S40200-021-00949-2/FIGURES/2
47. Khanam JJ, Foo SY. A comparison of machine learning algorithms for diabetes prediction. *ICT Express* 2021;7:432–9. https://doi.org/10.1016/J.ICTE.2021.02.004

48. Sakthivel A, Chandrasekaran A, Sadasivam M, Manickam P, Alwarappan S. Sulphur doped graphitic carbon nitride as a dual biosensing platform for the detection of cancer biomarker CA15–3. *J Electrochem Soc* 2021;168:017507. https://doi.org/10.1149/1945-7111/ABD927
49. Jin P, Ji X, Kang W, Li Y, Liu H, Ma F, et al. Artificial intelligence in gastric cancer: A systematic review. *J Cancer Res Clin Oncol* 2020;146:2339–50. https://doi.org/10.1007/S00432-020-03304-9/FIGURES/3
50. Fan L, Huang T, Lou D, Peng Z, He Y, Zhang X, et al. Artificial intelligence-aided multiple tumor detection method based on immunohistochemistry-enhanced dark-field imaging. *Anal Chem* 2022;94:1037–45. https://doi.org/10.1021/ACS.ANALCHEM.1C04000/ASSET/IMAGES/LARGE/AC1C04000_0005.JPEG
51. Dias R, Torkamani A. Artificial intelligence in clinical and genomic diagnostics. Genome Med 2019;11. https://doi.org/10.1186/s13073-019-0689-8
52. Esteva A, Robicquet A, Ramsundar B, Kuleshov V, DePristo M, Chou K, et al. A guide todeeplearninginhealthcare.*NatMed*2019;25:24–9.https://doi.org/10.1038/s41591-018-0316-z
53. Leung MKK, Delong A, Alipanahi B, Frey BJ. Machine learning in genomic medicine: A review of computational problems and data sets. *Proc IEEE* 2016;104:176–97. https://doi.org/10.1109/JPROC.2015.2494198
54. Adegbola PI, Aborisade AB, Adetutu A. Liver disease prediction in rats exposed to environmental toxicants using Machine-learning techniques. *Inform Med Unlocked* 2023;42. https://doi.org/10.1016/j.imu.2023.101369
55. Xiao Y, Ma D, Yang YS, Yang F, Ding JH, Gong Y, et al. Comprehensive metabolomics expands precision medicine for triple-negative breast cancer. *Cell Res* 2022;32:477–90. https://doi.org/10.1038/s41422-022-00614-0
56. Shi R, Bao X, Unger K, Sun J, Lu S, Manapov F, et al. Identification and validation of hypoxia-derived gene signatures to predict clinical outcomes and therapeutic responses in stage I lung adenocarcinoma patients. *Theranostics* 2021;11:5061–76. https://doi.org/10.7150/thno.56202
57. Gungor I, Gunaydin B, Buyukgebiz Yeşil BM, Bagcaz S, Ozdemir MG, Inan G, et al. Evaluation of the effectiveness of artificial intelligence for ultrasound guided peripheral nerve and plane blocks in recognizing anatomical structures. *Ann Anat* 2023;250. https://doi.org/10.1016/j.aanat.2023.152143
58. Bowness JS, Morse R, Lewis O, Lloyd J, Burckett-St Laurent D, Bellew B, et al. Variability between human experts and artificial intelligence in identification of anatomical structures by ultrasound in regional anaesthesia: A framework for evaluation of assistive artificial intelligence. *Br J Anaesth* 2023. https://doi.org/10.1016/j.bja.2023.09.023
59. Yadav S, Singh A, Singhal R, Yadav JP. Revolutionizing drug discovery: The impact of artificial intelligence on advancements in pharmacology and the pharmaceutical industry. *Intell Pharm* 2024. https://doi.org/10.1016/j.ipha.2024.02.009
60. Dara S, Dhamercherla S, Jadav SS, Babu CM, Ahsan MJ. Machine learning in drug discovery:Areview.*ArtifIntellRev*2022;55:1947–99.https://doi.org/10.1007/s10462-021-10058-4
61. Pandey H, Prabha S. *Smart Health Monitoring System using IOT and Machine Learning Techniques* 2020. *Sixth International Conference on Bio Signals, Images, and Instrumentation (ICBSII)*, Chennai, India, 2020, pp. 1–4. https://doi.org/10.1109/ICBSII49132.2020.9167660.
62. Yesevi A, Güler M, Yildiz MZ. Gömülü Sistem Tabanlı EKG Holter Cihazının Tasarlanması. *Acad Platform J Eng Sci* 2017:146–56. https://doi.org/10.21541/apjes.335275

63. Zikos D. A framework to design successful clinical decisionsupport systems. *ACM International Conference Proceeding Series*, vol. Part F128530, Association for Computing Machinery; 2017, p. 185–8. https://doi.org/10.1145/3056540.3064960
64. Esmaeilzadeh P. Challenges and strategies for wide-scale artificial intelligence (AI) deployment in healthcare practices: A perspective for healthcare organizations. *Artif Intell Med* 2024;151. https://doi.org/10.1016/j.artmed.2024.102861

9 Embedded Systems in Metabolic Bariatric Surgery *From Telemonitoring to Deep Learning Applications*

Athanasios G. Pantelis

9.1 INTRODUCTION

Obesity constitutes a pandemic and a health issue of major concern, given its prevalence: 988 million people were suffering from obesity, defined as body mass index ≥30 Kg/m^2, in the year 2020, which translates into 14% of the global population. More concerning is the fact that these numbers will almost double by the year 2035, according to projections officially issued by the World Obesity Federation Metabolic, with the prevalence of obesity reaching 24% [1]. In other words, almost one-fourth of the global population is predicted to be living within the next decade. Beyond its epidemiologic burden, the rise of obesity also imposes a considerable impact on the global economy: almost 2 trillion US dollars in 2020, i.e. 2.4% of total global GDP, projected to increase to more than 4 trillion US dollars (2.9% of global GDP) by the year 2035 [1].

Obesity has been characterized as a chronic, relapsing progressive disease [2, 3], and had been characterized as such by major professional and scientific bodies, including the World Health Organization (WHO), the American Medical Association (AMA), the American Association of Clinical Endocrinologists (AACE), and The Obesity Society (TOS) to name a few [4]. Most importantly, obesity is associated with a constellation of mechanical, metabolic, mental, and monetary problems, the so-called "4 Ms" of obesity, a term devised by Professor Arya Sharma and his colleagues in order to summarize the medical and practical sequelae that stem from obesity [5]. These issues include type 2 diabetes mellitus (T2DM), hypertension (HTN), dyslipidemia (DLP), metabolic dysfunction-associated fatty liver disease (MAFLD) [6], obstructive sleep apnea (OSA), osteoarthritis (OA) and joint pains, gastroesophageal reflux disease (GERD), infertility, and specific types of cancer (including esophageal adenocarcinoma, breast cancer in postmenopausal women, endometrial and ovarian cancers, kidney and colorectal cancers, and multiple myeloma, among others) [7], but also mood disorders, anxiety, sleep disorders, and

DOI: 10.1201/9781003508199-9

cognitive dysfunction, in addition to problematic access to education and employment, need for customized furniture, aids, and clothing, issues with life and health insurance, and long-lasting disability.

To date, metabolic bariatric surgery (MBS) constitutes the most effective treatment of obesity, with proven safety (90-day postoperative mortality: 0.2%) and sustainable results regarding weight control, management of associated health problems, and improvement of the quality of life [8–13]. There is an increasing body of evidence which supports that MBS is also effective in reducing mortality associated with two other major killers of our times, i.e. cardiovascular disease and cancer [14–19]. Most importantly, MBS has been shown to increase life expectancy, based on data from the SOS (Swedish Obese Subjects) Study, a high-volume (5182 patients allocated in the surgery, conservative treatment, and control groups) and long-standing (mean follow-up: 24 years) prospective study [20]. Of course, new, less invasive treatments are emerging, but they still need to sustain the challenge of long-term results [21].

Beyond its proven effectiveness, MBS is known to spearhead innovation among the array of minimally invasive procedures and swiftly endorse new technologies and novel techniques that will ensure better outcomes and improved safety for our patients. In the present chapter, we will examine the available evidence to date relevant to the usefulness and applicability of embedded systems in the perioperative period of MBS, focusing on telemonitoring and artificial intelligence (AI) applications in the preoperative, intraoperative, and postoperative periods.

9.2 TELEMONITORING

Telemedicine, in general, is not a new concept, however, its widespread adoption and implementation have been accelerated thanks to two pivotal circumstances, i.e. the COVID-19 pandemic with its ensuing mobility restrictions and the generalized use of smartphones that support a constellation of applications [22–26]. Telemonitoring is an indispensable part of telemedicine and refers to the remote monitoring of a patient's health status and vital signs using embedded systems. This can be in the form of wearable sensors, mobile applications, and home monitoring equipment that allow healthcare providers to track patient's health data remotely. The leverage of continuous monitoring outside of traditional healthcare settings and short-term encounters is that it facilitates prompt detection of health problems and deviations from the expected postoperative course, encourages better management of chronic conditions during the preoperative optimization, and allows timely interventions when needed.

As indicated, telemonitoring may occur during the preoperative phase, immediately postoperatively, and in the long run after MBS, serving different purposes on each occasion. Preoperative telemonitoring aims to achieve optimal physiologic reserves for patients who are by definition considered high-risk. One such example is the evaluation of adherence to CPAP (continuous positive airway pressure) therapy in candidates for bariatric surgery. As mentioned earlier, OSA is one of the major and most common associated health problems of obesity. During the preoperative evaluation, people who are candidates for MBS undergo screening for OSA by means of questionnaires [i.e. STOPBANG, an acronym formed by the initials of snoring, tiredness, observed apnea, high blood pressure, body mass index (BMI) >35 Kg/m^2, age >50 years, neck size ≥40 cm, male gender], polysomnography, or home sleep apnea testing (HSAT). In a prospective multicenter study from the Netherlands, the investigators implemented telemonitoring to determine the adherence to CPAP use of patients with newly diagnosed and pre-existing OSA (obstructive sleep apnea) [27]. The main outcome of the study was that adherence to CPAP usage was lower in the newly diagnosed OSA group as compared to the pre-existing one. The main strength of the study was the use of telemonitoring for assessing adherence (as opposed to questionnaires, which is another popular strategy), which renders the outcome quantifiable and the data more objective. OSA is an important parameter to consider and optimize preoperatively, as it can be linked directly to perioperative anesthesiologic parameters and most importantly may precipitate cardiac complications during the immediate postoperative course [28]. Similar methods could be implemented to monitor and optimize glycemic control in people living with obesity and type 2 diabetes mellitus who are scheduled to undergo MBS, as this might be important for preventing postoperative hypoglycemia and other complications [29]. Implementing telehealth services in the preoperative period might also have beneficial effects in a wider meaning, as it has been shown that it can increase access to bariatric surgery, particularly for minority populations, as well as decrease delay times from workup to operation itself [30, 31].

The main stem of the literature focuses on postoperative telemonitoring. For practical purposes, we will classify telemonitoring post-MBS into short-term and long-term. The former should serve as an early warning system (EWS) for postoperative complications, while the latter is supposed to be used as an objective means for recording progress on weight loss, resolution of associated health problems, improvement of the quality of life (QoL), and keeping up with dietary modifications and exercise.

Two of the most popular physiologic parameters measured in the context of telemonitoring are heart rate (HR) and respiratory rate (RR). Both can be measured by means of an accelerometer-based wearable biosensor called Healthdot (Philips Electronic Nederland BV). The device is placed on the patient's left lower rib in the care facility, the healthcare provider can monitor the patient remotely in real-time, and the patient is requested to return to the hospital in case the readings are indicative of deterioration [32]. According to the manufacturer, the accuracy of the device is ±1 rpm regarding RR and ±3% of the range regarding HR. The device is showerproof and can be worn and store recordings for up to 14 days, while its connectivity is accomplished via Wi-Fi. A study from the Netherlands examined the reliability of the measurements of Healthdot in a group of 30 consecutive post-MBS patients, by comparing them to the established method of vital sign monitoring that was available at the facility of the authors over 22 hours [33]. The comparison between the two methods was made using the Bland–Altman method for repeated measurements [34], and the agreement between the two methods of vital sign monitoring was determined to be 87.5% for HR, with a mean difference of –0.795 [95% CI (confidence interval) (–19.3)–17.8], and 92.3% for RR, with a mean difference of 1.3 [95% CI (–5.6)–8.2] [33]. The authors concluded that the device is a reliable method for accurately measuring HR and RR in post-MBS patients. In a similar study, the authors utilized both the Bland–Altman method and Clarke Error Grid analysis to visualize the differences between the wearable biosensor and the reference monitor during and after MBS [35]. The mean absolute difference was 1.26 ± 0.84 (standard deviation) during surgery and 1.84 ± 1.22 during the recovery phase for HR, and 1.78 ± 1.90 during surgery and 4.24 ± 2.75 at recovery for RR. According to the predefined criteria of the study, the difference did not exceed the limit for agreement regarding HR, but it did exceed them in 58% of the compared measurements of RR, rendering it unsuitable for respiratory monitoring in this setting. In another research from the Netherlands, the authors studied how the postoperative diurnal rhythm of HR (as measured by Healthdot) is affected by different types of surgery [36]. For instance, they compared 137 post-MBS patients with 100 post-surgical oncology ones and found that both groups showed recovery of diurnal disturbances, but in the latter group, both peak and nadir HRs were higher as compared to the post-MBS group. The limitation of the study is that deterioration in HR in the post-MBS group was a rare occurrence (only 3 patients), and even these cases were excluded from the study for various reasons. As such, the statistical interpretation of the results remains elusive.

The Healthdot device is capable of measuring more parameters than merely HR and RR. A group of investigators from the Netherlands has published a protocol for facilitating early discharge after MBS by implementing intensive telemonitoring for the first 7 postoperative days [37]. In this context, in addition to HR and RR, they will record the activity and body posture of the patient via the LoRaWan network, with the primary endpoints being 30-day mortality, mild and severe morbidity, readmission rate, and prolonged length of stay. Other groups of researchers have also investigated the potential of same-day discharge post-MBS with the use of telemonitoring as a surrogate of immediate and short-term postoperative follow-up. In a pilot retrospective study from the United States, Schaffer et al. compared 28 patients who underwent same-day laparoscopic sleeve gastrectomy (LSG) and were monitored by means of remote monitoring and self-recording of blood pressure with 53 peers who followed the routine inpatient postoperative trajectory [38]. The adherence rates in the early-discharge groups were 97% for the remote monitoring wearable and 80% for the blood pressure measurement. The investigators did not find significant differences between the two groups with regard to readmission rates (10% vs. 7.5%, $p > 0.05$). Most importantly, they conclude that the use of telemonitoring in this context has the potential to reduce costs, depending on the number of patients monitored per day, provided the healthcare system is capable of supporting this service. A similar feasibility of telemonitoring was demonstrated after Roux-en-Y gastric bypass (RYGB). In a prospective study of 50 patients post-RYGB, Nijland et al. showcased an adhesion rate to telemonitoring of 88%, which resulted in the presentation of 10 patients to the emergency department (10%) and a readmission rate of 4% (2 patients) within 30 days postoperatively, owing to the prompt recognition of a complication by the EWS of the telemonitoring device [39]. An interesting aspect of this study was the strict selection criteria that they implemented: the operation should have taken place before 11:00 AM, the case should have been the first or the second of the day, intraoperative or immediate postoperative complications should be absent, postoperative vital signs must have been normal, preoperative and postoperative blood hemoglobin levels must have differed <1 mmol/L, and the final decision for patient discharge belonged to the surgeon, depending on objective issues (vomiting, uncontrolled pain, wound problems, surgeon's doubt). This underscores that telemonitoring (and embedded systems in general) should be utilized as adjuncts to clinical judgment and evidence-based decision-making, instead of substitutes. One year earlier, the same group of investigators published another study in which they examined the feasibility of telemonitoring using a combination of video consultation and self-measurement of vital signs after both LSG and RYGB [40]. Interestingly, in this preliminary study, they concluded that their experience was "disappointing", owing to the poor compliance of the patients (56%) to the indicated measurements for 3 days after the bariatric operation. This denotes another important parameter of currently available telemonitoring systems, which is compliance. This might be a problem even in the case that the embedded system performs automatic measurements at predefined intervals because adherence and compliance might be a matter of correct application or dislocation of the device after the initial application at the healthcare facility. Consequently, it is imperative that these systems feature alarms of faulty application and malfunction that are distinguishable from alarms of physiologic disruption.

On the same wavelength, van Ede et al. published a series of articles on the use of Healthdot-based telemonitoring of HR and RR for the development of a continuous remote early warning score (CREWS). First, they described a concrete and stepwise protocol, which comprised an extensive literature search on the association of HR and RR with post-MBS complications, the organization of a series of multidisciplinary expert sessions, and the testing of the protocol performance [41]. The latter feature was further divided into the prompt detection of clinical deterioration, the alarm time setting optimization (i.e., the duration of the derangement), and the actual protocol performance testing by means of simulation via a programming language (Python). Their research concluded that at thresholds of 110 beats per minute (bpm), as far as HR is concerned, and 20 respirations per minute (rpm), regarding RR, the sensitivity for detecting post-MBS leak and hemorrhage was 75%. Most importantly, there was no clinically relevant impact of beta-blockers, an important type of antiarrhythmic and antihypertensive medication that is commonly prescribed to people living with obesity and relevant associated health problems. On a second level, they deployed telemonitoring in real-life clinical settings and compared the 30-day composite outcome after randomized allocation of patients between a same-day discharge telemonitoring group and a standard care group with discharge on postoperative day 1 [42]. There was a nonsignificant difference between the two groups [composite outcome achieved in 94% vs. 98% of patients, relative risk 2.9, 95% confidence interval (CI) 0.60–14.23, $p = 0.22$]. They also calculated that the decision for same-day discharge reduced hospitalization days by 61% ($p < 0.001$) overall and by 58% ($p < 0.001$) with readmission days included. On a third level, the investigators implemented the telemonitoring protocol according to patient preference, recruiting a total of 102 patients who were continuously monitored for 7 days based on the CREWS protocol [43]. HR data was missing in 14.7% of the patients, the specificity of the system reached 98%, while the false positive rate was 70%. The authors conclude that the implementation of the system is feasible and CREWS can detect serious complications, but in its current form, it is not mature enough to substitute nurses or physicians owing to its increased false negative rate.

Eventually, Caballero et al. investigated the effectiveness of same-day discharge using a different telemonitoring platform (REVITA®, HI Iberia SA) [44]. For this purpose, they recruited 14 consecutive post-MBS patients. The adherence rate was 71.4% and the visits to the emergency department reached 40%, without the need for readmissions or reoperations, and without serious complications. Consequently, they claimed that telemonitoring is effective and same-day discharge is feasible with this platform.

Beyond telemonitoring of the vital signs, another useful application is the remote detection and correction of post-MBS hypoglycemia, an issue presumably triggered by inappropriate hyperinsulinemia and increased sensitivity to insulin, and detected with increased frequency, particularly (but not exclusively) after bypass procedures [45, 46]. Among its potential but promising treatments is glucagon pump [47]. A group of investigators from the USA designed a double-blind, placebo-controlled, crossover trial to evaluate the efficacy of a closed-loop glucose-responsive automated glucagon delivery system [48]. The closed-loop glucagon system consists of 4 components: i) a glucose sensor that continuously measures interstitial glucose levels (which are indicative and directly related to blood levels), ii) a wireless receiver that receives the recordings from the continuous glucose monitor receiver; iii) a portable Artificial Pancreas System (pAPS) tablet that analyzes glucose patterns and henceforth predicts bouts of hypoglycemia; and iv) an infusion pump containing glucagon, which is connected to a wireless relay and releases glucagon into the bloodstream upon activation by the circuit. The primary objective of the study (and the device) is the prevention of postprandial hypoglycemia (glucose level <65 mg/dL), with secondary objectives being the prevention of severe hypoglycemia (<60 mg/dL), rebound hyperglycemia (>180 mg/dL), clinically significant hypoglycemia requiring rescue therapy (<55 mg/dL and/or severe neuroglycopenia), and improvement in glucose time (65–180 mg/dL). Twelve patients were recruited for the purpose of the study. People who received glucagon required no rescue glucose (versus 7 patients in the placebo group), experienced no severe hypoglycemia (versus 5 in the placebo group) and demonstrated significantly higher nadir glucose levels (67 ± 3 vs. 59 ± 2 mg/dL, $p = 0.004$). Complaints of local discomfort at the infusion site were similar in both groups (11/12 vs. 10/12). In conclusion, the system was effective in promptly detecting and averting postprandial hypoglycemia in patients who had undergone MBS and this constitutes another example of a promising embedded system that can effectively address a serious side effect of bariatric surgery.

Taking into consideration the aforementioned evidence, as well as established principles of EWS from other disciplines such as meteorology (risk knowledge, monitoring and warning, response capability, dissemination, and communication), the ideal early warning embedded system for post-bariatric complications should feature some baseline characteristics:

- **Continuous monitoring**: continuous monitoring of vital signs, including heart rate, respiratory rate, blood pressure, temperature, and oxygen saturation, is pivotal and feasible to some extent, as demonstrated in previous studies. Continuous data collection ensures that deviations from the normal range can be promptly detected and swiftly addressed.

- **Real-time alerts**: the device or system should be capable of acknowledging any deviation from normal in real time and prompt both the user (patient) and healthcare providers. These alerts should be timely and actionable, in order to trigger immediate intervention if necessary.
- **Statistical accuracy**: the device should be characterized by high sensitivity, in order not to miss any abnormality that might lead to detrimental complications, but at the same time should be specific, to avoid unnecessary expenditures in working hours and personnel with false alarms.
- **Customizable thresholds**: the device should allow for values at the extremes of the range that can be adjusted by the operator (healthcare provider), enabling them to set parameters specific to each patient's individual baseline and medical condition. This way will substantiate its objective of delivering individualized care and personalized medicine.
- **Integration with healthcare systems**: the system should have a function compatible with the existing hospital monitoring systems and should be seamlessly integrated into electronic health records (EHR), wherever these are available. This will ensure continuous and unhampered data transmission, will facilitate centralized monitoring by healthcare professionals, and will guarantee that relevant data is readily accessible by clinicians for timely decision-making.
- **User-friendly design**: such systems should come in a wearable form that is comfortable for patients to wear for extended periods, with a user-friendly interface that is easy to understand and operate. Intuitive controls and clear displays will ensure that patients will be able to interact with the device effortlessly. Presumably, this is the most important parameter for enhancing compliance with wearing the device continuously.
- **Long battery life**: a long battery life or the ability to recharge quickly and easily are *sine qua non* characteristics of a device that is destined for continuous monitoring. Additionally, this will ensure that patients can wear the device without frequent interruptions for charging, minimizing gaps in monitoring at the same time, which is of paramount importance.
- **Data analytics and predictive modeling**: advanced data analytic capabilities, including machine learning algorithms and predictive modeling, can help identify patterns and trends in patient data that may indicate and increased risk for postoperative complications. By analyzing historical data on patient-specific factors, the embedded system can provide early warning signs of potential issues before they escalate. The aforementioned closed-loop glucose-responsive automated glucagon delivery system is one such example. In a different context, Rozo et al. investigated patients who had undergone MBS and identified six different breathing patterns [49]. Consequently, they implemented data augmentation and transfer learning to increase the size of the training set. The next step was to analyze the data with two different machine/deep learning techniques [support vector machine (SVM) and convolutional neural network (CNN), respectively], a strategy that increased the performance of the system with

different combinations. The authors concluded that it is feasible to classify respiratory signals obtained with wearable systems using pre-trained AI models. For further and deeper insight into AI methods, please refer to the following Section ("Applications of artificial intelligence in metabolic bariatric surgery").

- **Multi-parameter monitoring**: as shown earlier, beyond HR and RR, the Healthdot device is capable of detecting changes in body posture and activity. Other parameters, such as sleep patterns, or fluid intake/output, can also be integrated into the recording. For example, a study investigated the role of monitoring physical activity, as documented by device-measured steps per day, in a cohort of 59 patients who had undergone catheter cardiac ablation for atrial fibrillation or MBS [50]. This comprehensive approach provides a holistic view of the patient's health status and enables early detection of complications that may not be evident from vital signs alone. This is very important in the case of bariatric surgery because the majority of patients are young, consequently, there may not be a deterioration of vital signs until late in the course of a potential complication such as an anastomotic or staple-line leak. Integration of multiple parameters with multiple readings (i.e. small changes in baseline temperature, reduced urine output) might facilitate the prompt detection of such potentially deleterious outcomes.
- **Secure data transmission**: robust encryption protocols and secure data transmission mechanisms will protect patient privacy and enhance the confidentiality of sensitive medical information. Compliance with regional healthcare regulations and standards, as well as general protocols such as the GDPR (general data protection regulation) is essential to safeguarding patient data.
- **Scalability and affordability**: the device should be scalable to accommodate varying patient populations and healthcare settings (from individual home use to hospital environments), thus increasing inclusiveness. Additionally, it should be affordable to ensure widespread adoption and accessibility across diverse patient demographics. This is also of increased significance in the population of patients living with obesity because at the initial postoperative phase when they have not lost enough weight, barriers to healthcare access are still applicable.

Table 9.1 summarizes the publications of embedded systems for the early postoperative period after MBS that have been mentioned in this Section.

While short-term monitoring post-MBS is mostly useful for promptly detecting and managing complications of the immediate postoperative period, medium- and long-term monitoring serves the purpose of optimizing outcomes, such as improving weight loss trajectories, retaining physical activity and fitness, and enhancing quality of life.

A couple of studies revolve around the role of telemedicine and embedded systems in effective weight loss. Goldstein et al. published a protocol on the implementation of a multi-sensor ecological momentary assessment (EMA) tool in order to locate the behavioral and psychological predictors of weight loss following MBS

TABLE 9.1
Publications of Embedded Systems for the Early Postoperative Period After MBS

First Author [Reference No.]	Country; Publication Year	Embedded System(s) Used	No. of Patients	Outcomes
Bartlett VL [50]	USA; 2021	Pedometer; scale	59 (29 MBS)	Post-MBS patients had fewer recorded steps than patients with AF post-catheter ablation.
Caballero A [44]	Spain; 2023	REVITA	14	Completion rate: 71.4%, ED visits 40%, serious complications-readmissions 0%.
Jacobs F [33]	The Netherlands; 2021	Healthdot	30	HR agreement: 87.5%; RR agreement: 92.3%
Kant N [35]	The Netherlands; 2021	Healthdot	94	HR–MAD (intraop) 1.26 bpm, (recovery) 1.84; RR–MAD (intraop) 1.78, (recovery) 4.24; data loss: 4.5%.
Mestrom EHJ [36]	The Netherlands; 2024	Healthdot	237 (137 MBS)	Peak and nadir HR: general surgery > MBS
Mulla CM [48]	USA; 2020	Closed-loop glucose res-ponsive auto-mated gluca-gon delivery system	12	Rescue glucose: 0 (glucagon delivery system) vs. 7 (placebo) (*p* 0.008); severe hypoglycemia: 0 vs. 5 (*p* 0.03); nadir plasma glucose: 67 vs. 59 (*p* 0.004); infusion site discomfort: 11 vs. 12.
Nijland LMG [40]	The Netherlands; 2020	Video consultation, measurement of vitals	84	Day 1: videoconference 92%, vitals 62%; Day 2: videoconference 88%, vitals 58%; Day 3: videoconference 90%, vitals 75%. All measurements on all days: 56%.
Nijland LMG [39]	The Netherlands; 2021	Video consultation, telemonitoring	50	Success rate: 88%; ED visits: 10%; readmissions: 4%.

(Continued)

TABLE 9.1 (CONTINUED)
Publications of Embedded Systems for the Early Postoperative Period After MBS

First Author [Reference No.]	Country; Publication Year	Embedded System(s) Used	No. of Patients	Outcomes
Schaffner TJ [38]	USA; 2023	Telemonitoring with wearable and blood pressure measurements	20 cases, 53 inpatient controls	Telemonitoring adherence: 97%; BP adherence: 80%; readmission rates: 10% vs. 7.5% (p >0.05).
Scheerhoorn J	The Netherlands; 2022	Healthdot	200	Pending (protocol phase)
van Ede ES [41]	The Netherlands; 2022	Healthdot	185	Detection of leak and bleeding: 75%; 0 alarms/day: 69.5%; 1 alarm/day: 1.6%.
van Ede ES [42]	The Netherlands; 2023	Healthdot	208	Textbook outcome: 94% (telemonitoring) vs. 98% (control), RR 2.9, 95% CI 0.60–14.23; reduced hospitalization days by 61% (total) and 58% (readmissions included).
van Ede ES [43]	The Netherlands; 2023	Healthdot	102	Missing data: 14.7%; specificity: 98%; false positive rate: 70%.

[51]. EMA is a study method originally stemming from clinical psychology that refers to the repeated sampling of patients' behaviors and experiences in real-time and in their natural environment, with the aim to minimize recall bias, maximize situational validity, and allow investigation of (largely unpredictable) processes that influence behavior in real-world conditions [52]. In the protocol of Goldstein et al., the EMA system consists of four components: an activity monitor, a bite counter, a smartphone application, and a mainframe through which data are transmitted to the research team in real-time. They targeted a sample of 100 post-MBS patients for a maximum follow-up period of 12 months, with the investigated parameters being meal frequency, physical activity, mood changes (including the development of depression), and type/quality of the food, along with weight changes during the same period. The final results of this study are still pending. In another study examining the role of fitness wearables in losing more weight postoperatively, the investigators recruited 37 patients, for whom they provided a wearable that kept track of the frequency of use, diet, weight, and sleep [53]. The adherence rate was 86.4%, whereas the reported satisfaction rate among those who adhered was 88.2%. Consequently, the group of fitness wearable (FW) users was compared to a matched non-user group (non-FW). The FW group demonstrated a nonsignificant greater reduction in the percentage of excess weight loss (%EWL; 65.2% vs. 52.4%, $p = 0.066$) and a significantly higher percentage of total weight loss (%TWL; 30.3% vs. 22.3%, $p = 0.02$) at 1-year follow-up, as compared to the non-FW group, suggesting that the use of the FW motivated patients after MBS to keep track of their physiologic changes and follow a healthier way of living, even after the cessation of the FW usage. On the contrary, in a randomized trial of 205 post-bariatric patients, the use of the eHealth platform or self-monitoring devices did not yield a significant impact on weight loss or QoL as compared to standard post-bariatric guidance [54]. Interestingly, the participation rate fell from a striking initial rate of 90–98% (depending on the chosen platform) to 62% in the first postoperative month and <20% after 2 years of follow-up.

Several relevant studies have examined the impact of device-based tracking on increasing physical activity and renouncing a sedentary lifestyle. With the use of wearable devices, a group of investigators from Australia found that, although MBS was effective regarding weight loss, neither the surgery on its own nor the use of wearables affected the increase of physical activity or reduction of sedentary time, suggesting that complementary behavioral interventions might be warranted for this purpose [55]. More recently, Hayotte et al. published a scoping review on the effects and acceptability by patients of the use of technology-based interventions regarding physical activity [56]. Their search yielded 7 studies on physical activity behavior, 6 of which (85.7%) showed improvement in physical activity with the use of technology (step counters or pedometers), although this effect did not reach statistical significance in the randomized trials of this group [57, 58]. More recently, a randomized trial from France of a telemedicine intervention program that collected data by means of a pedometer and connected scale failed to show any benefit on physical activity stemming from the use of the telemedicine intervention [59]. On the contrary, in another smaller-scale study from Canada, the use of telemedicine in conjunction with accelerometric recording of physical activity resulted in a significant increase of moderate-to-vigorous activity in patients awaiting MBS [60].

Yang et al. published a series of two papers on the use of a mobile application as a means of remote follow-up after MBS. The first publication was on the feasibility of implementation and the satisfaction on behalf of the users [61]. For this purpose, 52 post-MBS patients were recruited and were called to answer a series of multiple-choice and open-ended type questions. The application received favorable remarks on grounds of satisfaction, efficiency, learnability, and ease of use via the smartphone. With these initial repercussions, the researchers proceeded to the evaluation of the impact that this application had on weight loss and long-term complications, including micronutrient deficiencies [62]. For this purpose, they designed and implemented a prospective trial that included 44 patients in the interventional group and 43 patients in the control group (standard in-person follow-up). The investigators did not record significant differences between the two groups at 1 year postoperatively regarding weight loss (%EWL 47.1% vs. 50%, $p = 0.367$; %TWL 31.2% vs. 32.7%, $p = 0{,}459$), fat mass (32.8 vs. 33.2, $p = 0.902$), albumin levels ($p = 0.310$), calcium levels ($p = 0.181$), vitamin D, B12, and B1 levels ($p = 0.534$, 0.854, and 0.880, respectively), and readmission rates (13.6% vs. 2%, $p = 0.110$). As a result, the authors concluded that remote follow-up post-MBS by means of a smartphone application is equally effective with "traditional" postoperative surveillance, while it bears the additional benefits of reducing costs, saving patients' time, and allowing medical professionals to reallocate resources and focus on more severe medical problems. Undoubtedly, these results need to be validated in larger-scale studies with more patients and longer follow-up periods before widespread use.

The use of smartphone applications in MBS is paradoxically underdeveloped, regardless of the extensive use of smartphones and the familiarization of the population, particularly of the younger generations. A recent review retrieved 52 relevant applications [63]. More than half of them (56%) had payment-restricted content, whereas the vast majority (81%) necessitated the involvement of a medical/allied health professional. Their content comprised several categories, from clinic information (opening times, bookings, appointment administration) to patient information (description of different operations, pathways, and postoperative diets), from support (two-way communication with healthcare professional, chat functions, patient-specific dietary advice, push notifications) to tracking (BMI, weight loss, calories/diet, steps, exercise, fitness wearables support), and from education (guidelines, links to evidence, videos of surgical techniques, risk calculators) to dietary tools. The quality of the applications was evaluated by means of the Silberg score [64], and on a scale from 0 to 9, the mean score was 5.2.

As a closing remark of this section, it could be stated that the usefulness of embedded systems is more prominent in the immediate postoperative period rather than the long term, as documented by the existing literature. This could be attributed to the fact that short-term systems utilize easily countable attributes, such as the heart rate or the respiratory rate, while at the same time are intended to be utilized for a rather short period of time. The need for sustainable use presumably attenuates the effect of devices that record long-term results. In any case, research in both fields is at its beginning, and larger-scale usage of wearables and other embedded systems will elucidate their usefulness in assisting patients to assume healthier eating and lifestyle habits, with the ultimate goal being the minimization of weight recurrence in a clinically meaningful way.

9.3 APPLICATIONS OF ARTIFICIAL INTELLIGENCE IN METABOLIC BARIATRIC SURGERY

Artificial intelligence (AI) is the process followed by computer systems that emulate human cognitive functions, including learning and problem-solving, by means of algorithms and decision trees [65]. AI is an umbrella term that further covers methods that utilize input data to yield output categories utilizing specific feature extractors. These methods can be summarized as follows:

- Supervised machine learning (ML)—feature extractors are made by human operators and output categories are predefined also by human operators; the machine (i.e., the computer system) only learns to map the input data. Common "algorithms" that we all experience during our daily routine (i.e. product recommendations according to our web searches, financial accuracy, social media optimization and individualization, and predictive analytics based on previous events and experiences) belong to this category.
- Unsupervised ML—the machine creates its own output categories based on patterns of the input data.
- Natural language processing (NLP)—a process through which the machine extracts data from human language and makes decisions according to them. Chatbots, smart assistants, email automation and spam filtering, voice-to-text services and predictive text, as well as automated digital phone calls, are some relevant examples. NLP is considered a subcategory of unsupervised ML.
- Computer vision—the machine extracts data from still images or videos by means of segmentation of the digital input. Facial recognition, augmented reality applications, and traffic flow analysis constitute some examples. Computer vision is also considered a subordinate of unsupervised ML.
- Reinforced learning—outcomes are weighted based on the highest probability.
- Deep learning (DL)—its characteristic is that data are organized as a network of neurons with multiple layers, based on adjusted weighting that is determined by the machine. More frequently than not, layering and associations between input data and output outcomes are "invisible" by means of traditional statistical analysis. The most striking differentiation between ML and DL is that the latter "learns" from its own trial-and-error process, as such it demands a considerably larger amount of data (the so-called "big data"), which in turn translates into significantly more computational power.

An extensive analysis of the available evidence of the application of AI in MBS is beyond the scope of this chapter. Besides, there are several scoping and systematic reviews available that examine exactly this [66–68]. In brief, AI can be implemented in MBS in all phases of the care of the patient living with obesity, including preoperative evaluation, risk assessment, intra-operative management, clinical decision-making, prevention and management of complications, prediction of outcomes (weight loss, remission of associated health problems including T2DM, improvement of QoL), estimation of the duration of surgery, and quality improvement and education [67]. Regardless of the purpose of each specific AI application, every relevant study should follow some basic rules and requisites, including the mention of study design (retrospective or prospective), whether the target variable is numerical or not (regression in case it is continuous vs. classification in case it is categorical), and whether the evaluated algorithm was prognostic or diagnostic [69]. Additionally, they should include a training and a testing dataset appropriately allocated and ideally an external validation dataset. Finally, they should quantify the performance of the examined algorithm by reporting one or more metrics, including sensitivity, specificity, accuracy, precision, or the more sophisticated F1-score and area under the receiver operating characteristic curve (AUC or AUROC) [70]. Here, we will focus on the most clinically meaningful applications, which are connected more or less to embedded systems.

9.3.1 Intra-Operative Video Analysis

In 2019, Hashimoto et al. published their initial experience with using computer vision for analyzing intraoperative videos for LSG [71]. For this purpose, they used videos from 88 cases of LSG as their source of input data, with 70% randomly selected as the training set and the remaining 30% as the test set. The AI system was named as "SleeveNet" and it consisted of 2 DL components, a visual model based on Residual Neural Network and a temporal one based on long short-term memory (LSTM) neural networks. The 2-model system identified 7 discrete steps of the operation, based on the data of the digital videos: i) port placement, ii) liver retraction, iii) liver biopsy, iv) dissection of the gastrocolic ligament (i.e. mobilization of the greater curvature), v) stapling of the (remaining) stomach, vi) bagging (collection) of the specimen, and vii) final inspection of the staple line. Any deviation from these steps was registered as an "event". There were 4 types of events: bleeding (documented in 23.9% of cases), adhesiolysis (required in 8% of cases), additional steps (e.g. hiatal hernia repair, takedown of previous Nissen fundoplication) (17% of cases), and others (staple misfire in 1 case, 1.1%). The steps and events that were identified by the algorithm were compared to the assessment of human expert annotators and the mean concordance correlation coefficient was 0.862. In other words, there was good agreement between the AI model and the human experts. The mean accuracy of the combined temporal-spatial model in identifying the steps of LSG was 82% and the maximum accuracy reached 85.6%. In brief, this was considered a successful model of computer vision for evaluating the performance of surgical trainees in LSG.

9.3.2 Prediction of Leak and Venous Thromboembolism After MBS

Nudel et al. developed three AI prediction models for leak and venous thromboembolism (VTE) after MBS, based on artificial neural networks (ANN), gradient boosting machines (XBG), and conventional logistic regression (LR) [72]. Their source data included 436,807 patients from the MBSAQIP (Metabolic and Bariatric Surgery Accreditation and Quality Improvement Program) database over a two-year period, which was split into a training set (50%), a validation set (25%), and a testing population (25%). In the case of VTE, the AI algorithms were compared with BariClot, an established VTE risk assessment tool. Their software analysis was based on the Python programming language (version 3.6). As far as leak was concerned, the best performing predictive model was ANN [AUC 0.75 (fair performance), 95% CI 0.73–0.78], followed by XGB [AUC 0.70 (poor), 95% CI 0.68–0.72)], and LR [AUC 0.63 (poor), 95% CI 0.61–0.65]. Regarding VTE, the performance of all AI models was similar (AUC 0.65, 0.67, and 0.64 for ANN, XGB, and LR, respectively), however, it is noteworthy that all AI models significantly outperformed BariClot (AUC 0.56, $p<0.001$ for all 3 AI models). Moreover, the XGB model identified age, preoperative BMI, change in BMI, weight, hematocrit, height, a trainee as the first assistant, and albumin (in declining order of significance) as the most important factors predisposing to leak. The respective factors for VTE were preoperative BMI, age, weight, height, hematocrit, albumin, change in BMI, and past history of VTE. The authors concluded that the AI models had a better performance compared to traditional LR for predicting leaks. The performance of the AI algorithms was not as effective in the case of VTE, but still, they surpassed the established risk stratification method of BariClot.

9.3.3 Prediction of Complications After One-Anastomosis Gastric Bypass

One-anastomosis gastric bypass (OAGB) is a relatively old procedure that has been endorsed only recently by both official bariatric surgery organizations, IFSO (International Federation for the Surgery of Obesity and metabolic disorders) and ASMBS (American Society for Metabolic and Bariatric Surgery) [73, 74]. Sheikhtaheri et al. developed a clinical decision support system for predicting complications in the early postoperative period after OAGB. The study population consisted of patients who had undergone the operation in multiple bariatric centers in Iran over a 5-year period. The algorithm they selected for building their clinical decision tool was multilayer perceptron (MLP) network, an ANN model (DL). They built different MLPs in order to assess the incidence of complications at 10 days, 1 month, and 3 months postoperatively. The source data were randomly allocated into the training (70%), testing (15%), and validation (15%) datasets. Data balancing was achieved with the synthetic minority over-sampling technique (SMOTE) and the implemented programming language was R (version 3.2.3). Table 9.2 summarizes the performance of the algorithm in the test dataset by time point and performance metric.

TABLE 9.2
Performance of the Algorithm in the Test Dataset by Time Point and Performance Metric

Parameter	10 Days	3 Months	6 Months
Sensitivity	98.6%	93%	86.6%
Specificity	98.3%	98.4%	91.5%
Accuracy	98.4%	96%	89.3%
AUC	0.996	0.995	0.921

In brief, the algorithms achieved excellent performance (based on AUC) in predicting complications in the immediate postoperative period, as well as at 3 and 6 months.

9.3.4 Five-Year Weight Trajectory post-MBS (SOPHIA)

The SOPHIA study (and the ensuing clinical tool and smartphone application) is maybe one of the few examples that AI has found direct and realistic application in clinical practice to date [75]. This multinational study by Saux et al. utilized patient data from 10 prospective cohorts (including the Swedish Obese Subjects database, the largest bariatric database available with the longest-term surveillance) and two seminal randomized trials [the SleevePass (NCT00793143) and the SM-BOSS (NCT00356213)]. The training cohorts included patients from 2 centers in France. The total number of patients used to extract data was 10,231 and the total number of patient-years was 30602. These data were collectively used to develop an ML-based model that predicts weight loss for the first 5 postoperative years regarding the 3 most widely used bariatric operations (LSG, RYGB, and adjustable gastric band). Among 434 baseline characteristics, the authors selected 7 variables to build their predictive trajectories upon: height, weight, type of intervention, age, T2DM status, T2DM duration, and smoking status. The performance of the model was assessed by means of median absolute deviation (MAD), root mean squared error (RMSE), and mean difference between predicted and observed BMI, which were 2.8 Kg/m^2 (95% CI 2.6–3.0), 4.7 Kg/m^2 (95% CI 4.4–5.0), and –0.3 Kg/m^2 ± 4.7 (standard deviation – SD), respectively at the end of the 5 years. Consequently, the authors developed and released a handy smartphone application to which the user (clinician or patient) can upload the relevant information and get in return the predicted trajectory with minimum and maximum SD values at monthly increments.

9.3.5 Remission of T2DM post-RYGB

Cao et al. developed a DL-based model (convolutional neural network—CNN) to predict the remission of T2DM, based on 8.057 patients from the Scandinavian Obesity Surgery Registry (SOReg) [76]. For this purpose, the population was randomly divided into a training set (80%) and a test set (20%). The predictive capability of the model was compared to traditional currently available scores, including

DiaRem, Ad-DiaRem, DiaBetter, and IMS (individualized metabolic surgery). The model achieved an AUC of 0.83 for pharmacological remission and 0.82 for complete remission. The respective AUC values in the test dataset for the traditional tools were 0.75 (DiaRem), 0,74 (Ad-DiaRem), 0.74 (DiaBetter), and 0.76 (IMS). In other words, the DL algorithm achieved 9–11% better predictive performance than the established tools.

9.3.6 Prediction of Gastroesophageal Reflux Disease After LSG

The development of gastroesophageal reflux disease (GERD) is one of the most feared long-term complications of this operation. Emile et al. developed and validated an AI-based model for predicting the manifestations of this complication after examining a series of algorithms on data from 441 patients [77]. The best-performing algorithm among the examined ones was the Ensemble model, which reached an AUROC of 0.92, a sensitivity of 79.2%, a specificity of 86.1%, a positive predictive value of 85.1%, and a negative predictive value of 80.5%. The predictors for GERD with their respective numerical cutoff values were the following: age (42 years, OR 1.03, 95% CI 0.94–0.99); weight (140.1 Kg, OR 1.02, 95% CI 0.99–1.04); BMI (52.1 Kg/m^2, OR 1.1, 95% CI 0.86–0.98); distance from the pylorus (3 cm, OR 1.25, OR 0.66–0.98); and bougie size (38 Fr, OR 1.74, 95% CI 1.39–2.18). Among these factors, some are non-modifiable (low- vs. high-risk patients *a priori*), whereas others (notably the bougie size and the distance from the pylorus) are modifiable. As such, the "risky" thresholds of these factors are determined by the AI model in order to minimize the presentation of GERD in the future. The model is available online and free to download (https://www.dropbox.com/sh/z1nqd7jtpmp97z2/AADhgez0bY-tkhOqixSl0MMca?dl=0).

9.4 FUTURE PERSPECTIVES AND ETHICAL CONSIDERATIONS

The advent of AI paves the way for new endeavors, particularly in combination with embedded systems, which will be able to transmit a wealth of data in real time. For example, there are commercially available kits that comprise a water bottle sensor to remind the post-MBS patient to drink water, a pill bottle sensor to remind the patient to take their vitamin and mineral supplements, a wearable that quantifies daily activity and measures HR, RR, and even blood pressure and oxygen saturation, and a scale which measures weight, BMI, and fat mass [78]. All these components are interconnected via Bluetooth and further linked to a smartphone application, which prompts the user at regular intervals throughout the day to keep up with their post-operative scheme.

A more advanced example of the combination of AI with embedded systems is the integration of AI applications in robotic surgery platforms, with an emphasis on computer vision. To date, there are no publications specifically referring to MBS, but we can extrapolate from relevant applications in general surgery [79]. In this context, data pertaining to patient characteristics, intraoperative digital video, robotic instrument kinematics, and robotic sensors can be integrated and analyzed by one or more AI algorithms and consequently provide intraoperative feedback, navigation, and

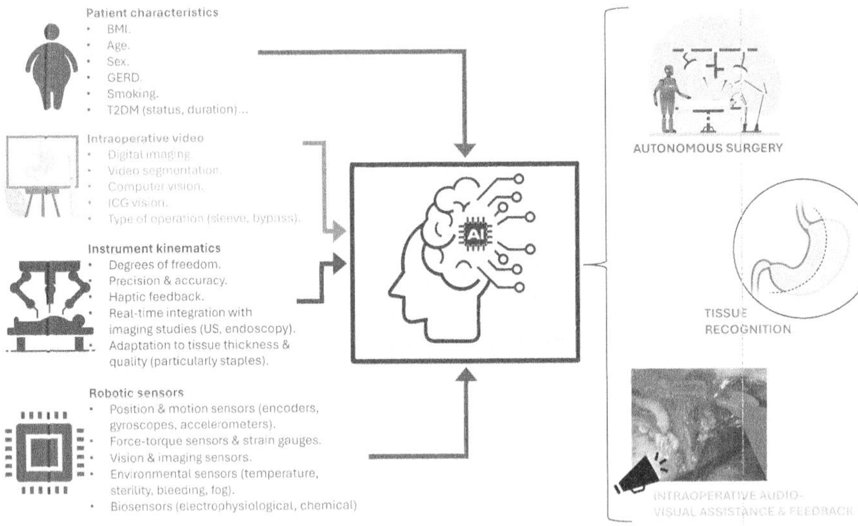

FIGURE 9.1 Graphical representation of potential collaborations between embedded systems and artificial intelligence in metabolic bariatric surgery.

assistance (by real-time annotation, for example), surgical skills assessment, and a scaffold toward autonomous surgery. Figure 9.1 graphically depicts these concepts in MBS.

The SAGES (Society of American Gastrointestinal and Endoscopic Surgeons) recently published a white paper on the definition of digital surgery, which is the epitome of the integration of embedded systems in the practice of surgery [80]. According to it, digital surgery, "in its simplest form, inserts a computer interface between the surgeon and the patient". In turn, this has multiple ramifications, from advanced visualization to enhanced instrumentation, from data capture to data analytics by means of AI/ML, and from connectivity via teleconference to robotic surgical platforms. In essence, it captures the concepts analyzed in this chapter, which apply specifically to MBS.

Another currently developing concept is that of collaborative intelligence [81, 82]. The starting point for this concept is the assumption (or the recognition) that neither humans nor machines are capable of carrying out all types of tasks with the same high-quality efficiency. Consequently, based on the interacting principles of complementarity, sustained interaction, and shared objective, collaborative intelligence might achieve better, upgraded results than the sum of human ingenuity and machine consistency.

Amidst these fascinating developments awaiting to be conquered anytime soon, the responsible clinician and investigator has the moral and professional obligation to endorse the ethical dimensions of routinely combining embedded systems and AI in clinical practice. Parameters such as human autonomy, explicability and transparency, patient privacy and data protection, fairness (which additionally includes bias and discrimination, as well as unemployment and workforce displacement), and ultimately prevention of harm (the cornerstone of Medicine that had been recognized since the era of Hippocrates), are indispensable components of the ethics governing AI [83]. These principles, of course, do not apply exclusively to the field of MBS but are universal across the spectrum of Surgery and Medicine. Most importantly, these principles give rise to a whole new academic field, i.e., digital humanism [84, 85], which has philosophical, political, and above all scientific extensions.

Finally, one should take into consideration the medicolegal repercussions of the increasing penetration of AI and embedded systems into clinical practice, the more prominent issues among them being accountability and liability [86]. Let's take for example the case that an AI algorithm recommends a specific bariatric operation in a patient living with obesity, who suffers from GERD at the same time, with the aim to maximize weight loss and simultaneously minimize the risk of short- and long-term complications. Subsequently, depending on the AI recommendation, the accuracy of the prediction of the algorithm, the eventual decision of the surgeon, and the patient outcome, there are eight possible scenarios. In the first four scenarios, the AI algorithm recommends the "standard of care", that is, let's say, RYGB. The surgeon decides to follow the AI recommendation and the patient has an uneventful postoperative course. The outcome is no injury and no liability. In case the surgeon decides to do an alternative operation (let's say LSG), based on their own experience and personal bias, and the patient develops Barrett's esophagus and esophageal cancer after some years, then there is clearly injury (cancer) and liability of the surgeon (they acted against the standard of care and the recommendations of the AI algorithm). Conversely, if the surgeon follows the recommendation of the algorithm and the patient develops esophageal cancer again after some years, then there is injury, but no liability, since they acted based on evidence-based recommendations. Finally, if the surgeon refuses to follow the recommendation of the algorithm but the patient is healthy after many years, there is neither injury nor liability. The situation gets more perplexing in case the AI algorithm recommends a nonstandard care operation, i.e. LSG in this very patient with pre-existing GERD. If the surgeon follows the recommendation and the patient loses weight without major complications, then neither injury nor liability is set. The same holds true in case the surgeon decides to reject the recommendation of the algorithm and the outcome is still favorable. But who will be considered liable in case the surgeon accepts the algorithmic recommendation and the patient develops esophageal cancer? Even worse, what will happen in the scenario that the same adverse outcome occurs after the surgeon has rejected the suggestion of the algorithm and has performed a standard-of-care RYGB operation? The same scenarios can be reproduced if we consider the readings of an embedded system in place of the recommendation of the AI algorithm. These simplified and crude examples with a multitude of outcomes denote that the road from conceptualization to the actual implementation of embedded systems and AI into clinical practice is far more complicated than simply considering it as a Swiss army knife ready to solve all our problems. Above all, they remind us that clinical judgment is the ultimate determinant of our professional integrity as surgeons. But this takes again back to the Hippocratic aphorism: *ars longa, vita brevis*.

REFERENCES

1. World Obesity Federation [Internet]. [cited 2023 Oct 23]. *World Obesity Atlas* 2023. Available from: https://www.worldobesity.org/resources/resource-library/world-obesity-atlas-2023
2. Bray GA. Beyond BMI. *Nutrients*. 2023 May 10;15(10):2254.
3. De Lorenzo A, Gratteri S, Gualtieri P, Cammarano A, Bertucci P, Di Renzo L. Why primary obesity is a disease? *J Transl Med*. 2019 May 22;17(1):169.
4. Rosen H. Is obesity a disease or a behavior abnormality? Did the AMA get it right? *Mo Med*. 2014;111(2):104–8.
5. Sharma AM. M, M, M & M: A mnemonic for assessing obesity. *Obes Rev Off J Int Assoc Study Obes*. 2010 Nov;11(11):808–9.
6. Gofton C, Upendran Y, Zheng MH, George J. MAFLD: How is it different from NAFLD? *Clin Mol Hepatol*. 2023 Feb;29(Suppl):S17–31.
7. Patel AV, Patel KS, Teras LR. Excess body fatness and cancer risk: A summary of the epidemiologic evidence. *Surg Obes Relat Dis Off J Am Soc Bariatr Surg*. 2023 Jul;19(7):742–5.
8. Courcoulas AP, King WC, Belle SH, Berk P, Flum DR, Garcia L, et al. Seven-year weight trajectories and health outcomes in the longitudinal assessment of bariatric surgery (LABS) study. *JAMA Surg*. 2018 May;153(5):427.
9. Courcoulas AP, Gallagher JW, Neiberg RH, Eagleton EB, DeLany JP, Lang W, et al. Bariatric surgery vs lifestyle intervention for diabetes treatment: 5-year outcomes from a randomized trial. *J Clin Endocrinol Metab*. 2020 Mar 1;105(3):866–76.
10. Kirwan JP, Courcoulas AP, Cummings DE, Goldfine AB, Kashyap SR, Simonson DC, et al. Diabetes remission in the alliance of randomized trials of medicine versus metabolic surgery in type 2 diabetes (ARMMS-T2D). *Diab Care*. 2022 Jul 7;45(7):1574–83.
11. Schauer PR, Bhatt DL, Kirwan JP, Wolski K, Aminian A, Brethauer SA, et al. Bariatric surgery versus intensive medical therapy for diabetes – 5-year outcomes. *N Engl J Med*. 2017 Feb 16;376(7):641–51.
12. Alghamdi S, Mirghani H, Alhazmi K, Alatawi AM, Brnawi H, Alrasheed T, et al. Roux-en-Y gastric bypass and laparoscopic sleeve gastrectomy effects on obesity comorbidities: A systematic review and meta-analysis. *Front Surg*. 2022;9:953804.
13. Nielsen HJ, Nedrebø BG, Fosså A, Andersen JR, Assmus J, Dagsland VH, et al. Seven-year trajectories of body weight, quality of life and comorbidities following Roux-en-Y gastric bypass and sleeve gastrectomy. *Int J Obes 2005*. 2022 Apr;46(4):739–49.
14. Aminian A, Zajichek A, Arterburn DE, Wolski KE, Brethauer SA, Schauer PR, et al. Association of metabolic surgery with major adverse cardiovascular outcomes in patients with type 2 diabetes and obesity. *JAMA*. 2019 Oct 1;322(13):1271–82.
15. Sutanto A, Wungu CDK, Susilo H, Sutanto H. Reduction of major adverse cardiovascular events (MACE) after bariatric surgery in patients with obesity and cardiovascular diseases: A systematic review and meta-analysis. *Nutrients*. 2021 Oct 12;13(10):3568.
16. Aminian A, Wilson R, Al-Kurd A, Tu C, Milinovich A, Kroh M, et al. Association of bariatric surgery with cancer risk and mortality in adults with obesity. *JAMA*. 2022 Jun 28;327(24):2423–33.
17. Wilson R, Aminian A. Obesity-associated cancer risk reduction after metabolic surgery: insights from the SPLENDID study and the path forward. *Surg Obes Relat Dis Off J Am Soc Bariatr Surg*. 2023 Jul;19(7):788–93.
18. Kim MS, Kim JY, Song YS, Hong S, Won HH, Kim WJ, et al. Association of bariatric surgery with indicated and unintended outcomes: An umbrella review and meta-analysis for risk-benefit assessment. *Obes Rev Off J Int Assoc Study Obes*. 2024 Mar;25(3):e13670.

19. Doumouras AG, Hong D, Lee Y, Tarride JE, Paterson JM, Anvari M. Association between bariatric surgery and all-cause mortality: A population-based matched cohort study in a universal health care system. *Ann Intern Med.* 2020 Nov 3;173(9):694–703.
20. Carlsson LMS, Sjöholm K, Jacobson P, Andersson-Assarsson JC, Svensson PA, Taube M, et al. Life expectancy after bariatric surgery in the Swedish obese subjects study. *N Engl J Med.* 2020 Oct 15;383(16):1535–43.
21. Pantelis A, Lapatsanis DP. Metabolic bariatric surgery in face of new anti-obesity medications-10 + 1 challenges. *Metab Target Organ Damage.* 2023 Oct 16;3(4), 1–18.
22. Ali OI, Abdelraouf OR, El-Gendy AM, Abdelgalil AA, Abdelaal AK, Dahlawi HA, et al. Efficacy of telehealth core exercises during COVID-19 after bariatric surgery: A randomized controlled trial. *Eur J Phys Rehabil Med.* 2022 Dec;58(6):845–52.
23. Lodewijks Y, Nienhuijs S. Bariatric tele-screening during the COVID-19 pandemic: Holding back for direct approval? *Obes Surg.* 2022 Apr;32(4):1072–6.
24. Parnell KE, Philip J, Billmeier SE, Trus TL. The effects of using telemedicine for introductory bariatric surgery seminars during the COVID-19 pandemic. *Surg Endosc.* 2023 Jul;37(7):5509–15.
25. Sockalingam S, Leung SE, Ma C, Tomlinson G, Hawa R, Wnuk S, et al. Efficacy of telephone-based cognitive behavioral therapy for weight loss, disordered eating, and psychological distress after bariatric surgery: A randomized clinical trial. *JAMA Netw Open.* 2023 Aug 1;6(8):e2327099.
26. Daouadji-Ghazouani A, Aron-Wisnewsky J, Torcivia A, Irigoin-Guichandut M, Poitou C, Faucher P, et al. Follow-up, safety, and satisfaction with tele-bariatric follow-up implemented during the COVID-19 French lockdown: A 2-year follow-up study. *Obes Surg.* 2023 Apr;33(4):1083–91.
27. van Veldhuisen SL, van Boxel MF, Wiezer MJ, van Veen RN, de Castro SMM, Swank DJ, et al. Evaluation of CPAP adherence in bariatric patients diagnosed with obstructive sleep apnea: Outcomes of a multicenter cohort study. *Sleep Breath Schlaf Atm.* 2023 Dec;27(2):535–44.
28. Katasani T, Holt G, Al-Khyatt W, Idris I. Peri- and postoperative outcomes for obstructive sleep apnoea patients after bariatric surgery – A systematic review and meta-analysis. *Obes Surg.* 2023 Jul;33(7):2016–24.
29. Morey-Vargas OL, Aminian A, Steckner K, Zhou K, Kashyap SR, Cetin D, et al. Perioperative management of diabetes in patients undergoing bariatric and metabolic surgery: A narrative review and the Cleveland Clinic practical recommendations. *Surg Obes Relat Dis Off J Am Soc Bariatr Surg.* 2022 Aug;18(8):1087–101.
30. Schlottmann F, Dreifuss NH, Masrur MA. Telehealth: Increasing access to bariatric surgery in minority populations. *Obes Surg.* 2022 Apr;32(4):1370–2.
31. Mills J, Liebert C, Pratt J, Earley M, Eisenberg D. Complete telehealth for multidisciplinary preoperative workup does not delay time to metabolic and bariatric surgery: A pilot study. *Obes Surg.* 2022 Nov;32(11):3605–10.
32. Philips [Internet]. [cited 2024 May 12]. *Philips Healthdot.* Available from: https://www.philips.com.tr/healthcare/e/healthdot
33. Jacobs F, Scheerhoorn J, Mestrom E, van der Stam J, Bouwman RA, Nienhuijs S. Reliability of heart rate and respiration rate measurements with a wireless accelerometer in postbariatric recovery. *PloS One.* 2021;16(4):e0247903.
34. Bland JM, Altman DG. Statistical methods for assessing agreement between two methods of clinical measurement. *Lancet Lond Engl.* 1986 Feb 8;1(8476):307–10.
35. Kant N, Peters GM, Voorthuis BJ, Groothuis-Oudshoorn CGM, Koning MV, Witteman BPL, et al. Continuous vital sign monitoring using a wearable patch sensor in obese patients: A validation study in a clinical setting. *J Clin Monit Comput.* 2022 Oct;36(5):1449–59.

36. Mestrom EHJ, van der Stam JA, Nienhuijs SW, de Hingh IHJT, Boer AK, van Riel NAW, et al. Postoperative circadian patterns in wearable sensor measured heart rate: A prospective observational study. *J Clin Monit Comput*. 2024 Feb;38(1):147–56.
37. Scheerhoorn J, van Ede L, Luyer MDP, Buise MP, Bouwman RA, Nienhuijs SW. Postbariatric early discharge controlled by healthdot (PEACH) trial: study protocol for a preference-based randomized trial. *Trials*. 2022 Jan 21;23(1):67.
38. Schaffner TJ, Wilkes M, Laverty R, Schwab SD, Zahradka N, Pugmire J, et al. Remote patient monitoring to facilitate same-day discharge after laparoscopic sleeve gastrectomy: A pilot evaluation. *Surg Obes Relat Dis Off J Am Soc Bariatr Surg*. 2023 Sep;19(9):1067–74.
39. Nijland LMG, de Castro SMM, Vogel M, Coumou JWF, van Rutte PWJ, van Veen RN. Feasibility of same-day discharge after laparoscopic roux-en-Y gastric bypass using remote monitoring. *Obes Surg*. 2021 Jul;31(7):2851–8.
40. Nijland LMG, van Veen RN, Ruys AT, van Veldhuisen CL, Geerdink TH, de Castro SMM. Feasibility of postoperative home monitoring using video consultation and vital sign monitoring of bariatric patients. *Obes Surg*. 2020 Jun;30(6):2369–74.
41. van Ede ES, Scheerhoorn J, Bonomi AG, Buise MP, Bouwman RA, Nienhuijs SW. Continuous remote monitoring in post-bariatric surgery patients: Development of an early warning protocol. *Surg Obes Relat Dis Off J Am Soc Bariatr Surg*. 2022 Nov;18(11):1298–303.
42. van Ede ES, Scheerhoorn J, Buise MP, Bouwman RA, Nienhuijs SW. Telemonitoring for perioperative care of outpatient bariatric surgery: Preference-based randomized clinical trial. *PloS One*. 2023;18(2):e0281992.
43. van Ede ES, Scheerhoorn J, Schonck FMJF, van der Stam JA, Buise MP, Nienhuijs SW, et al. Lessons learned from telemonitoring in an outpatient bariatric surgery pathway-secondary outcomes of a patient preference clinical trial. *Obes Surg*. 2023 Sep;33(9):2725–33.
44. Caballero A, Tarascó J, Moreno P, López-Vendrell L, Pellitero S, Martínez E, et al. Implementation of a same-day discharge bariatric surgery program and follow-up with a telemonitoring platform. *Cirugia Espanola*. 2023 Dec;101(12):841–6.
45. Ostrovsky V, Knobler H, Lazar LO, Pines G, Kuniavsky T, Cohen L, et al. Persistent post-bariatric-surgery hypoglycemia: A long-term follow-up reassessment. *Nutr Metab Cardiovasc Dis*. 2023 Jun 1;33(6):1197–205.
46. Athavale A, Ganipisetti VM. Postbariatric surgery hypoglycemia. In: *StatPearls* [Internet]. Treasure Island (FL): StatPearls Publishing; 2024 [cited 2024 May 13]. Available from: https://www.ncbi.nlm.nih.gov/books/NBK592417/
47. Carpentieri GB, Gonçalves SEAB, Mourad WM, Pinto LGC, Zanella MT. Hypoglycemia post bariatric surgery: Drugs with different mechanisms of action to treat a unique disorder. *Arch Endocrinol Metab*. 2023;67(3):442–9.
48. Mulla C, Zavitsanou S, Laguna Sanz A, Pober D, Richardson L, Walcott P, et al. A randomized, placebo-controlled double-blind trial of a closed-loop glucagon system for postbariatric hypoglycemia. *J Clin Endocrinol Metab* [Internet]. 2020 Apr 1 [cited 2024 May 13];105(4). Available from: https://pubmed.ncbi.nlm.nih.gov/31714583/
49. Rozo A, Moeyersons J, Morales J, Garcia van der Westen R, Lijnen L, Smeets C, et al. Data augmentation and transfer learning for data quality assessment in respiratory monitoring. *Front Bioeng Biotechnol*. 2022;10:806761.
50. Bartlett VL, Ross JS, Shah ND, Ciaccio L, Akar JG, Noseworthy PA, et al. Physical activity, patient-reported symptoms, and clinical events: Insights into postprocedural recovery from personal digital devices. *Cardiovasc Digit Health J*. 2021 Aug;2(4): 212–21.

51. Goldstein SP, Thomas JG, Vithiananthan S, Blackburn GA, Jones DB, Webster J, et al. Multi-sensor ecological momentary assessment of behavioral and psychosocial predictors of weight loss following bariatric surgery: Study protocol for a multicenter prospective longitudinal evaluation. *BMC Obes.* 2018;5:27.
52. Shiffman S, Stone AA, Hufford MR. Ecological momentary assessment. *Annu Rev Clin Psychol.* 2008;4:1–32.
53. Huang EY, Chung D, Hollandsworth HM, Goldhaber NH, Robles L, Horgan M, et al. Bite by byte: Can fitness wearables help bariatric patients lose more weight after surgery? *Surg Endosc.* 2023 Aug;37(8):6526–31.
54. Versteegden DPA, Van Himbeeck MJJ, Luyer MD, van Montfort G, de Zoete JPJGM, Smulders JF, et al. A randomized clinical trial evaluating eHealth in bariatric surgery. *Surg Endosc.* 2023 Oct;37(10):7625–33.
55. Zabatiero J, Smith A, Gucciardi DF, Hamdorf Am JM, Taylor SF, Hill K. Patterns of change in device-based physical activity and sedentary time following bariatric surgery: A longitudinal observational study. *Obes Surg.* 2021 Jul;31(7):3015–25.
56. Hayotte M, Gioda J, d'Arripe-Longueville F. Effects and acceptability of technology-based physical activity interventions in bariatric surgery: A scoping review. *Obes Surg.* 2022 Jul;32(7):2445–56.
57. Wiklund M, Sundqvist E, Fagevik Olsén M. Physical activity in the immediate postoperative phase in patients undergoing roux-en-Y gastric bypass-a randomized controlled trial. *Obes Surg.* 2015 Dec;25(12):2245–50.
58. Creel DB, Schuh LM, Reed CA, Gomez AR, Hurst LA, Stote J, et al. A randomized trial comparing two interventions to increase physical activity among patients undergoing bariatric surgery. *Obes Silver Spring Md.* 2016 Aug;24(8):1660–8.
59. Lurbe I Puerto K, Bruzzi M, Rives-Lange C, Poghosyan T, Bretault M, Chatellier G, et al. My good trip, a telemedicine intervention for physical activity recovery after bariatric surgery: Randomized controlled trial. *JMIR Form Res.* 2023 Mar 28;7:e26077.
60. Baillot A, St-Pierre M, Lapointe J, Bernard P, Bond D, Romain AJ, et al. Acceptability and feasibility of the telehealth bariatric behavioral intervention to increase physical activity: Protocol for a single-case experimental study. *JMIR Res Protoc.* 2022 Sep 29;11(9):e39633.
61. Yang C, Kessler M, Taebi N, Moorthy P, Reissfelder C, Otto M, et al. Smartphone application-based follow-up care of patients after bariatric surgery: A mixed-method study of usability. *Digit Health.* 2022;8:1–8.
62. Yang C, Kessler M, Taebi N, Hetjens M, Reissfelder C, Otto M, et al. Remote follow-up with a mobile application is equal to traditional outpatient follow-up after bariatric surgery: The BELLA pilot trial. *Obes Surg.* 2023 Jun;33(6):1702–9.
63. Thomas C, Simmons E, Musbahi A, Small P, Courtney M. A contemporary review of smart phone applications in bariatric and metabolic surgery: An underdeveloped support service. *Obes Surg.* 2023 Jun;33(6):1866–75.
64. Eunjoo J, Park HA, Min YH, Kim HY. Analysis of the information quality of Korean obesity-management smartphone applications. *Healthc Inform Res.* 2014 Jan 3;20:23–9.
65. Loftus TJ, Tighe PJ, Filiberto AC, Efron PA, Brakenridge SC, Mohr AM, et al. Artificial intelligence and surgical decision-making. *JAMA Surg.* 2020 Feb 1;155(2):148–58.
66. Pantelis AG, Stravodimos GK, Lapatsanis DP. A scoping review of artificial intelligence and machine learning in bariatric and metabolic surgery: Current status and future perspectives. *Obes Surg.* 2021 Oct 1;31(10):4555–63.
67. Bellini V, Valente M, Turetti M, Del Rio P, Saturno F, Maffezzoni M, et al. Current applications of artificial intelligence in bariatric surgery. *Obes Surg.* 2022 Aug 1;32(8):2717–33.

68. Bektaş M, Reiber BMM, Pereira JC, Burchell GL, van der Peet DL. Artificial intelligence in bariatric surgery: Current status and future perspectives. *Obes Surg*. 2022 Aug 1;32(8):2772–83.
69. Luo W, Phung D, Tran T, Gupta S, Rana S, Karmakar C, et al. Guidelines for developing and reporting machine learning predictive models in biomedical research: A multidisciplinary view. *J Med Internet Res*. 2016 Dec 16;18(12):e323.
70. Shah NH, Milstein A, Bagley SC. Making machine learning models clinically useful. *JAMA*. 2019 Oct 8;322(14):1351–2.
71. Hashimoto DA, Rosman G, Witkowski ER, Stafford C, Navarette-Welton AJ, Rattner DW, et al. Computer vision analysis of intraoperative video: Automated recognition of operative steps in laparoscopic sleeve gastrectomy. *Ann Surg*. 2019 Sep;270(3):414–21.
72. Nudel J, Bishara AM, de Geus SWL, Patil P, Srinivasan J, Hess DT, et al. Development and validation of machine learning models to predict gastrointestinal leak and venous thromboembolism after weight loss surgery: An analysis of the MBSAQIP database. *Surg Endosc*. 2021 Jan;35(1):182–91.
73. De Luca M, Piatto G, Merola G, Himpens J, Chevallier JM, Carbajo MA, et al. IFSO update position statement on one anastomosis gastric bypass (OAGB). *Obes Surg*. 2021 Jul;31(7):3251–78.
74. Ghiassi S, Nimeri A, Aleassa EM, Grover BT, Eisenberg D, Carter J, et al. American society for metabolic and bariatric surgery position statement on one-anastomosis gastric bypass. *Surg Obes Relat Dis Off J Am Soc Bariatr Surg*. 2023 Nov 23;S1550–7289(23):00793–1.
75. Saux P, Bauvin P, Raverdy V, Teigny J, Verkindt H, Soumphonphakdy T, et al. Development and validation of an interpretable machine learning-based calculator for predicting 5-year weight trajectories after bariatric surgery: A multinational retrospective cohort SOPHIA study. *Lancet Digit Health*. 2023 Oct 1;5(10):e692–702.
76. Cao Y, Näslund I, Näslund E, Ottosson J, Montgomery S, Stenberg E. Using a convolutional neural network to predict remission of diabetes after gastric bypass surgery: Machine learning study from the Scandinavian obesity surgery register. *JMIR Med Inform*. 2021 Aug 19;9(8):e25612.
77. Emile SH, Ghareeb W, Elfeki H, El Sorogy M, Fouad A, Elrefai M. Development and validation of an artificial intelligence-based model to predict gastroesophageal reflux disease after sleeve gastrectomy. *Obes Surg* [Internet]. 2022 Aug [cited 2023 Nov 14];32(8). Available from: https://pubmed.ncbi.nlm.nih.gov/35596915/
78. Sheth A, Jaimini U, Thirunarayan K, Banerjee T. Augmented personalized health: How smart data with IoTs and AI is about to change healthcare. *RTSI Int Forum Res Technol Soc Ind*. 2017 Sep;2017. https://doi.org/10.1109/RTSI.2017.8065963
79. Knudsen JE, Ghaffar U, Ma R, Hung AJ. Clinical applications of artificial intelligence in robotic surgery. *J Robot Surg*. 2024 Mar 1;18(1):102.
80. SAGES Digital Surgery Working Group, Ali JT, Yang G, Green CA, Reed BL, Madani A, et al. Defining digital surgery: a SAGES white paper. *Surg Endosc*. 2024 Feb;38(2):475–87.
81. Bhatt AB, Bae J. Collaborative Intelligence to catalyze the digital transformation of healthcare. *Npj Digit Med*. 2023 Sep 25;6(1):1–4.
82. Schleiger E, Mason C, Naughtin C, Reeson A, Paris C. Collaborative intelligence: A scoping review of current applications. *Appl Artif Intell*. 2024 Dec 31;38(1):2327890.

83. The ethical issues of the application of artificial intelligence in healthcare: A systematic scoping review | AI and Ethics [Internet]. [cited 2024 May 16]. Available from: https://link.springer.com/article/10.1007/s43681-021-00131-7
84. Digital Humanism [Internet]. [cited 2024 May 16]. Available from: https://link.springer.com/book/10.1007/978-3-031-12482-2
85. Introduction to Digital Humanism [Internet]. [cited 2024 May 16]. Available from: https://link.springer.com/book/10.1007/978-3-031-45304-5
86. Price WN II, Gerke S, Cohen IG. Potential liability for physicians using artificial intelligence. *JAMA*. 2019 Nov 12;322(18):1765–6.

10 Integration of Machine Learning Techniques with Multi-Criteria Decision-Making for a Better Treatment

Inci Albayrak, Jale Sade, and Hale Gonce Kocken

10.1 INTRODUCTION

Health is one of the most valuable assets that humanity possesses. A healthy body, mind, and living environment have a significant impact on a person's happiness, well-being, productivity, and overall quality of life. Medicine offers a variety of health services, including preventive, developmental, and rehabilitative health services, as well as diagnostic and treatment services. In the medical field, the most crucial factor in diagnosis, treatment, and all other processes that determine people's health is the decision-making process that prioritizes up-to-date and reliable information and medical ethics. Medical professionals and decision-makers frequently struggle with decision-making problems when it comes to enhancing the provision of healthcare or arriving at accurate and reliable decisions that will benefit patients. Enhancing this decision-making process can significantly improve both individual and societal health. Accurate and reliable information, combined with appropriate decision-making processes, can elevate all areas of health, from individual to public health, to the highest possible level [1].

Decision-making in medicine is a relatively new area of study that has gradually developed over time, much like all processes in the healthcare field [2]. Conscious and sometimes unconscious decision-making processes primarily carry out the diagnosis and treatment of illnesses. These processes involve identifying the patient's most significant complaints, ordering the necessary tests, evaluating the results, and ultimately determining the appropriate treatment. Improving decision-making processes can make important contributions to both individual and public health in the body, soul, and environment.

The decision-making process entails selecting the most beneficial option from a set of available options while considering multiple factors at the same time. Problems from the real world often involve numerous crucial factors or criteria that can have an

DOI: 10.1201/9781003508199-10

impact on decision-making outcomes either directly or indirectly. When human life is at stake, the importance of making the right decision increases manifold. Deciding which drug, treatment, or medical equipment to utilize can be a complex problem with multiple criteria, and the effects can deeply impact multiple parties. The MCDM approach has been evolving since the early 1970s and has emerged as an important research topic for addressing complex decision-making issues that involve multiple criteria [3]. MCDM theory is a computational method that involves evaluating and selecting the finest option among a range of alternatives based on preferences and multi-criteria. It is used in a variety of fields to identify the optimal solution to a problem where more than one parameter needs to be taken into account and user experiences alone cannot decide the solution. The approach provides a ranking outcome depending on the chosen criteria, their associated values, and allocated weights [4]. The MCDM analysis follows a general procedure, which is illustrated in Figure 10.1. Patients, physicians, hospital administrators, and engineers can all benefit greatly from the application of MCDM theory in biomedical engineering and healthcare [5–10].

In today's era, AI is one of the most often utilized methods for making decisions. AI comprises algorithms using machine to demonstrate human abilities including creativity, learning, reasoning, and classification. AI algorithms use ML and deep learning (DL) to try to replicate human intellect [11]. The healthcare sector's increased data availability has enabled recent successes with AI applications. AI technology can reveal clinical information buried behind large, complex data sets, which greatly aids physicians' judgment and decision-making. This process expedites the diagnosis of diseases and the reporting of pertinent examinations, thereby reducing the time patients spend in healthcare institutions. Recent studies have demonstrated that AI holds promise to contribute significantly to the diagnosis, treatment, monitoring, and classification of various diseases, as well as identifying risky

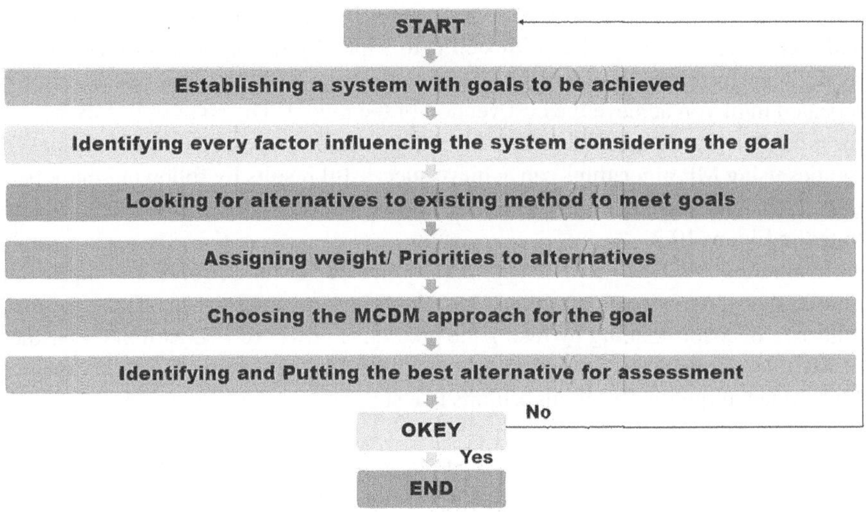

FIGURE 10.1 Standard operating procedure for MCDM analysis.

situations [12–21]. Furthermore, AI has proven to be useful in drug, device, and vaccine production, medical education, and health management [22–26].

Many researchers are conducting experiments using ML algorithms to diagnose diseases. The reason why ML algorithms are preferred is that they provide more accurate and faster results at a lower cost for diagnosing different diseases. ML algorithms combine data from various sources and increase their predictive power thanks to their capacity for handling vast volumes of data.

Essentially, ML algorithms fall into two broad categories: supervised and unsupervised learning [27]. The unsupervised learning algorithms do not predefine the classes. Automatically creating classification labels is the primary goal of unsupervised learning. These algorithms search for similarities between data pieces to determine their potential for grouping and classification. Known as clusters, these groups embody an entire variety of machine-learning approaches for clustering. Supervised algorithms predefine the classes. Humans create these classes from a limited set, assigning a label to a specific portion of the data that corresponds to one of these classifications. Finding patterns and creating mathematical models is the job of the ML algorithm. After that, these models are assessed according to how well they can forecast variances in the actual data [28]. Supervised learning is a useful tool for identifying the connections between patient data (input) and predetermined outcomes (output) to find solutions for healthcare issues. A supervised ML model divides the learning process into six steps. In the first step, the data is collected, cleaned, and organized; feature engineering is performed as needed, and statistical analyses and visualizations are conducted to enhance the data. The second step involves dividing the prepared data set. Typically, the data is separated into two groups: testing and training. While the model is learning from the training data, the performance of the overall model is measured using test data. The third step is to select an appropriate ML model depending on the data type, problem type, and performance goals. The fourth step is that the selected model starts to learn from the training data. In this process, the model evolves by extracting patterns from the data and predicting outcomes. The fifth step is to adjust hyperparameters to improve the model's performance or solve problems such as overfitting. This process can be repeated until you achieve the best version of the model. The sixth step is to evaluate the model on test data, and then reliable results can be presented to decision-makers. Studies using ML algorithms can achieve successful results by following these basic steps [29]. The supervised ML process follows a general procedure, which is illustrated in Figure 10.2.

Integrating MCDM and ML techniques can be useful in solving complex and multidimensional decision-making problems more effectively. This approach improves decision-making by fusing the predictive power of ML with the robustness of MCDM. To increase prediction accuracy and decision support, we can integrate MCDM techniques with ML algorithms like support vector machines, decision trees, and neural networks.

The process of evaluating and comparing ML techniques can be considered to be a very complex and qualitative problem, and the role of the created ML models can remain limited while making decisions. Many advanced hybrid models obtain various metric outcomes, but the trade-offs and conflicts between the criteria make it

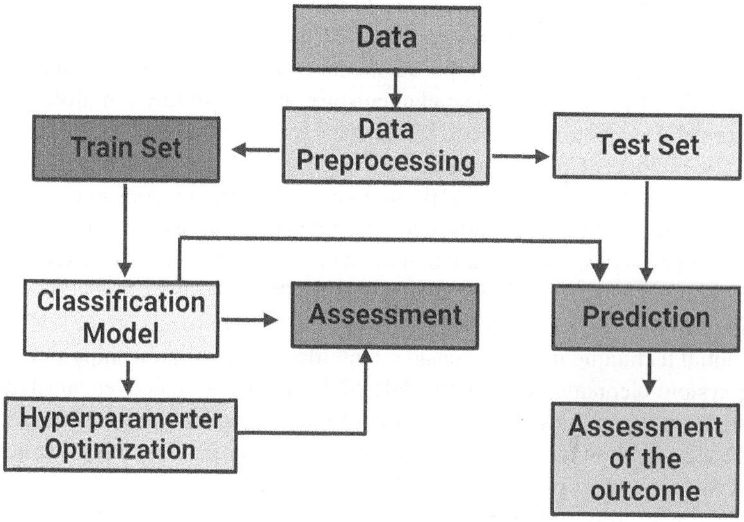

FIGURE 10.2 Supervised ML process.

challenging to choose the best model. On that account, the MCDM approach is a necessary and effective approach to overcome problem complexities such as the difficulty of having more than one evaluation criterion, criterion trade-offs, and criterion importance. Thus, this integration can offer a more consistent and rational way of making complex and multidimensional decisions. That is, MCDM techniques improve the performance of ML algorithms [30]. Combining these two approaches can achieve better results, especially in areas such as health, finance, and industry [31–35].

10.2 MCDM TECHNIQUES IN MEDICAL DECISION-MAKING

A decision in the realm of health holds immense importance due to its procedure and subsequent outcomes. For example, while treating an illness, the correct selection of the most effective treatment strategy can prevent the disease's progression, incorrect selection can result in the patient's death. Healthcare decisions are complex and involve multiple factors. Accordingly, the decision-making process can be made better by employing multiple-criteria approaches. At this stage, MCDM's capacity to assess numerous options based on a range of criteria for the selection of the best alternative makes it an excellent technique for addressing and evaluating complicated problems in real time [36]. Researchers have created several MCDM methods to deal with decision-making challenges in application fields. These techniques include Analytic Hierarchy Process (AHP), Analytic Network Process (ANP), Technique for Order of Preference by Similarity to Ideal Solution (TOPSIS), VlseKriterijumska Optimizacija I Kompromisno Resenje (VIKOR), Elimination and Choice Translating Reality (ELECTRE), and Preference Ranking Organization Method for Enrichment Evaluation (PROMETHEE), frequently employed in literature.

AHP, structures pairwise comparisons to establish the weights of the criteria and alternative priorities, is a widely used MCDM method developed by Saaty [37]. In AHP, a decision problem is decomposed into its component elements based on shared characteristics. Furthermore, these elements are represented by a multilayer hierarchical model. Decision-makers can create sub-levels within levels according to their needs. The method helps decision-makers rank and choose challenging issues with accuracy. While the strengths of AHP are that it is adaptable, does not contain complex mathematical structures, and each criterion is more transparent due to its hierarchical structure, its weaknesses are that the data is collected based on expert opinion, and the problem can become more complicated [38].

ANP is an MCDM model created by Saaty [39] that expands on the AHP. ANP is a substantial technique in that it considers interdependent relationships and feedback among system elements. Similar to AHP, ANP organizes objectives, attributes, and alternatives in hierarchies. The benefit of ANP is its applicability in different fields; nevertheless, its drawbacks are the complexity and time-consuming nature of the process for non-expert participants [40].

TOPSIS was proposed by Yoon and Hwang [41] as the distance-based technique. This method's general principle is that the optimal choice should be the one that is most near the ideal solution and most distant from the negative ideal solution. TOPSIS employs basic ranking, fully utilizes the information that is provided and does not require extra information. However, it essentially ignores the distinction between positive and negative values because it operates based on Euclidian distance. The attribute values should also be rising or decreasing monotonically [42].

Opricovic [43] developed the VIKOR approach as an MCDM method to address a problem where several criteria are incompatible. This approach mainly focuses on selecting and ranking alternatives and finding solutions that compromise conflicting criteria. By guiding decision-makers toward a solution that meets all criteria, this approach can aid in the process of reaching a final judgment. A compromise is described as an agreement established via the exchange of compromises from both parties and in this case, a compromise solution is a workable solution that approaches the ideal the closest. VIKOR is an upgraded version of TOPSIS that calculates the ratio of positive and negative ideal solutions, thereby eliminating their impact. The weakness of the method is that it becomes challenging to create a real-time model when a contradictory scenario occurs and requires adjustment when working with sparse data [44].

Benayoun et al. first introduced the ELECTRE MCDM method [45]. The method establishes a superiority relationship between preferred and non-preferred alternative forms, considering indicators of conformance and non-compliance. These indicators allow decision-makers to determine which alternative is more prominent. The ELECTRE method is a helpful strategy since it considers both utility and ambiguity [46]. Its drawback, however, is that its internal workings can be challenging to understand.

The PROMETHEE is a member of the outranking method family introduced by Brans and Vincke [47], which also includes the PROMETHEE II for complete ranking of the alternatives and the PROMETHEE I for partial ranking [48]. The PROMETHEE method relies on pairwise correlations between options for each criterion. PROMETHEE has advantages such as being simple to use due to its outranking strategy, effectively applied to real-world planning challenges, and providing a comprehensive ranking. The PROMETHEE method lacks a clear method for assigning weights [49], which is a disadvantage.

The review article [50] provides a detailed overview of the techniques. Also, an extensive assessment of the advantages and disadvantages of each MCDM approach can offer valuable insights into their suitability for various decision-making scenarios.

10.3 ML TECHNIQUES IN MEDICAL DECISION-MAKING

ML's contribution to medical science is undeniable in many fields. When healthcare systems apply ML to clinical decision-making, patient health information can be gathered and analyzed, then recommended the most effective way to improve the patient's condition[51]. The most commonly used ML algorithms that contribute to healthcare are K-Nearest Neighbour (KNN), Support Vector Machine (SVM), Decision Tree (DT), Random Forest (RF), Naive Bayes (NB), and Logistic Regression (LR) [52].

KNN is an algorithm used in regression and classification problems, where predictions are made based on the similarities of data points to each other. When given an unclassified data point, the KNN algorithm assigns it to a related class by observing which class its nearest k different neighbors belong to [53]. Its computational and memory costs are significantly higher since KNN must load all training data into memory and determine the distance between each new point and all of the training data.

For classification and regression, SVM is a very straightforward and effective ML technique. The SVM builds a hyperplane in infinite or high-dimensional space, or a group of hyperplanes. Intuitively, the hyperplane that is farthest from the nearest training data points in each class achieves a significant separation since the bigger the margin, the lower the classifier's generalization error. Its performance in high-dimensional spaces is good, and its behavior varies according to the kernel—a group of mathematical functions. The typical kernel functions used in SVM classifiers are linear, polynomial, radial basis function (RBF), and sigmoid. However, SVM's performance suffers when the dataset has more noise in it, including target class overlap [54].

DT, a well-liked non-parametric method for supervised learning, applies to regression and classification applications. The instances are categorized by DT, which is the tree from a few leaf nodes to the base. By looking at the attribute that each node defines and moving down the branch that corresponds to the attribute value, DT classifies instances. When dividing data, "entropy" is most frequently used for information gain and "gini" for Gini impurity. However, if the decision tree has many layers or more training samples, its calculation complexity may increase [55].

RF is a common ensemble classification approach for many applications. Multiple decision tree classifiers are fitted in parallel on different subsamples of the data set using a technique known as "parallel ensembling", and the outcomes are decided by a majority vote or average. It therefore lessens the overfitting problem and enhances control and forecast accuracy. Because of this, RF learning models based on many DTs typically exhibit higher accuracy than models based on a single DT. RF does not require feature scaling because it employs a rule-based methodology as opposed to a distance-based one. It is also incredibly effective at managing nonlinear parameters. However, creating a RF is difficult, and training is time-consuming [56].

NB is another technique for supervised learning, as well as a statistical approach to classification. The NB method relies on the premise of independence between every pair of features, which is based on Bayes' theorem. It is fast and effective in many real-world applications, such as document or text classification and spam filtering, for both binary and multi-class categories. However, its feature independence assumptions may impact its performance in different directions. NB classifiers are commonly available in Gaussian, Multinomial, and Bernoulli variations [57].

LR, a widely used statistical ML model, is commonly employed to tackle classification due to its probabilistic framework. Typically, LR estimates the probabilities using a logistic function, which is also known as the sigmoid function. It performs successfully at splitting datasets linearly and managing large-scale datasets. By employing regularization techniques, overfitting can be avoided in these kinds of circumstances. A key flaw in LR is the linearity assumption between the independent and dependent variables [58].

The review article [59] provides a detailed overview of the ML techniques.

10.4 INTEGRATION FRAMEWORK OF ML WITH MCDM FOR TREATMENT OPTIMIZATION

An unscientific decision regarding health may cause patient and healthcare professional dissatisfaction, increased costs, incorrect diagnosis and treatment, and consequent patient losses. A complete understanding of all available options and consideration of future repercussions are necessary to make the greatest selection feasible while handling the decision. When selecting a treatment, one may evaluate criteria like effectiveness, side effects, patient preferences, and cost. MCDM methods can help determine the relative importance of these criteria and make the best decision. MCDM is a potentially useful approach for evaluating several elements of contradictory and unrelated data to make better decisions. Additionally, AI-based ML algorithms can greatly benefit doctors' judgment and decision-making by surfacing clinical information hidden beneath the increasingly complex and big data in the healthcare industry. For example, an algorithm can forecast a patient's likelihood of contracting a specific illness if they exhibit particular symptoms, or it can learn from data to optimize the effectiveness of a treatment plan. In this regard, the integration of ML and MCDM techniques can contribute to the decision-making process in health.

To make a comprehensive analysis of publications on MCDM and ML integration in the medical field, queries were conducted using the data provided in Table 10.1. After conducting the queries, a total of 16 articles related to the issue were found. Furthermore, it has been noted that there were no prior publications on the subject before 2020. This review, which concentrated on the integration of MCDM and ML techniques, excluded DL techniques.

TABLE 10.1
Search Procedure

Admissions	Description
Query 1	"Disease" AND "Machine Learning" AND "Multi Criteria Decision Making"
Query 2	"Health" AND "Machine Learning" AND "Multi Criteria Decision Making"
Query 3	"Better Treatment" AND "Machine Learning" AND "Multi Criteria Decision Making"
Query 4	"Supervised Learning" AND "Multi-criteria" AND "Decision-making" AND "Diagnoses"
Acceptance Standards	Publications found in the Scopus database
Rejection Standards	Non-English articles

The most cited publications covering the integration of MCDM and ML can be presented as follows:

Albahri et al. [60] put forth a rescue plan that would provide the most critically ill COVID-19 patients with the best convalescent plasma (CP) to save the most severe COVID-19 patients using ML and MCDM methods. The presented framework classifies patients in the most urgent need using ML methods, based on four blood groups, and matches them with a donor-tested CP list. We then applied MCDM methods to the tested CP list using the CP decision matrix to select the most appropriate CP. Mohammed et al. [61] initially applied DL-based feature extraction and 12 well-known ML techniques to a total of 50 lung X-ray images, of which 25 were positive COVID-19 cases and the other 25 were normal cases. Regarding the choice of the best COVID-19 diagnostic model and their evaluation, they have accepted criteria such as accuracy, f1 score, ROC curve, and time complexity. In order to determine the best-performing ML technique, they weighted the criteria with the entropy method, which is one of the MCDM approaches, and ranked them with TOPSIS. Sharma and Sharma [62] tried to determine the ML techniques that provide the best classification for an accurate and timely diabetes diagnosis. This study initially preprocessed the data using well-known Kaggle (Pima Indian) data [68]. They apply and compare various ML classification techniques, including SVM, RF, KNN, LR, and NB, based on performance evaluation parameters like accuracy, specificity, and sensitivity. Additionally, they use Evaluation Based on Distance to Average Solution (EDAS), one of the MCDM methods, to compare techniques' performance. They rank NB as the best classifier and RF as the second-best alternative. Chowdhury et al. [63] studied finding the best ML technique for classifying COVID-19 from cough sounds as COVID-19 or non-COVID-19. They proposed an ensemble-based MCDM method to select top-performing ML models. They applied entropy to calculate evaluation criteria weights and used TOPSIS for ranking purposes. They found that the Extra-Trees classifier showed promising results. Mustapha et al. [64] conducted a binary classification study of 569 breast cancer cases (212 malignant or 357 benign tumors) and 30 input features using ML techniques for early breast cancer diagnosis. Additionally, they first used Principal Component Analysis (PCA) to reduce the dimension of the 30 features before classification. To select the best ML result, they resorted to MCDM methods by adding various additional criteria, such as the impact of hyperparameters on feature scaling, as well as performance metrics. For model evaluation, preference ranking was made with the fuzzy PROMETHEE method, using fuzzy numbers instead of exact numbers, which are more sensitive to real-world difficulties. Alqaysi et al. [65] developed hybrid diagnostic models to diagnose patients with autistic spectrum disorders based on medical tests and sociodemographic characteristics. After performing various preprocessing on the data, they created 15 diagnostic models using three different feature selection techniques and classified them separately in five different ML algorithms. Since the performance results obtained from ML methods consist of multiple metrics (precision, F1 score, recall, test time, train time, and AUC), the MCDM technique was required. To choose the best ML technique, criterion weighting used the fuzzy weighted zero discrepancy (FWZIC) method, while FDOSM (fuzzy decision by opinion score method) was used for ranking. Jassim et al. [66], in order to diagnose autistic spectrum disorder in adults, dual-classified 189 cases diagnosed with autism and 515 non-autistic cases according to 20 characteristics, including 10 behavioral characteristics as well as 10 personality characteristics. They first preprocessed the data to correct the data class imbalance, then classified it with various ML algorithms and suggested using VIKOR, one of the MCDM methods, to determine the most accurate way to diagnose autism. While acquiring the classification outcomes, they used the AHP method, assigning weights to each classification performance criterion (accuracy, f1 score, precision, recall, and specificity) based on expert evaluation. In order to effectively predict cervical cancer, Kuanr et al. [67] suggested finding particular risk indicators and applying specific ML algorithms. Using the Cervical Risk Classification dataset, they evaluated the performance of the suggested system using a variety of MCDM ranking methods. Precision, recall, F1-score, and mean reciprocal rank (MRR) were all higher with the MCDM algorithm's multi-objective optimization on the basis of ratio analysis (MOORA) than with the other techniques. Kumar and Kaur [68] presented an MCDM-based framework to assess ML methods used in diabetes prediction. Using 8 performance metrics for diabetes prediction, the performance of 10 ML approaches on the Diabetes Pima Indian Dataset was evaluated in order to validate the suggested strategy. Initially, utilizing a variety of comparable performance criteria, the specific ranks of ML techniques in terms of performance of diabetes prediction were determined using Weighted Aggregated Sum (WSM), TOPSIS, and VIKOR from MCDM methods. The ultimate ranking of the ML techniques was then ascertained using a fusion approach (rank position method), with LR being found to be the most effective prediction modeling for diabetes. Salih et al. [69] used FDOSM from MCDM methods to determine which ML methods were best for classifying COVID-19 according to chest X-ray (CXR) images. In the first stage, eight different ML methods were used on images, and a new decision matrix was constructed to assess the ML methods. In the second stage, the FDOSM method was used to solve MCDM problems. The result is that ANN was the best ML method among the used methods. Sharma et al. [70] suggested a system that uses ML, DL, metaheuristics, and an MCDM algorithm to find problems with the thyroid in images from ultrasound and histopathology. After applying feature extraction and feature transformation to the dataset, using the altered dataset, five distinct machine learning classifiers were assessed the 5-fold stratified cross-validation technique. For determining and ranking the best ML model from the MCDM techniques, the Method Based on the Removal Effects of Criteria (MEREC) for defining weights and TOPSIS for ranking were used. By feature selection based on optimization, the RF model received the highest rating. The authors of [71] suggested using MOORA from the MCDM method to find the best ML regression model for predicting early detection of breast cancer by using important data from tumor cells. With an RMSE value of 0.0483, it has been found that the Extreme Gradient Boosting (XGB) Regressor is the most appropriate for predicting breast cancer. The second most effective ML regressor is MLP, with an RMSE value of 0.0322. Akdag et al. [35] proposed integrating Pythagorean fuzzy MCDM with ML to assess patients' cervical cancer risk levels. Using a cervical cancer behavior risk data set first, feature selection in ML was used to select the best parameters for estimating the risk of cancer. Secondly, the MCDM methods used the Criteria for Importance Through Inter-criteria Correlation (CRITIC) method to give the criteria objective priority levels. Finally, we prioritized patients' risk levels using the TOPSIS and EDAS techniques. Hongliang et al. [72] utilized the integration of ML and MCDM methods for forecasting influenza outbreaks using weekly influenza-like illness (ILI) rates in southern and northern China. The study started with feature selection using XGB and ML techniques for determining important factors. Then, various ML regression models were evaluated and the evaluated ML regression models were ranked using the MARCOS (measurement of alternatives and ranking according to compromise solution) method from MCDM and determined to be the best ML regression model for predicting ILI rates. Kumar et al. [73] suggested an MCDM technique known as the Combined Compromise Solution (CoCoSo) to assess ML techniques for heart disease prediction while taking into account a variety of performance metrics. An experimental study was carried out to evaluate the efficacy of 15 ML approaches for heart disease prediction across three datasets related to heart disease, taking into consideration six performance indicators in total. The findings indicate that, when six performance metrics are taken into account at once, the LR and SVM are suggested as the best ML algorithms for heart disease prediction. Zhang and Li [74] presented a heterogeneous ensemble classification approach to forecast rectal cancer patients' chances of survival. The model generated sample sets for training component classifiers using a bagging technique and four different classifier types as component classifiers. They employed fuzzy TOPSIS from MCDM methods to evaluate the results of component classifiers and selected RF and Gradient Boosting Trees as the best algorithms.

10.5 EVALUATION AND RECOMMENDATIONS

The number of studies has gradually increased in recent years integrating ML and MCDM for medical decision-making. The articles [35, 60–74] integrate ML and MCDM in medical application areas such as COVID-19 diagnosis, cancer detection, autism prediction, and diabetes prediction. The distribution of relevant articles

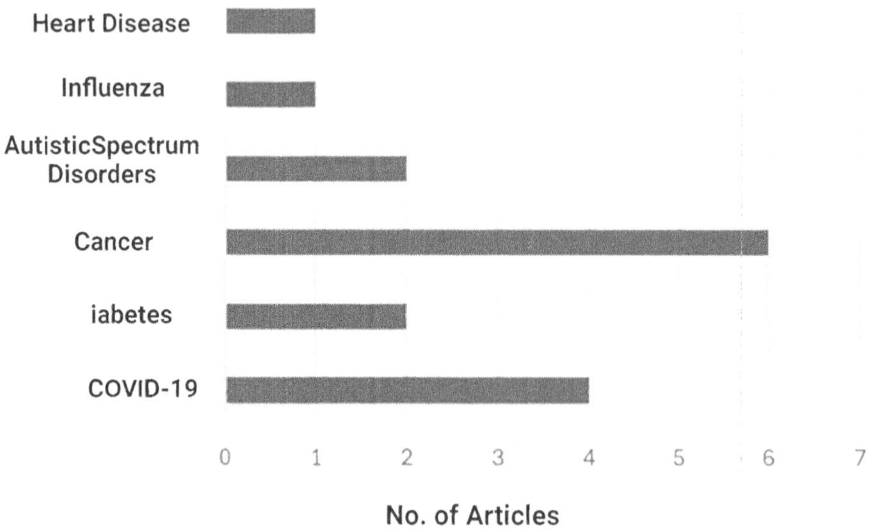

FIGURE 10.3 Distribution of the articles that include integration based on various health issues.

according to various health issues is presented in Figure 10.3. Different performance criteria are used when evaluating the performance of ML algorithms. None of these criteria alone are sufficient to determine the performance of the algorithms. Therefore, taking more than one performance criterion into consideration and selecting the algorithm based on the most effective performance criteria would be a more in-depth approach. Studies on the integration of ML and MCDM have determined that the most common form of integration involves evaluating the performances of ML algorithms using MCDM algorithms. The use of MCDM algorithms in feature selection is another form of integration. The increasing number of these studies in recent years demonstrates how promising this integration is, and it will be important for researchers to turn to this approach. Moreover, Figure 10.4 shows the publication trend for each year. It was observed that there were no publications related to the subject prior to the year 2020.

10.6 FUTURE RESEARCH DIRECTIONS

This review investigates scientific articles to highlight the importance of the integration of MCDM and ML methods in healthcare fields. Determining the visionary scientific studies and new developments, this review will be crucial. There is a lot of promise for improving decision-making processes by combining MCDM with cutting-edge technologies like blockchain, AI, and the Internet of Things. Further research and development opportunities include resolving ambiguity and vagueness, investigating uncharted realms, and strengthening the robustness and adaptability of MCDM approaches.

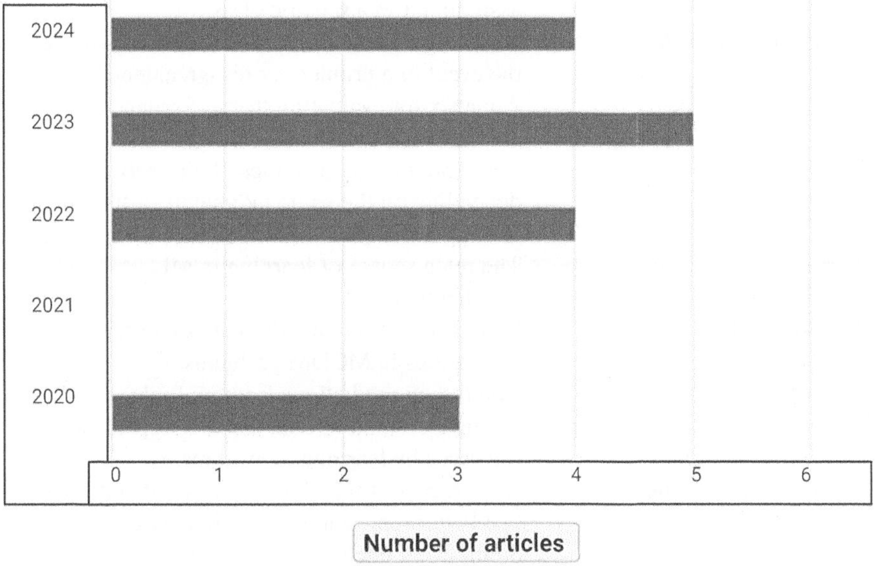

FIGURE 10.4 Distribution of articles that include integration based on years.

10.7 CONCLUSION

Studies demonstrate that integrating ML approaches with MCDM methods can significantly improve decision-making abilities. It is observed that the integration of the MCDM approach with ML algorithms in medical decision-making has enhanced the depth of research in selecting the most appropriate ML algorithm by analyzing performance criteria and also in feature selection. Given this comprehension, our review presents notable articles that offer solutions by integrating ML and MCDM techniques for complex decision-making problems in the field of medical decision-making. Thus, our review, aiming to guide future research on this dynamic topic, offers a thorough of the integration of MCDM and ML methods. Furthermore, the aim of this investigation is to establish a framework for future research endeavors that will employ this integration by examining existing literature and highlighting areas that require further investigation.

KEY TERMS AND DEFINITIONS

Alternative Available choices.

Accuracy A measure of the rate of correct predictions of a classification model.

Binary Classification A type of learning problem in which the model attempts to distinguish between two different classes.

Class Category within the classification problem.

Classification Model	A model that uses input data to classify it by assigning it to a specific class.
Compromise Solution	Reaching a common point between the choices in the event of a problem or disagreement.
Confusion Matrix	A matrix for evaluating the performance of a classification model.
Criteria	The fundamental attributes of alternatives depending on the value judgments of those making decisions.
Data	The main source of learning in ML.
Dataset	A collection of data.
Decision matrix	Matrix for displaying alternatives, criteria, and evaluations in MCDM problems.
Ensemble	Combining predictions from multiple models.
Feature	A single column of data that is accepted as a reference by learning algorithms.
Feature Engineering	The process of transforming raw data into features that better represent the problem based on predictive models.
Goal	The aim that the decision-maker hopes to accomplish.
Hyperparameter	Parameters set during training of the model.
Hyperplane	A plane that divides space between two subdomains.
Instance	A single row of data in a dataset.
Learning	Predicting future actions based on past facts or observations.
Machine Learning Model	A model that can learn from training data and make predictions on new data.
Negative Ideal Solution	The solution that maximizes the cost criterion and minimizes the benefit criterion.
Normalization	The process of converting values to a standard range.
Objective	Decision-makers' requests.
Overfitting	A situation where the model greatly fits the training data and performs poorly on new data.
Pairwise Comparison Matrix	Matrix for determining the importance levels of criteria among themselves.
Positive Ideal Solution	The solution that minimizes the cost criterion and maximizes the benefit criterion.
Ranking	A structure in which the alternatives are ordered from best to worst.
Training	The learning process of the ML model over the dataset.
Validation Set	The part of the dataset where its hyperparameters are tuned and the model is validated.

Variance A statistic measure that the degree to which data points deviate from the mean.

WEIGHT Relative importance for each criterion.

REFERENCES

1. Vordermark II JS. *An introduction to medical decision-making: Practical insights and approaches*. Springer International Publishing. 2019. https://doi.org/10.1007/978-3-030-23147-7
2. Trimble M, Hamilton P. The thinking doctor: Clinical decision making in contemporary medicine. *Clin Med.* 2016;16:343–6. https://doi.org/10.7861/clinmedicine.16-4-343
3. Abdel-Basset M, Chakrabortty RK, Gamal A. *Multi-criteria decision making theory and applications in sustainable healthcare*. CRC Press. 2023:1–256. https://doi.org/10.1201/9781003343462
4. Ozsahin I, Ozsahin D, Uzun B. *Applications of multi-criteria decision-making theories in healthcare and biomedical engineering*. Academic Press. 2021. https://doi.org/10.1016/B978-0-12-824086-1.00021-9
5. Pesode P, Barve S, Wankhede S V., Jadhav DR, Pawar SK. Titanium alloy selection for biomedical application using weighted sum model methodology. *Mater Today Proc.* 2023;72:724–8. https://doi.org/10.1016/j.matpr.2022.08.494
6. Yadav R, Singh M, Meena A, Lee SY, Park SJ. Selection and ranking of dental restorative composite materials using hybrid Entropy-VIKOR method: An application of MCDM technique. *J Mech Behav Biomed Mater.* 2023;147:106103. https://doi.org/10.1016/J.JMBBM.2023.106103
7. Amran ME, Aziz SA, Muhtazaruddin MN, Masrom M, Haron HN, Bani NA, et al. Critical assessment of medical devices on reliability, replacement prioritization and maintenance strategy criterion: Case study of Malaysian hospitals. *Qual Reliab Eng Int.* 2024;40:970–1001. https://doi.org/10.1002/QRE.3447
8. Jeon J, Suvitha K, Arshad NI, Kalaiselvan S, Narayanamoorthy S, Ferrara M, et al. A probabilistic hesitant fuzzy MCDM approach to evaluate India's intervention strategies against the COVID-19 pandemic. *Socioecon Plann Sci.* 2023;89:101711. https://doi.org/10.1016/J.SEPS.2023.101711
9. Menekşe A, Camgöz Akdağ H. Medical waste disposal planning for healthcare units using spherical fuzzy CRITIC-WASPAS. *Appl Soft Comput.* 2023;144:110480. https://doi.org/10.1016/J.ASOC.2023.110480
10. Salehi V, Moradi G, Omidi L, Rahimi E. An MCDM approach to assessing influential factors on healthcare providers' safe performance during the COVID-19 pandemic: Probing into demographic variables. *J Saf Sci Resil.* 2023;4:274–83. https://doi.org/10.1016/J.JNLSSR.2023.05.002
11. Secinaro S, Calandra D, Secinaro A, Muthurangu V, Biancone P. The role of artificial intelligence in healthcare: A structured literature review. *BMC Med Inform Decis Mak.* 2021;21. https://doi.org/10.1186/S12911-021-01488-9
12. Zebari DA, Ibrahim DA, Zeebaree DQ, Mohammed MA, Haron H, Zebari NA, et al. Breast cancer detection using mammogram images with improved multi-fractal dimension approach and feature fusion. *Appl Sci.* 2021;11:12122. https://doi.org/10.3390/APP112412122
13. Said Y, Alsheikhy AA, Shawly T, Lahza H. Medical images segmentation for lung cancer diagnosis based on deep learning architectures. *Diagnostics.* 2023;13:546. https://doi.org/10.3390/DIAGNOSTICS13030546

14. Wang Z, Keane PA, Chiang M, Cheung CY, Wong TY, Ting DSW. Artificial intelligence and deep learning in ophthalmology. *Artif Intell Med.* 2022. https://doi.org/10.1007/978-3-030-64573-1_200
15. Sakagianni A, Feretzakis G, Kalles D, Koufopoulou C, Kaldis V. Setting up an easy-to-use machine learning pipeline for medical decision support: A case study for COVID-19 diagnosis based on deep learning with CT scans. *J MantasPublic Health Dur Pandemic.* 2020;272:13–6. https://doi.org/10.3233/SHTI200481
16. Stoel BC. Artificial intelligence in detecting early RA. *Semin Arthritis Rheum.* 2019. https://doi.org/10.1016/j.semarthrit.2019.09.020
17. Nguyen D, Pham T, Batchuluun G, Yoon HS, Park KR. Artificial intelligence-based thyroid nodule classification using information from spatial and frequency domains. *J Clin Med.* 2019. https://doi.org/10.3390/jcm8111976
18. Hwang Y, Lee HH, Park C, Tama BA, Kim JS, Cheung DY, et al. Improved classification and localization approach to small bowel capsule endoscopy using convolutional neural network. *Digest Endosc.* 2021;33:598–607. https://doi.org/10.1111/DEN.13787
19. Hart S, Flotte W, Andrew F, Shah KK, Buchan ZR, Mounajjed T, Flotte TJ. Classification of melanocytic lesions in selected and whole-slide images via convolutional neural networks. J *Pathol Inform.* 2019; 10:1–5. https://doi.org/10.4103/jpi.jpi_32_18
20. Kosaraju S, Hao J, Koh H, Kang M. Deep-Hipo: Multi-scale receptive field deep learning for histopathological image analysis. *Methods.* 2020;179:3–13 https://doi.org/10.1016/j.ymeth.2020.05.012
21. Navarrete-Welton A, Hashimoto DA. Current applications of artificial intelligence for intraoperative decision support in surgery. *Front Med.* 2020;14:369–81. https://doi.org/10.1007/s11684-020-0784-7
22. Radanliev P, De Roure D. Disease X vaccine production and supply chains: Risk assessing healthcare systems operating with artificial intelligence and industry 4.0. *Health Technol (Berl).* 2023;13:11–5. https://doi.org/10.1007/S12553-022-00722-2/FIGURES/2
23. Li VOK, Lam JCK, Han Y, Chow K. A big data and artificial intelligence framework for smart and personalized air pollution monitoring and health management in Hong Kong. *Environ Sci Policy.* 2021;124:441–50. https://doi.org/10.1016/J.ENVSCI.2021.06.011
24. Anitha C, Komala CR, Vivekanand CV, Lalitha SD, Boopathi S, Revathi R. Artificial Intelligence driven security model for Internet of Medical Things (IoMT). *3rd International Conference on Innovative Practices in Technology and Management, ICIPTM.* 2023;1–7. https://doi.org/10.1109/ICIPTM57143.2023.10117713
25. Bordukova M, Makarov N, Rodriguez-Esteban R, Schmich F, Menden MP. Generative artificial intelligence empowers digital twins in drug discovery and clinical trials. *Expert Opin Drug Discov* 2024;19:33–42. https://doi.org/10.1080/17460441.2023.2273839
26. Zhang W, Cai M, Lee HJ, Evans R, Zhu C, Ming C. AI in Medical Education: Global situation, effects and challenges. *Educ Inf Technol (Dordr)* 2024;29:4611–33. https://doi.org/10.1007/S10639-023-12009-8/METRICS
27. Ahsan MM, Luna SA, Siddique Z. Machine-learning-based disease diagnosis: A comprehensive review. *Healthcare.* 2022;10:541. https://doi.org/10.3390/HEALTHCARE10030541
28. Brownlee J. Machine learning mastery with Python: Understand your data, create accurate models, and work projects end-to-end. Machine Learning Mastery. 2016.
29. Janiesch C, Zschech P, Heinrich K. Machine learning and deep learning. *Electron Markets.* 2021;31:685–95. https://doi.org/10.1007/S12525-021-00475-2
30. Sharma M, Sehrawat R. A hybrid multi-criteria decision-making method for cloud adoption: Evidence from the healthcare sector. *Technol Soc.* 2020;61:101258. https://doi.org/10.1016/J.TECHSOC.2020.101258

31. Chowdhury SJ, Mahi MI, Saimon SA, Urme AN, Nabil RH. An integrated approach of MCDM methods and machine learning algorithms for employees' churn prediction. *International Conference on Robotics, Electrical and Signal Processing Techniques.* 2023:68–73. https://doi.org/10.1109/ICREST57604.2023.10070079
32. Dohale V, Kamble S, Ambilkar P, Gold S, Belhadi A. An integrated MCDM-ML approach for predicting the carbon neutrality index in manufacturing supply chains. *Technol Forecast Soc Change.* 2024;201:123243. https://doi.org/10.1016/J.TECHFORE.2024.123243
33. Maniatis Y, Doganis A, Chatzigeorgiadis M. Fire risk probability mapping using machine learning tools and multi-criteria decision analysis in the GIS environment: A case study in the National Park Forest Dadia-Lefkimi-Soufli, Greece. *Appl Sci.* 2022;12:2938. https://doi.org/10.3390/APP12062938
34. Kadkhodazadeh M, Anaraki MV, Morshed-Bozorgdel A, Farzin S. A new methodology for reference evapotranspiration prediction and uncertainty analysis under climate change conditions based on machine learning, multi criteria decision making and Monte Carlo methods. *Sustainability.* 2022;14:2601. https://doi.org/10.3390/SU14052601
35. Akdag HC, Menekse A, Sahin F. Cervical cancer risk assessment using machine learning integrated fuzzy MCDM methodology. *J Intell Fuzzy Syst.* 2024;46:4573–92. https://doi.org/10.3233/JIFS-234647
36. Yilmaz BÖ, Tozan H, Karadayi MA. Multi-criteria decision making (MCDM) applications in military healthcare field. *J Health Syst Pol.* 2020;2:149–181
37. Saaty TL. What is the analytic hierarchy process? *Math Models Decis Sup.* 1988: 109–21. https://doi.org/10.1007/978-3-642-83555-1_5
38. Ishizaka A, Labib A. Analytic hierarchy process and expert choice: Benefits and limitations. *OR Insight.* 2009;22:201–20. https://doi.org/10.1057/ORI.2009.10
39. Saaty TL, Vargas LG. The analytic network process. *Int Ser Oper Res Manag Sci.* 2013;195:1–40. https://doi.org/10.1007/978-1-4614-7279-7_1/COVER
40. Asadabadi M, Chang E, Saberi M. Are MCDM methods useful? A critical review of analytic hierarchy process (AHP) and analytic network process (ANP). *Taylor & Francis.* 2018;3. https://doi.org/10.1080/23311916.2019.1623153
41. Yoon K, Hwang CL. TOPSIS (technique for order preference by similarity). In *Multiple Attribute Decision Making: An Introduction* Sage Publications. 1995. 38
42. Zhang H, Gu C, Gu L. The evaluation of tourism destination competitiveness by TOPSIS & information entropy–A case in the Yangtze River Delta of China. *Tour Manag Elsevier.* 2011. https://doi.org/10.1016/j.tourman.2010.02.007
43. Opricovic S. Programski paket VIKOR za visekriterijumsko kompromisno rangiranje. In *17th International Symposium on Operational Research SYM-OP-IS.* 1990.
44. Liao H, Xu Z, Zeng XJ. Hesitant fuzzy linguistic VIKOR method and its application in qualitative multiple criteria decision making. *IEEE Trans Fuzzy Syst.* 2014. https://doi.org/10.1109/TFUZZ.2014.2360556
45. Benayoun R, Roy B, Sussmann B. ELECTRE: Une méthode pour guider le choix en présence de points de vue multiples. *Note de Travail.* 1966:2–120.
46. Konidari P, Mavrakis D. A multi-criteria evaluation method for climate change mitigation policy instruments. *Energy Policy.* 2007;35:6235–57. https://doi.org/10.1016/J.ENPOL.2007.07.007
47. Brans JP, Vincke Ph. *Note—A Preference Ranking Organisation Method.* 1985;31: 647–56. https://doi.org/10.1287/MNSC.31.6.647
48. Behzadian M, Kazemzadeh RB, Albadvi A, Aghdasi M. PROMETHEE: A comprehensive literature review on methodologies and applications. *Eur J Oper Res Elsevier.* 2009;200:198–215. https://doi.org/10.1016/j.ejor.2009.01.021

49. Murat S, Kazan H, Coskun S. An application for measuring performance quality of schools by using the PROMETHEE multi-criteria decision making method. *Proc-Soc Behav Sci Elsevier*. 2015. https://doi.org/10.1016/j.sbspro.2015.06.344
50. Chakraborty S, Raut RD, Rofin TM, Chakraborty S. A comprehensive and systematic review of multi-criteria decision-making methods and applications in healthcare. *Healthcare Anal.* 2023;4:100232. https://doi.org/10.1016/J.HEALTH.2023.100232
51. Kushwaha P, Kumaresan M. Machine learning algorithm in healthcare system: A Review. *IEEE International Conference on Technological Advancements and Innovations (ICTAI)*. 2021. https://doi.org/10.1109/ICTAI53825.2021.9673220
52. Ferdous M, Debnath J, Chakraborty NR. Machine learning algorithms in healthcare: A literature survey. *11th International Conference on Computing, Communication and Networking Technologies, ICCCNT*. 2020. https://doi.org/10.1109/ICCCNT49239.2020.9225642
53. Guo G, Wang H, Bell D, Bi Y, Greer K. KNN model-based approach in classification. *On the Move to Meaningful*. 2003;2888:986–96. https://doi.org/10.1007/978-3-540-39964-3_62
54. Pedregosa F, Michel V, Grisel O, Blondel M, Prettenhofer P, Weiss R, et al. Scikit-learn: Machine learning in Python. *J Mach Learn Res*. 2011;12:2825–30.
55. Rokach L, Maimon O. *Data mining with decision trees: Theory and applications*. 2014;61: 77–81.
56. Biau G, Scornet E. A random forest guided tour. *Test*. 2016;25:197–227. https://doi.org/10.1007/S11749-016-0481-7/FIGURES/4
57. Balaji VR, Suganthi ST, Rajadevi R, Krishna Kumar V, Saravana Balaji B, Pandiyan S. Skin disease detection and segmentation using dynamic graph cut algorithm and classification through Naive Bayes classifier. *Measurement*. 2020;163:107922. https://doi.org/10.1016/J.MEASUREMENT.2020.107922
58. Musa AB. Comparative study on classification performance between support vector machine and logistic regression. *Int J Mach Learn Cybern*. 2013;4:13–24. https://doi.org/10.1007/S13042-012-0068-X/TABLES/5
59. Sarker IH. Machine learning: Algorithms, real-world applications and research directions. *SN Comput Sci*. 2021;2. https://doi.org/10.1007/S42979-021-00592-X
60. Albahri O, Al-Obaidi J, Zaidan A, Albahri AS, Zaidan BB, Salih MM, et al. Helping doctors hasten COVID-19 treatment: Towards a rescue framework for the transfusion of best convalescent plasma to the most critical patients based on. *Comput Meth Programs Biomed*. 2020. https://doi.org/10.1016/j.cmpb.2020.105617
61. Mohammed M, Abdulkareem K, Al-Waisy AS, Mostafa SA, Al-Fahdawi S, Dinar A, et al. Benchmarking methodology for selection of optimal COVID-19 diagnostic model based on entropy and TOPSIS methods. *IEEE Access* 2020. https://doi.org/10.1109/ACCESS.2020.2995597
62. Sharma S, Sharma B. EDAS based selection of machine learning algorithm for diabetes detection. *9th International Conference System Modeling and Advancement*. 2020. https://doi.org/10.1109/SMART50582.2020.9337118
63. Chowdhury NK, Kabir MA, Rahman MM, Islam SMS. Machine learning for detecting COVID-19 from cough sounds: An ensemble-based MCDM method. *Compu Biol Med*. 2022. https://doi.org/10.1016/j.compbiomed.2022.105405
64. Mustapha M, Ozsahin D, Ozsahin I, Uzun B. Breast cancer screening based on supervised learning and multi-criteria decision-making. *Diagnostics*. 2022. https://doi.org/10.3390/diagnostics12061326

65. Alqaysi ME, Albahri AS, Hamid RA. Hybrid diagnosis models for autism patients based on medical and sociodemographic features using machine learning and multi-criteria decision-making. *Comput Math Methods Med.* 2022. https://doi.org/10.1155/2022/9410222
66. Jassim MM, Ali MH, Elamer AS, Jaber MM, Mohammed MQ, Alkhayyat A. Multi-criteria decision making for machine learning algorithms using AHP-VIKOR techniques: Case study adult autism diagnosis. *5th International Conference on Engineering Technology and Its Applications (IICETA).* 2022. https://doi.org/10.1109/IICETA54559.2022.9888273
67. Kuanr M, Mohapatra P. Outranking relations based multi-criteria recommender system for analysis of health risk using multi-objective feature selection approach. *Data Knowl Eng.* 2023;145. https://doi.org/10.1016/j.datak.2023.102144
68. Kumar A, Kaur K. A novel MCDM-based framework to recommend machine learning techniques for diabetes prediction. *Int J Eng Technol Innov.* 2024;14. https://doi.org/10.46604/ijeti.2023.11837
69. Salih MM, Ahmed MA, Al-Bander B, Hasan KF, Shuwandy ML, Al-Qaysi ZT. Benchmarking framework for COVID-19 classification machine learning method based on fuzzy decision by opinion score method. *Iraqi J Sci.* 2023:922–43. https://doi.org/10.24996/ijs.2023.64.2.36
70. Sharma R, Mahanti GK, Panda G, Rath A, Dash S, Mallik S, Hu R. A framework for detecting thyroid cancer from ultrasound and histopathological images using deep learning, meta-heuristics, and MCDM algorithms. *J Imaging.* 2023;9:173. https://doi.org/10.3390/jimaging9090173
71. Debnath A, Tarafdar A, Bhattacharya P, Shaikh A. MOORA MCDM based optimal machine learning regression techniques for breast cancer prediction. *IEEE Silchar Subsection Conference (SILCON).* 2023:1–7. https://doi.org/10.1109/SILCON59133.2023.10404380
72. Hongliang G, Zhiyao Z, Ahmadianfar I, Escorcia-Gutierrez J, Aljehane NO, Li C. Multi-step influenza forecasting through singular value decomposition and kernel ridge regression with MARCOS-guided gradient-based optimization. *Comput Biol Med.* 2024;169:107888. https://doi.org/10.1016/j.compbiomed.2023.107888.
73. Kumar A, Singh AK, Garg A. Evaluation of machine learning techniques for heart disease prediction using multi-criteria decision making. *J Intell Fuzzy Syst.* 2024;46:1259–73. https://doi.org/10.3233/JIFS-233443
74. Zhang F, Li X. HBagging-MCDM: An ensemble classifier combined with multiple criteria decision making for rectal cancer survival prediction. *Ann Oper Res.* 2024;335:469–90. https://doi.org/10.1007/S10479-023-05642-6

11 Embedded Systems in Developing Advanced Strategies in Healthcare Management

Selcan Karakuş, Elif Tüzün, Magdy M. Elnashar, and Sinem Özlem Enginler

11.1 INTRODUCTION

Environmental monitoring, control, and processing capabilities frequently converge within embedded systems, albeit not universally. The term "embedded" underscores their integration into broader products. Following are several examples for elucidation:

- Several components, such as carburation and brake control mechanisms, are found in modern vehicles.
- The administration panel for a building's intelligent air conditioning system.
- Microcontrollers were intended to be used in electronic devices such as smart stop-and-go lights.
- Platforms for monitoring health.

A system having a narrowly defined goal, clear internal communication methods, and comparatively few, well-specified external communication methods is called an embedded system. Generally, one team or a group of teams who collaborate intensively to develop a clearly defined solution produce embedded systems.

Embedded systems are essential for improvements in patient care, diagnosis, and medical treatment in biomedical applications. These systems are crucial for precisely and effectively dispensing medications, monitoring patient status, and regulating medical equipment. By utilizing diagnostic tools and software to identify and fix faults, healthcare instrument designers guarantee the security and dependability of their products. Prior to being deployed in medical facilities, embedded systems are thoroughly tested using emulators that mimic actual conditions. Because they offer the processing and control methods required to carry out image collection, processing, and presentation tasks effectively, embedded systems are critical to the design of imaging devices. These systems are the silent engines of accuracy and dependability in healthcare and monitoring systems, coordinating vital tasks with the least amount

DOI: 10.1201/9781003508199-11

of human involvement. They work instantly, quickly deciphering information from pictures to provide accurate diagnosis and research. Additionally, they precisely time the acquisition and control the functioning of image sensors and medical apparatus.

It's crucial to have a solid understanding of digital electronics gear. Logic gates are used in the construction of the products under study, and microchips and electronic components house every facet of digital electronics, including all basic circuits. Partially understanding these technologies is inadequate due to their intricacy. A plethora of knowledge is required in electronic devices; even building aesthetically pleasing boards for electronics necessitates deep understanding. Writing software for embedded devices won't work as well without a thorough grasp. In actuality, programming is being used more and more for purposes beyond the conventional management of embedded systems, including internet servers, operating systems, computation of images, and graphical user interfaces. Embedded system programming is distinguished by certain elements that set it apart from other programming languages. Applications for embedded systems should prioritize minimal memory usage. Embedded systems must perform their tasks without extra slowdown and at a crucial speed. When interacting with software that is embedded, intelligibility and ease of change are also key. Support initiatives ensure high efficiency and regulatory compliance by assisting with embedded systems' lifetime maintenance and operation. Integrating these approaches for the embedded development of software helps physicians to provide individualized, effective therapy that ultimately enhances patient results and standard of life. Embedded systems are customized components that unite the CPU with the operating system of a machine to do a particular task. These systems, which are composed of both hardware and software, allow machines that comprise both digital and physical parts to work with an operating system or chip for specific uses. In order to produce imaging equipment that are efficient in regards to imagine capture, processing, and presentation, embedded systems are essential. They improve smartphone battery life, simplify low-power activities, and combine fault tolerance and redundancy to ensure constant performance. While translators convert high-level coding into commands that a computer can comprehend, integrated development environments enable it to be easier to develop distinctive embedded programs. Systems for imaging in medicine make significant use of embedded systems. Tools such as magnetic resonance imaging (MRI), computed tomography (CT) examinations, positron emission tomography (PET), and ultrasonography (USG) share the characteristic of being embedded systems, despite operating on different platforms. Embedded systems are characterized by low-power processors housed within high-speed processing units, operating under a software operating system or direct administration architecture. They possess the capability to control detectors and operators. While financial transactions in embedded systems traditionally remain smaller than those of computing devices, studies in Industry 4.0 and advancements in technology are gradually narrowing this gap in size. However, executing operation-based functions such as automated rationalization, artificial intelligence (AI), and machine learning (ML) requires significant space in embedded system design. Prior research has shown that the most significant components, ranked in order, are software libraries, Linux tools, In-Circuit Emulator (ICE), configuration management tools, Static Analysis tools, and program drivers. In terms of hardware, key components include the Oscilloscope, Debugger, Compiler/assembler, Integrated Development Environment (IDE), Logic analyzer, and Joint Test Action Group/ Background Debug Mode (JTAG/BDM). The seamless integration of embedded technologies has revolutionized image processing and capture in the digital age. These technologies play an essential role in shaping the entire imaging experience, from the moment light strikes an image detector to the final presentation on a user interface. To illustrate the impact of embedded systems on modern imaging technology, this chapter covers their various roles in image capture, processing, compression, feature extraction, user interface management, networking, power management, and customization (Table 11.1).

11.1.1 Embedded Systems in Healthcare Technology

Many people's lives are becoming better as a result of technological advancements, particularly in the area of illness management. The most serious of these illnesses is obesity, which is becoming a serious problem. A social issue that affects people of all demographics, obesity is subtle and quickly spreading to a global scale. More than three hundred million individuals worldwide are obese, with emerging nations bearing a disproportionately large load on the healthcare system. As such, it is critical that the industry combat obesity (1). In the United States of America, among other countries, the young population is experiencing excessive weight gain, leading to an inevitable increase in obesity. Consequently, the state is actively seeking solutions to address this issue (2). Similarly, in France, the prevalence of obesity is rapidly rising, albeit at a rate of 6–11 percent (3). Preventing obesity, a condition with such a significant global increase, and conducting studies on this subject are becoming

TABLE 11.1
Embedded Systems Functions in Modern Imaging Technology

Function	Components
Image capture	Detector, shutter speed, lens control, exposure time, adjustments to the white balance, digital data conversion, and image capture.
Image processing	Deformation correction, quality enhancement, interference reduction, color adjustment, noise reduction, and sharpening.
Compression	JPEG, PNG, image compression, storage capacity reduction, bandwidth optimization, real-time extraction, and real-time compression.
Feature extraction	Data extraction, edge detection, object recognition, face detection, advanced imaging systems, robotic focusing, environment monitoring, and image stabilization.
User interface	LCD monitors, knobs, smartphones, tablets, and imaging devices.
Networking and connectivity	Wi-Fi, USB, and Bluetooth, remote management, software updates, and electronic image transfer.
Power management	Cameras, photographic instruments, and battery.
Customization and flexibility	Detectors, monitors, and information technology units.

increasingly crucial. Romania, ranking third in Europe in terms of obesity rates, is also combating this condition, which contributes to numerous diseases. The most concerning aspect of this ailment is its association with a range of chronic conditions, from depression to diabetes, and from high blood pressure to sleep apnea, as well as heart diseases. It is vital to improve the quality of life of these patients, make lifestyle improvements and, if necessary, take their health under control with surgical interventions. As a result of increasing inappropriate nutrition, the need for practical ways that patients can apply at home to control problems such as weight control (such as obesity) is increasing day by day. Embedded systems are becoming increasingly important in the treatment of diseases that threaten the quality of life. Thanks to embedded systems, patients will be able to easily find solutions to their medical problems, save time and live in their own living spaces under economic conditions. It is of great importance in the treatment of people whose lives are at risk for health problems such as obesity, which can cause serious problems in vital organs such as the heart and brain, thanks to devices that monitor their movements at home. These embedded devices play an important role in treatment with functions such as early warning systems, emergency plans, and location detection in monitoring pulse and blood pressure. Additionally, having the ability to transfer health-related information on the online platform integrated into these systems is extremely beneficial for individuals at risk (4, 5).

Embedded systems use special monitors to digitally process health data and ensure the security of the data. These systems aim to securely collect, interact, and evaluate patient data in the biomedical field. The use of embedded systems in healthcare has increased with high sensitivity, high selectivity, cost-effectiveness, flexibility, reliability, simple use, energy efficiency, excellent data processing units, and rapid problem-solving capabilities, as well as interactions such as ML calculations, AI systems, specialist software, Bluetooth and Wi-Fi (6, 7). Such devices are required for different types of applications, such as electrocardiograms, mobile devices, and personal health (8). In the medical domain, where devices leveraging embedded systems are employed, ensuring device reliability and conducting accurate tests are paramount. While embedded systems offer numerous conveniences in biomedical applications, they also pose challenges. Devices utilized for ECG/EEG, CT scans, blood pressure, and glucose measurement benefit from embedded systems, each requiring tailored computing solutions to address distinct needs. Consequently, meticulously designing and executing every stage of device development, encompassing aspects such as battery life, performance, and reliability, holds significant value (9). In the latest technology, the number of useful devices in the field of biomedical medicine is increasing by combining different engineering fields with the convergence of a wide variety of fields for embedded systems. Studies in this field are very promising for developing easily portable, affordable, and high-quality devices in embedded systems. For these systems, issues such as data collection, processing, and sensor sensitivity require great attention. Research and development studies are gaining importance to improve these details (10).

The integration of numerous devices facilitating insulin level, movement, blood pressure, pulse, and heart rate measurements into monitors via microcontrollers, enabled by embedded systems, enhances medical application fields (Figure 11.1).

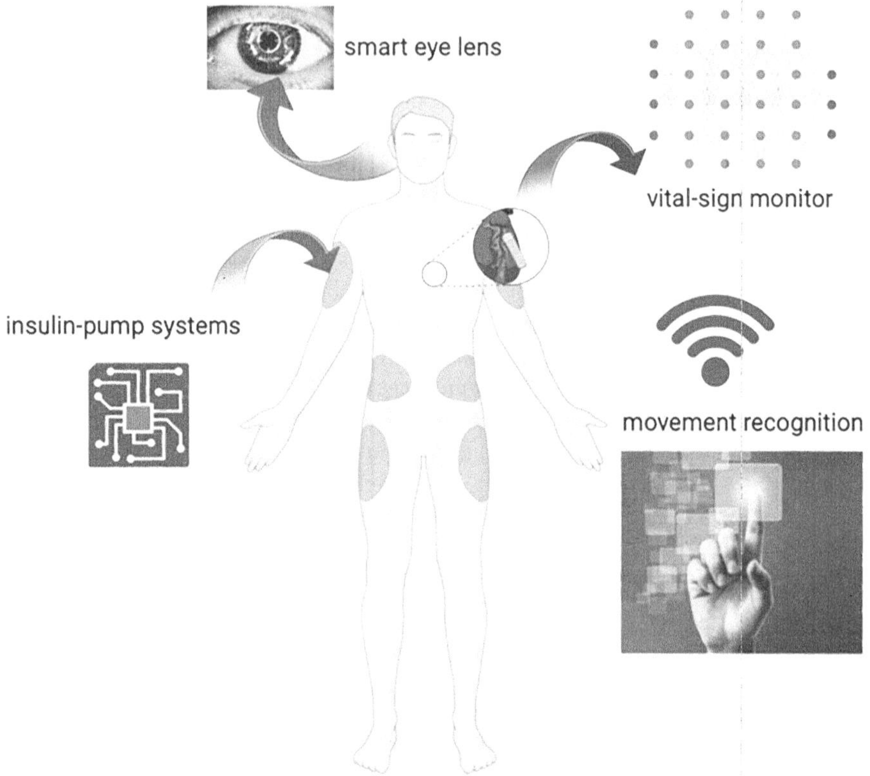

FIGURE 11.1 The integration of numerous devices facilitating insulin level, movement, and heart rate measurements into monitors by embedded systems.

A specialized process is required to process the signals with the assistance of these microprocessors until the data reaches the monitors (11). Consequently, chip technology must be enhanced and performance increased for embedded systems. The advancement of this technology, along with chip production and the integration of processors, memory, and interfaces, is gaining importance for cost reduction. This not only offers benefits such as ease of use, extended battery life, and improved performance but also facilitates treatment and subsequent challenging processes by embedding embedded systems in diseases requiring numerous surgical operations, such as epilepsy and Parkinson's, as well as brain and heart diseases. Sensor applications of microelectronic systems enabling medical electronic implantation are rapidly increasing and developing in the biomedical field for common diseases, as they can be utilized in numerous diagnostic methods and subsequently for treatment (12). Examples of microelectronic systems include microfluidic chips, pressure sensors, acceleration measurement devices, microphones, gyroscopes, strain sensors, and imaging sensor systems. (13–16). It's crucial for these devices to be compact for ease of use. Advancements in semiconductor technology can aid in achieving this goal. An innovative approach is necessary to simplify and streamline the development of embedded systems software, making it user-friendly for practitioners. Consequently, to enhance efficiency in the biomedical field, new sensor systems must be developed, and their hardware and algorithms must be tailored accordingly (11).

Electronic devices known as embedded systems have been developed to allow for smart system integration in the use of products and services. In recent years, the healthcare industry has started to often adopt advanced embedded medical technology in both homes and clinics. Some of the embedded medical equipment includes defibrillators for cardiac problems, blood analysis components, diagnostic imaging instruments, monitors for cholesterol levels and blood sugar levels, fetal heart rate monitoring, oximeters for measuring the oxygen concentration of hemoglobin in blood, arrhythmia regulator devices such as pacemakers, drug delivery performance monitors by measuring liquid flow, smartphones, textile-based goods, and lenses. Wearable sensors also enable remote monitoring of body temperature, blood pressure, and oxygen saturation levels. The compact size of these medical devices enables them to transfer clinical data to computerized systems in clinics. Intelligent technology utilizes algorithms for diagnosis, which can enhance the quality of diagnosis when the data volume is sufficiently high. These devices detect vibrations in the vessel wall to provide signals, allowing changes in blood pressure to be identified. Most infrared measuring devices can monitor body temperature without contact, while smart pillows can measure it with contact. In 2006, Guerra et al. designed a hardware and software device using PET to detect gamma radiation in animals. When combined with small animal PET systems employing fewer rotating planar detection devices, this chip makes high-resolution imaging more cost-effective (17). The objective of the work is to integrate the coincidence unit and acquisition devices of a fully digital four-head PET detector onto one chip using advancements in the semiconductor industry. Commercially available industry components, such as a PC in a 6U cPCI setup and a computer-based fast-speed acquisition board, are utilized in the proof of concept. The acquisition of electronic segments, coincidental logic, and networking interface uses approximately thirty percent of the resources, allowing for potential system upgrades. In the study by Arandia et al., artificial vision systems are essential to the growth of healthcare technology because they make it simpler to create complex structures in a variety of medical disciplines, including the fields of radiology surgery, gastroenterology, and ophthalmatology (18). Embedded vision research has created intelligent image analysis possible in lightweight applications by simply incorporating specialized camera components into surgical instruments. Eye monitoring devices are one major application that is addressed; these systems offer an opportunity to diagnose and treat patients. These devices assist in discovering retinal conditions including strabismus by using computerized vision algorithms to detect eye motion. In recent years, research studies on the development of eye-tracking devices integrated with embedded systems, such as the special Irisbond system, have increased to evaluate the arithmetic skills of children with cerebral palsy. Ultrasound (USG) systems play a role in disease assessment, treatment guidance, and overall health monitoring in both human and veterinary healthcare. USG method is used for a number of factors in the treatment of injuries to the skeletal system, monitoring pregnancy, early detection of tumors, and health services. On the other hand, the USG technique is used in the treatment of both domestic and cattle.

Additionally, this technique can be used to diagnose ovarian and uterine pathologies, estimate the length of the reproductive cycle, and evaluate the effectiveness of treatment. The application of ultrasound imaging systems in both veterinary and human medicine represents a significant advancement in medical research and promotes health on a broad scale. In 2012, El-Tager et al. developed a new ultrasound imaging system, which is a small embedded Doppler ultrasound equipment that utilizes a multiple-core computing system to rapidly obtain information from variables (19). When abnormal albumin excretion or a decrease in renal function persists for more than three months, chronic kidney disease is diagnosed. The glomerular filtration rate can directly assess kidney function. This illness poses significant community health challenges as it increases the risk of fatalities, elevates overall mortality and morbidity rates, and enhances the likelihood of cardiovascular conditions. The National Kidney Foundation has established stage criteria based on kidney damage and glomerular filtration rate values to measure the level and risk of the disease. In 2021, Gudigar et al. investigated the application of visual processing and image fusion techniques to automatically recognize ultrasound images for use in chronic kidney disease (20). In another study, Liu et al. developed an electromagnetic sensor with GPS-like properties with an innovative approach to improve laparoscopic ultrasound navigation (21). This strategy had a potential to significantly improve surgical results by providing a more accurate surgical strategy. The investigations focused on the assessment of the clinical effects and broader relevance of embedded electronic imaging systems in laparoscopic surgical procedures, underscoring the need for additional research and validation in clinical settings.

More portability and versatility in healthcare monitoring and diagnostic equipment have been made possible by the shrinking of electronic systems, improvements in battery technology (potential and size), the expansion of mobile technology, and the falling prices of necessary technologies. Machine designers are depending more and more on remote monitoring platforms as essential tools for controlling operator connections and improving their digital brand representation as industrial and small-scale producers want to expand their product offerings. Still, dispersed settings are incompatible with the conventional approach of remote monitoring for groups. As a result, the business sector needs novel approaches to develop virtual interpersonal connections. Developments in network technology have expanded the potential of smart image gadgets to connect with one another, even though embedded systems have provided dependable controllers for this purpose. These days, embedded devices connected to servers thousands of kilometers distant can broadcast real-time information. Furthermore, biomedical remote monitoring and diagnostic solutions, which transform medical care delivery, are built on embedded systems. Embedded systems advance healthcare technologies and improve patient care by enabling real-time information transfer and analysis. To sum up, imaging systems depend on embedded systems to function properly. These systems provide crispy, clear images, easy user interfaces, and seamless integration in small, effective packaging.

It advances the concept of Bluetooth systems with embedded devices, enabling the examination of more essential activities by the systems. Workload and stress factors can be assessed, along with the emotional and physical stress levels of the individual being detected, by analyzing the monitored factors. It also enables the analysis of the person's response to environmental modifications. The system can respond rapidly to unanticipated modifications when utilizing internet monitoring. These alterations could be physiological in nature, such as stress or altered behavior, or they could be responses to external changes. An adequate reaction to any variation or loss of essential activities can frequently prevent potentially fatal conditions or unfavorable medical effects.

The integration of embedded systems and ML techniques to augment wearable sensors is of significant significance for use in healthcare. The physical and chemical aspects, which are now the most prevalent mechanisms for soft sensors, are the primary focal point of wearable sensor operating principles. The data collected by these kinds of sensors serves as crucial for building ML systems that work. Unlike ML which relies on image or video data, the mechanism of soft sensors frequently generates time-series data. Research specifically addresses novel models intended for signal reception and processing from flexible wearable sensors. Both contemporary artificial neural networks (ANNs) and conventional embedded ML models can benefit from these techniques. In addition, the features that fall into three application areas—monitoring, connection, and resource harvesting—are the subject of research. These domains depend on the employment of mobile devices, soft sensors, along with appropriate ML models. Investigation on the drawbacks and difficulties of embedded ML in flexible systems, as well as possible solutions, is still underway. Embedded system-based ML becomes an effective tool for quick data processing when combined with flexible sensor technologies. Research focuses on the assistance of ML algorithms in the data analysis process. The precision and generalizability of the data are impacted by crucial processes, including preprocessing and feature extraction. Evaluation, validation, and training sets of data are separated accordingly. While the validation set assesses the model's suitability and adjusts the parameters, ML models utilize the training set to determine parameter values. Model parameters cannot be altered at this stage; instead, the actual effectiveness is assessed using an experimental set. The accuracy score, confusion matrix, and loss index are typical indicators of performance. Occasionally, to expand the training set, researchers may omit the validation set. When selecting appropriate smart algorithms, the format and structure of the data are significant factors. In comparison to previous traditional approaches, recently published studies have investigated ML models in greater detail. According to the latest research, the integration of flexible wearable sensors and ML in smart wearable devices has led to potential advancements in the healthcare sector.

11.1.2 Deep Learning for Embedded Vision Systems

The efficacy and advantages of embedded vision systems have been demonstrated in various applications over the past few years. Advances in image technology and the accessibility of powerful devices capable of integrating with deep learning algorithms are driving the integration of vision capabilities into electronics, such as embedded healthcare devices. However, performing image analysis on embedded devices is challenging and often requires significant CPU power, even for simple tasks like object recognition. Improved outcomes may be achieved by implementing deep learning algorithms and evaluating them on task-specific databases. Previous studies have proposed and analyzed a deep learning-based method for enhancing the image processing design of embedded vision platforms. Successful results were achieved by implementing and evaluating these deep learning algorithms on embedded images. Finding the essential elements is the primary goal of recognition of patterns and categorization of images. Over the last few years, a number of AI-based embedded systems have been invented to function comparable to humans. Humans are typically inclined to recognize and identify significant factors. Deep learning networks can be combined with a class of embedded vision model integrations to learn many levels of data representation. Through a computer system, any kind of knowledge, including written material, voice, and photographic images could be sent. This might be trained in an unsupervised manner to get started, and then refined under supervision. Effective comprehension of upper-level characteristics is facilitated by a low-level characteristic. Target identification and classification for embedded vision systems are only two of the many tasks that might be produced with the use of this kind of learning by identifying the invariant and abstract properties.

Another rapidly developing technology in AI, known as deep learning, is a subset of ML. It consists of several networks that may learn from collected data, which may be unstructured or unorganized. More specifically, deep learning analyses the raw data at multiple levels of description in order to perform tasks such as identification and categorization ANNs are computerized algorithms and methods used in ML that simulate neural networks found in the human brain. An ANN is a structure made up of interrelated nodes which make up the hierarchical segments. Measurements are continuously adjusted by each network node during the exercise period, and outcomes are subsequently transmitted to an activity function. Three basic layers comprise ANNs: the input layer, hidden layer or layers, and output layer. Each node in the input layer, which acts as the data entering point, reflects a distinctive characteristic or output factor. After that, the hidden layer(s) modify this data in a number of techniques, using activation algorithms and connected weights to draw out complicated relationships and patterns from the information. The network may learn extensive ways to represent the input variables thanks to these intermediate layers, which improves its capacity for generalization and precise prediction-making. In order to deliver the intended results or groups, the output layer produces the data that has been analyzed from the hidden levels. Collectively, these steps are the basis of ANNs, enabling them to successfully and automatically handle a wide range of operations, including identification of patterns, regression analysis, and classification (22).

Deep learning was primarily created to improve the functionality of the traditional ANN, which is made up of multiple hidden layers that manage the network's identification in a comprehensive manner. The conventional neural network, or CNN, is reportedly quite well-liked in AI systems. CNN assists in creating the map of features which employs the weighted convolution matrices to calculate each pixel's value in the initial photo as well as its adjacent pixel. AI-based strategy is a key component of healthcare image processing that is revolutionizing patient care standards and diagnostic accuracy (Figure 11.2). To meet particular application needs, a variety of matrix operations—such as edge detection, image blurring, and sharpening—are used.

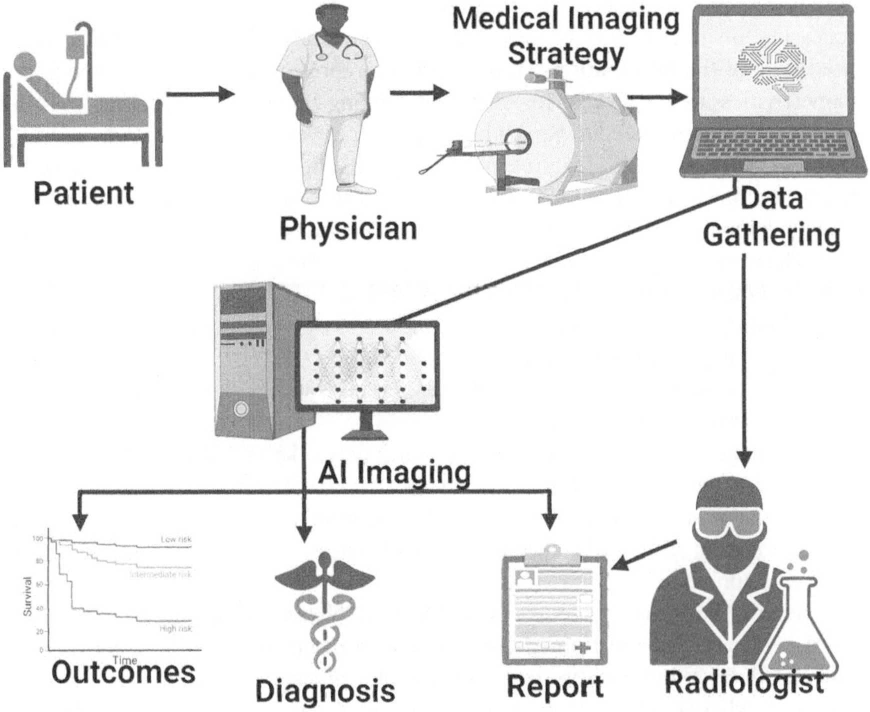

FIGURE 11.2 Revolutionizing healthcare through AI-enabled image processing.

As a branch of AI, ML consists of algorithms that can extract significant details from raw data and apply that data to self-learn in order to produce predictions or precise classifications. Because ML is reliable and credible, it has become more and more widespread. ML algorithms are able to analyze inputs rapidly and offer accurate findings in a shorter amount of time thanks to improvements in the software and hardware parts of machine technologies. ML utilizes trends found in datasets to complete tasks rather than relying solely on direct coding. Individuals input characteristics and guidelines using conventional computer programming, sometimes referred to as rules-based coding or classic learning algorithms. Statistical techniques are then applied to organize or identify information based on these characteristics. Ultimately, this method produces the required output outcomes. However, the process of ML networks often encounters challenges in achieving closure and avoiding overfitting in the learning set. Additionally, the complexity of acquiring data dimensions and resource computations presents challenges for deep learning networks. Deep learning is rapidly advancing in its sector, primarily due to the advancement of computer components such as the graphics processing unit (GPU). However, during the training stage, several variables must be optimized to enable complex nodes to identify the connections and depth within the dataset's structures. As a result, deep learning networks require a significant amount of training data, which increases the processing capacity needed to analyze such datasets. During the training period, the dataset is preprocessed to extract its significant properties. Feature extraction, similar to preprocessing, involves tasks like image enhancement and noise reduction based on the initial state of the information. Through feature representation, accurate and unique characteristics are retrieved. However, generalizing this process becomes challenging, as these features need to be newly designed for every new application, a practice known as "hand-crafting" features in deep learning methodology. Consequently, this process becomes increasingly difficult to generalize, requiring the construction of these functionalities from scratch each time a completely new application is developed. The deep learning approach refers to this procedure as "hand-crafting" components. Healthcare, imagine deep learning algorithms have been used for four different kinds of computer image tasks: segmentation of instances, segmentation based on semantics, recognition of objects, and classification (23, 24).

The predominant methodologies of deep learning architectures in healthcare:

Deep Learning Architectures:

Ronneberger's U-Net: Convolutional neural networks including U-Net are made primarily for the segmentation of biomedical image tasks. It is composed of an expanding symmetrical path for accurate localization and a contracted route to capture environment. Biomedical segmentation of images is one area where U-Net has found widespread use.

Generative Adversarial Networks (GANs): GANs are formed up of two kinds of neural networks that are trained concurrently: a discriminator and a network that generates data. The algorithm that discriminates assesses the accuracy of the data generated, whereas the generator creates artificial data, such as visuals. Realistic images are produced frequently using this type of construction.

Autoencoders are neural networks that compress inputs into a latent-space image and then restore the results from this model. They are employed for unsupervised training tasks, especially in the processing of images, for learning effective models for data.

Google's Inception Network: The Inception Network of Google, also referred to as GoogLeNet, is an advanced CNN architecture developed specifically for visual recognition purposes. It is distinguished by its adoption of inception sections, which carry out operations on convolution at multiple levels within a single layer, and by its deep structure.

The predominant methodologies utilizing image processing techniques in healthcare:

Image Processing Techniques:

Fuzzy C-Means (FCM): FCM is a clustering method that is frequently applied to work involving image segmentation. Based on the pixel's resemblance to the cluster centroids, and it allocates each of the pixels in an image to any number of clusters.

K-Nearest Neighbors (KNN): For regression and classification tasks, KNN is a fundamental machine learning approach. In the medical imaging field, KNN can be used to classify images based on the predominant class among neighboring images in the feature space.

Convolutional Neural Network (CNN): Convolutional neural networks, or CNNs, are particular deep learning models developed to handle organized grid data, such as images. CNNs are frequently employed for applications including recognizing objects, the process of segmentation and classification of images in the healthcare field.

Expectation Maximization (EM) Algorithm: An approach for quantitatively predicting predictive models is the EM method. When it comes to image analyzing, EM is frequently used for applications including picture rebuilding, in which the elements of a mathematical model are repeatedly calculated based on the data that was observed.

In the field of healthcare image processing, where accurate imagine evaluation and comprehension are essential for diagnosis and treatment strategy, these structures and approaches are particularly significant.

A different branch of ML, deep learning, has showcased remarkable results in identifying various products in images. With sufficient training, deep learning models can even surpass humans in certain circumstances. ML algorithms are commonly employed to evaluate product quality. In biomedical applications, various ML techniques such as support vector machines (SVM), Naive Bayes, ANN, decision trees, fuzzy logic, k-nearest neighbor (k-NN), k-means clustering, random forest (RF), and others have been extensively utilized (24).

In 2022, Pally et al. demonstrated the beneficial effects of deep learning techniques, particularly CNNs, in assessing emergency preparedness and examining flood-related data in the field of imaging (25). This study exemplifies the diverse applications of intelligent technologies. These ML approaches are commonly utilized in computer vision to effectively analyze flood images by assigning learnable weights to various elements. Their research underscored the importance of utilizing integrated vision technologies, including communication capabilities, image processing methods, and video, to enable flood signal detection. To facilitate flood image analysis and object identification, they compiled a training dataset of over nine thousand images from social media platforms, live river sensors from the US Geological Survey, five hundred eleven highway surveillance cameras from the Department of Transportation, and search engine results. Additionally, they developed the Python package "FloodImageClassifier," which integrates several CNN architectures, including SSD MobileNet, Fast R-CNN, EfficientDet, YOLOv3, and Mask R-CNN, to enable simultaneous object recognition and classification. In this study, Pally et al. demonstrated that deep learning algorithms are valuable tools for flood image evaluation and flood preparedness planning. Their work underscores the importance of networked vision algorithms in image identification and flood signal recognition.

SARS-CoV-2 is the origin of COVID-19, which has presented serious challenges since the worldwide pandemic was declared in March 2020. As of May 6, 2024, seven million fatalities and nearly 705 million cases, with 675 million recoveries, had been recorded. Lockdowns, travel limitations, and infection prevention protocols are examples of present-day management techniques. In the absence of specialized treatments, therapeutic intervention remains the major course of therapy. Hospitalization and mortality are examples of undesirable outcomes, with severe cases exhibiting a variety of clinical parameters. The fact that many infected people have no symptoms makes diagnosis more difficult. Although rRT-PCR is the most common method for diagnosis, results have been delayed due to insufficient supplies. Quick and efficient diagnostic methods are vital for controlling the spread of the pandemic due to these complications. Unlike conventional model-based strategies, ML algorithms are capable of modeling data without making rigid mathematical assumptions. The modeling of clinical data for predicting the medical diagnosis or prognosis of numerous diseases, including COVID-19, has advanced significantly. By using ML approaches, two kinds of patient information are typically used to create COVID-19 predictive models, including image data and/or organized information. The boundary data may consist of statistics, medical records, signs and symptoms, health indicators, and laboratory results; picture information can include chest X-rays (CXR) and/or lung CT scans. Predicting COVID-19 results is largely dependent on predictive algorithms, especially when utilizing various forms of datasets. Numerous case reports, reviews, and meta-analyses have shown the high clinical reliability of imaging data, especially CT scans, for SARS-CoV-2. Nonetheless, ML algorithms can effectively include organized medical data, which is readily available subsequent to individuals' first interactions with frontline healthcare providers. Through this combination, the statistical accuracy of these mathematical models is increased, improving their capacity to determine the presence of COVID-19, thus averting further fatalities and managing the global epidemic. In 2022, A meta-analysis on the precision of ML techniques utilizing non-image data for COVID-19 prediction in healthcare applications was published by Kuo et al. (26). In their report, Ulutas et al. highlighted the use of a unique deep learning approach for COVID-19 diagnosis on embedded systems by utilizing CT images (27). Because of the novel COVID-19-caused pandemic pneumonia epidemic, professionals are desperately required to develop a computer to assist procedures using CT images to quickly identify patients who have COVID-19. Their study's goal was to introduce a completely controlled automatically cutting-edge deep-learning approach for COVID-19 predictive evaluation and diagnosis on embedded systems. In their study, they reported that the CT images were utilized in this investigation to determine whether a subject had respiratory infections, COVID-19, or belonged to an ordinary category. Two pre-trained CNN algorithms, ResNet50 and MobileNetv2, commonly used for the image software, were employed for detection. Additionally, a novel CNN structure, known as CovidxNet-CT, was introduced specifically for COVID-19 diagnosis using three different types of CT images. To assess the performance of the proposed approach, a popular technique for determining deep learning performance, k-fold cross-validation, was applied. Furthermore, this research evaluated the proposed approach on the Jetson Nano and Tx2 embedded systems, demonstrating its applicability in situations with limited resources. This work recommended an AI-based, fully automated strategy for COVID-19 prognostic evaluation and diagnosis that is especially intended for usage with deep learning-based embedded devices.

11.1.3 Embedded Systems in the Internet of Intelligent Things

With the advent of Internet technology, data across various domains such as industrial processing and healthcare has experienced rapid growth. Both academia and business sectors acknowledge the significance of big data technology, particularly with AI at its core, which has seen rapid advancement due to large-scale computing capabilities. Government agencies and academic circles have shown considerable interest in the applications of the Internet of Medical Things (IoMT) and Industrial Internet of Things (IIoT). Traditional IIoT encompasses communication, automation, computer science, information technology, and other disciplines. Essential for the widespread adoption of IIoT are numerous technological advancements including data processing, network design, and the development of devices and sensors.

Setting a threshold to choose embedded devices that will constitute the basis application platform for the Internet of Intelligent Things is important. It suggests three essential factors to guide this selection process (28):

Energy Efficiency: Guaranteeing long-term, adaptable, environmentally friendly, and ultimately safe use.

Affordability: Targeting affordability to enable large-scale adoption is affordability.

Sufficient Processing Power: Enables ML and deep learning algorithms to be executed efficiently.

Manufacturers are integrating cyber-physical components within production facilities by linking virtual computer networks to real-world facilities via the web. Real-time monitoring of commercial data from manufacturing processes using monitors enhances productivity. IoMT applications are primarily found in three main domains (29):

i) A secure healthcare system built on IoMT enables real-time tracking of individuals' well-being and provides healthcare professionals with easier tools for assessing various bodily indicators.
ii) Continuous monitoring of temperature, electrical conditions, and moisture in pharmaceutical environments ensures accurate tracking.
iii) The integration of the Internet of Things with healthcare devices facilitates the creation of smart healthcare platforms through device connections, significantly altering the pharmaceutical and medical products industry model.

Recognizing the significance of increasing the error sensitivity rate for system accident testing and enhancing data transmission security throughout the IoMT network, the incorporation of proven wireless communication technology from IIoT is proposed as a means to achieve these objectives. Aimed at meeting the specific needs of the medical field, studies are focused on establishing a fundamental IoMT concept. Through the utilization of Bluetooth networks and resource allocation techniques, this approach seamlessly connects medical resources with a variety of biomedical services.

Mainframe computer systems commanded the processing of data in the 1980s, but the advent of personal computers (PCs) and their increased capability and availability ushered in the era of customized programming. PCs were first used for office work but have since developed to manage work settings. The term "ubiquitous computing" was invented by Mark Weiser, who saw computers processing data anytime and everywhere with ease. He anticipated the incorporation of machines into common goods, influencing their widespread use in embedded systems, automobiles, homes, and other devices nowadays (28).

The concept of the Internet of Intelligent Things (IoIT) has been addressed in great detail in recent years, with a focus on comprehensive perspectives that include the topics of embedded systems, cutting-edge computing, and neural networks. These fields are developing at a rapid rate, which means that in order to fix problems that haven't been addressed before, novel approaches for advancement and study are needed. Previous studies have concentrated on the emerging trend of AI-powered embedded systems in an attempt to fill important research gaps in this area. In order to achieve this, a great deal of these studies have concentrated on how the most recent advancements in wireless communication and embedded device solutions have assisted in the rise of IoIT applications in a variety of biomedical sectors (28).

11.1.4 ML and AI-based Systems for Advanced Biotechnological Purposes

Most experts now concur that a large portion of data processing will eventually take place at the boundary. In order to accommodate external factors dimensions, sizes, and energy limitations, embedded systems will be used in hardware acceleration devices for ML and AI-based neural networks. Relocating signals and their analysis near to the point of origin not only reduces reliance on the internet or basic use of resources but also speeds up decision-making by addressing issues related to privacy and security. By nature, embedded systems are usually customized for certain applications and have unique features. Significant breakthroughs in a variety of fields have been driven by the biotechnological advancement in the embedded area, which has been powered by the integration of AI into powerful microcontrollers. One of the main areas of research for computer-aided diagnosis (CAD) is imaging for medical purposes. Using automated diagnostic imaging, the ultimate decision is made by the healthcare professional using the results of the computational evaluation as a "second opinion". This approach can aid with the diagnosis process itself or analyze the findings of the assessment. It can also be used to monitor the success rate of the therapy over time. For instance, molecular imaging was created to investigate how cellular structures and molecules change as an illness progresses, whereas medical USG is frequently utilized to identify interior body structure defects non-destructively or to direct the course of treatment. In the past, skilled dermatologists have made errors because of their personal views while analyzing the color of the skin and interpreting clinical illnesses based on their expertise and knowledge. Medical researchers are becoming more and more interested in computer-assisted techniques for skin cancer detection in an effort to make diagnosis results less subjective. Particularly, the ideal features of the lesion area are quantified and the observation of human vision is minimized through the use of certain computerized imaging techniques.

In order to identify spatial and optical (color) data from the target areas using a red-green-blue (RGB) image in the spectrum of visible light, a dual visible/IR camera combination was developed. In the meantime, temporal and thermal characteristics are derived from the infrared results.

With great accuracy and precision, malignant tumors can be identified by using these characteristics from the standpoint of mathematical modeling. This testing approach is a potent instrument to lessen the effect of skin tumors on the population because individuals with cancerous lesions have an almost one hundred percent survival chance if they detect it earlier. In this specific scenario, one of the initial challenges to address is the temporal and spatial synchronization of images taken concurrently with both sensors. While a setup with two cameras enables precise opto-mechanical positioning, it significantly increases the cost of the medical device and limits the individual's actions. Since there is minimal object mobility and the process only takes a couple of minutes, image identification emerges as the superior choice in this case. However, the RGB and infrared photos, captured at various wavelengths and in close proximity to the body, lacked recognizable identifiable characteristics that could guide the registration method. Consequently, traditional methods typically did not yield excellent results in this situation. Numerous publications address the issue of image authorization and suggest multiple strategies, including those that rely on sharing data or the sum of squared discrepancies. Nevertheless, particularly in heterogeneous images, these techniques frequently depend on relationships that take advantage of surface similar characteristics, which aren't always present. As a substitute, strategies including Speeded-Up Robust Features (SURF) and Scale Invariant Feature Transform (SIFT) based on image data have been employed. Certain techniques have been utilized to examine thermal and visual images in order to estimate optical motion from affine changes or identify diseases of plants. Several programs that combine optical and thermal images have been implemented in industrial products, including FLIR ONE, and platforms like the Compute Unified Device Architecture. However, many of these methods depend on elements that have been manually chosen among images with varied spectra, which can be unsuccessful in various conditions. Additionally, certain approaches compute control points for photo registration by using edge detection in both samples. However, because this method is performed one image at a time, it may not be especially precise and is only applicable to images based on linear sections, which may not be common in numerous uses. This is because there are frequently not enough corresponding locations to obtain correct findings. Since image registration methods are computationally expensive, they are often used off-line, where the video is first obtained, and the resulting information is then analyzed on a computing device. While some research has explored using GPUs to accelerate image registration, the computational workload is still predominantly handled offline and requires substantial computing resources, making the development of a lightweight scanning tool more challenging. The increased computational capacity required for strategies that locate and link data across various spectral components exacerbates these issues, particularly for multimodal registration (30). To put it briefly, the future application of ML and AI in the biotechnological field essentially consists of leveraging embedded systems, cutting-edge computing, and cutting-edge imaging ways to change diagnostic and therapeutic models and enhance the treatment and care of patients' effects.

REFERENCES

1. NHLBI Obesity Education Initiative TAUB RC 628 .P73 2000 The Practical Guide Identification, Evaluation, and Treatment of Overweight and Obesity in Adults.
2. Seasonal [Internet]. Available from: www.veterinaryworld.org
3. Mezghani N, Ammar A, Boukhris O, Abid R, Hadadi A, Alzahrani TM, et al. The Impact of Exercise Training Intensity on Physiological Adaptations and Insulin Resistance in Women with Abdominal Obesity. *Healthcare (Switzerland).* 2022 Dec 1;10(12): 2533.
4. Gavrilas M. Institutul Politehnic din Iași. Faculty of Electrical Engineering, IEEE Romania Section, Institutul Politehnic din Iași. Societății Absolvenților Facultății de Electrotehnică din Iași, Institute of Electrical and Electronics Engineers. *EPE 2016: Proceedings of the 2016 International Conference and Exposition on Electrical and Power Engineering (EPE).*
5. Medical Applications User Guide Home Portable Medical Diagnostic and Therapy Devices Medical Imaging Wearables [Internet]. Available from: www.nxp.com/healthcare
6. Shi F, Wang J, Shi J, Wu Z, Wang Q, Tang Z, et al. Review of Artificial Intelligence Techniques in Imaging Data Acquisition, Segmentation, and Diagnosis for COVID-19. *IEEE Reviews in Biomedical Engineering.* Institute of Electrical and Electronics Engineers Inc. 2021;14:4–15.
7. Ding X, Clifton D, Ji N, Lovell NH, Bonato P, Chen W, et al. Wearable Sensing and Telehealth Technology with Potential Applications in the Coronavirus Pandemic. *IEEE Reviews in Biomedical Engineering.* 2021;14:48–70.
8. Nandini KP, Seshikala G. Role of Embedded Computing Systems in Biomedical Applications-Opportunities and Challenges. In: *2021 IEEE International Conference on Distributed Computing, VLSI, Electrical Circuits and Robotics, DISCOVER 2021 – Proceedings.* Institute of Electrical and Electronics Engineers Inc.; 2021:332–5.
9. Agarwal K, Jegadeesan R, Guo YX, Thakor N V. Wireless Power Transfer Strategies for Implantable Bioelectronics. *IEEE Reviews in Biomedical Engineering.* Institute of Electrical and Electronics Engineers. 2017;10:136–61.
10. Firouzi F, Rahmani AM, Mankodiya K, Badaroglu M, Merrett GV Wong P, et al. *Internet-of-Things and Big Data for Smarter Healthcare: From Device to Architecture, Applications and Analytics.* Vol. 78, Future Generation Computer Systems. Elsevier B.V.; 2018:583–6.
11. Farahani B, Firouzi F, Chang V, Badaroglu M, Constant N, Mankodiya K. Towards Fog-driven IoT eHealth: Promises and Challenges of IoT in Medicine and Healthcare [Internet]. 2017. Available from: https://www.elsevier.com/open-access/userlicense/1.0/
12. Yaqoob T, Abbas H, Atiquzzaman M. Security Vulnerabilities, Attacks, Countermeasures, and Regulations of Networked Medical Devices-A Review. *IEEE Communications Surveys and Tutorials.* 2019 Oct 1;21(4):3723–68.
13. https://www.marketdataforecast.com/market-reports/asia-pacifichealthcare-cybersecurity-market
14. https://www.thebusinessresearchcompany.com/report/medical-devicesmarket
15. https://www.marketreportsworld.com/16547658. https://www.marketreportsworld.com/16547658
16. https://www.medicaldesignbriefs.com/component/content/article/mdb/features/articles/38147
17. Guerra, P., Sportelli, G., Ortuño, J., Ledesma-Carbayo, M. J., Member, I., Vaquero, J. J., Desco, M., Ieee, A. S., & Member, S. (2007). *PETonCHIP: Architecture of a on-chip High-Resolution, Fully Digital Positron Emission Tomography Scanner for Small Animal Imaging.*

18. Arandia N, Garate JI, Mabe J. Embedded Sensor Systems in Medical Devices: Requisites and Challenges Ahead. *Sensors*. 2022 Dec 1;22(24).
19. El-Tager MA, El-Alamy EA, Mahdy AS, Youssef I, El-Dien MN, Kadah YM. K10. Embedded real time ultrasound system. *National Radio Science Conference, NRSC, Proceedings*. 2012;699–704.
20. Gudigar A, Raghavendra U, Samanth J, Rohit Gangavarapu M, Kudva A, Paramasivam G, et al. Automated detection of chronic kidney disease using image fusion and graph embedding techniques with ultrasound images. *Biomedical Signal Processing and Control* [Internet]. 2021 [cited 2024 May 9];68:102733. Available from: https://doi.org/10.1016/j.bspc.2021.102733
21. Liu X, Kane TD, Shekhar R. GPS Laparoscopic Ultrasound: Embedding an Electromagnetic Sensor in a Laparoscopic Ultrasound Transducer. *Ultrasound in Medicine and Biology* [Internet]. 2019 Apr 1 [cited 2024 May 9];45(4):989–97. Available from: https://www.umbjournal.org/article/S030156291830526X/fulltext
22. Udendhran R, Balamurugan M, Suresh A, Varatharajan R. Enhancing Image Processing Architecture Using Deep Learning for Embedded Vision Systems. *Microprocessors and Microsystems* [Internet]. 2020 [cited 2024 May 5];76:103094. Available from: https://doi.org/10.1016/j.micpro.2020.103094
23. Udendhran R, Balamurugan M, Suresh A, Varatharajan R. Enhancing Image Processing Architecture Using Deep Learning for Embedded Vision Systems. *Microprocessors and Microsystems* [Internet]. 2020 [cited 2024 May 6];76:103094. Available from: https://doi.org/10.1016/j.micpro.2020.103094
24. Tomihama RT, Dass S, Chen S, Kiang SC. *Machine Learning and Image Analysis in Vascular Surgery*. Vol. 36, Seminars in Vascular Surgery. W.B. Saunders; 2023. p. 413–8.
25. Pally RJ, Samadi S. Application of Image Processing and Convolutional Neural Networks for Flood Image Classification and Semantic Segmentation. *Environmental Modelling & Software*. 2022 Feb 1;148:105285.
26. Kuo KM, Talley PC, Chang CS. The Accuracy of Machine Learning Approaches Using Non-image Data for the Prediction of COVID-19: A Meta-analysis. *International Journal of Medical Informatics* [Internet]. 2022 [cited 2024 May 6];164:104791. Available from: https://doi.org/10.1016/j.ijmedinf.2022.104791
27. Ulutas H, Sahin ME, Karakus MO. Application of a Novel Deep Learning Technique using CT Images for COVID-19 Diagnosis on Embedded Systems. [cited 2024 May 6]; Available from: https://doi.org/10.1016/j.aej.2023.05.036
28. Oliveira F, Costa DG, Assis F, Silva I. Internet of Intelligent Things: A Convergence of Embedded Systems, Edge Computing and Machine Learning. *Internet of Things* [Internet]. 2024 [cited 2024 May 6];26:2542–6605. Available from: https://creativecommons.org/licenses/by/4.0/
29. Ding X, Zhang Y, Li J, Mao B, Guo Y, Li G. A Feasibility Study of Multi-mode Intelligent Fusion Medical Data Transmission Technology of Industrial Internet of Things Combined with Medical Internet of Things. 2023 [cited 2024 May 7]; Available from: https://doi.org/10.1016/j.iot.2023.100689
30. Inostroza F, Díaz S, Cárdenas J, Godoy SE, Figueroa M. Embedded Registration of Visible and Infrared Images in Real Time for Noninvasive Skin Cancer Screening. 2017 [cited 2024 May 8]; Available from: https://doi.org/10.1016/j.micpro.2017.09.006

12 Human Health Status Detection from the Tongue Image Using Embedded Image Processing

Mohit Bhandwal, Mukesh Roy, and Pratap Patil

12.1 INTRODUCTION

Rooted deeply in traditional medicine (e.g., Indian and Chinese) and with several thousands of years of history, tongue-based health diagnostics have been a time-tested and trusted way to gauge a person's well-being. It entails inspecting the color, shape, size, texture, and coating of the tongue as these are reported as significant indices of evidences of the condition of several internal organs and systems [1, 2]. The tongue can paint us a near-perfect picture of what someone's health is or will be without them even knowing it. Practitioners noted the color, shape, texture, and tongue coating for imbalance or health issue assessment. Different tongue regions correspond directly with different organs within our more extensive human body system, as shown in Figure 12.1. This centuries-old traditional practice gives an integral insight into what's happening inside the patient [3].

Recently, this traditional diagnostic tool has ignited the interest of physicians in integrating it into modern medical practices. Indeed, the greater attention to holistic health, or the study of the interconnectedness of the systems in the body, and the importance of non-invasive methods of early detection, is driving this interest.

The tongue as a "mirror" of the body can give diagnostic clues to a person's well-being, providing visual insight into physiological etiology. The tongue is divided into separate areas in Traditional Chinese Medicine and Ayurvedic Medicine, and these correspond to different organs: the tip corresponds to the heart-lungs, the center to the stomach-spleen, the sides to the liver-gallbladder, and the root to the kidneys-bladder [5]. This inscription of a detailed body map facilitates acupuncturists to relate changes in the tongue to afflictions in specific parts of the body. Though modern medicine values tongue-based diagnostics because they are non-invasive and offer immediate, subjective assessments of the patient's health, the tongue examination, unlike many diagnostic tests which are cumbersome or call for costly

 DOI: 10.1201/9781003508199-12

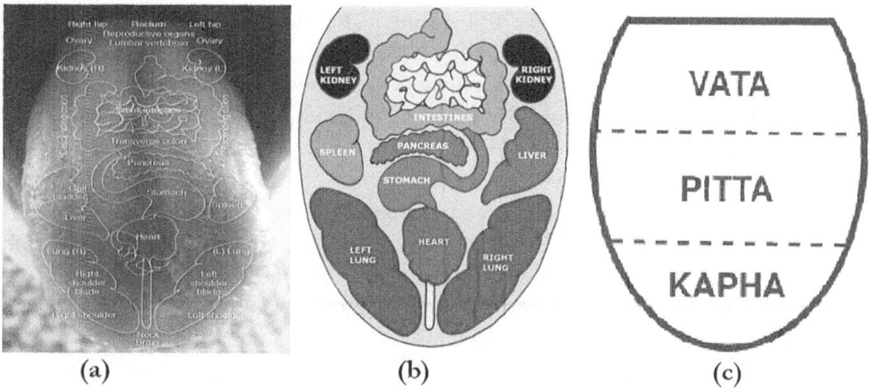

FIGURE 12.1 (a) Tongue image. (b) Representation of different parts of the body on the tongue. (c) Division of tongue according to the Ayurvedic medical system [4].

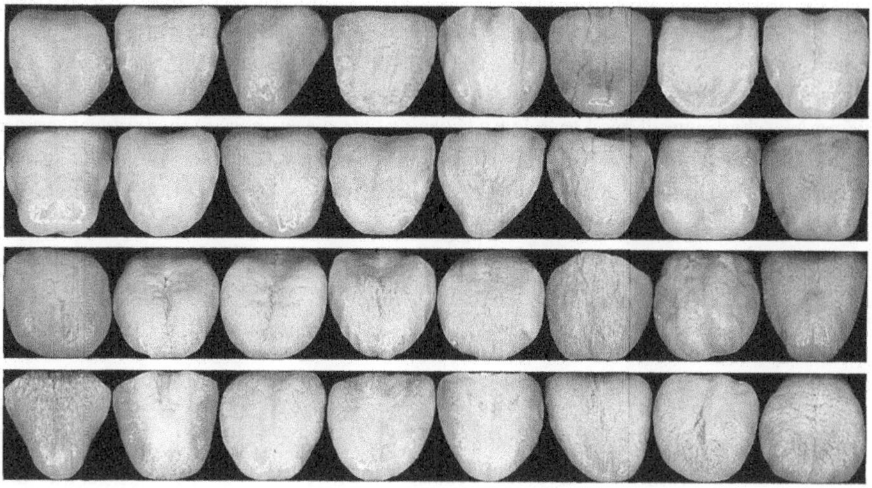

FIGURE 12.2 Different colors of the tongue [6].

equipment, can be easily and inexpensively done. Thus, simple tongue diagnostics criteria can be used as a first approach to health evaluation in situations where no other diagnosis tools are available. Also, the diagnostics of the language of the tongue will help you identify health problems as early as possible. The update is that the tongue may show subtle signs of abnormal appearance as a pre-symptom in these individuals before full-blown symptoms develop, this will give a window of contribution for early intervention. For example, a pale tongue can mean anemia or lack of essential nutrients, while a bright red tongue may suggest an infection or inflammation. A thick yellow coating on the tongue suggests digestive disturbances or toxicity within the body [2]. Tongue images of different colors are shown in Figure 12.2.

Moreover, given the uniqueness of the tongue, tongue diagnostics can help monitor the healing processes. For example, by checking the tongue, healthcare providers can see how the current status of the tongue compares with the history of the patient, and adapt treatment as necessary. An assessment continuing in this way can be very useful for the management of chronic disease in order to achieve better patient care. Through a non-invasive, efficient, and comprehensive approach that also includes the tongue examination, early diagnosis can be achieved, personalized treatment can be undertaken, and patient follow-up can be managed. As integrative healing approaches are gaining popularity, including features such as tongue diagnosis methods from traditional medicine into modern medicine, supports a hope that can significantly improve the quality of health as a whole.

It has been a breakthrough with the use of image processing and artificial intelligence (AI) in tongue diagnoses. The image processing techniques offer a dependable method to take snaps of the tongue with a high level of accuracy and yet it can be further processed into segments of information that are almost unnoticeable to the human eye. This gives practitioners a more concrete and measurable examination of tongue qualities by these methods [7]. However, taking this principle to the next level, machine learning tuned in artificial intelligence could analyze the vast tongue image data and therefore provide us with an opportunity to detect patterns and relationships to myriad different health conditions [8]. A model can thus be evolved by using AI, which would be able to learn those minute differences in the input of tongue characteristics and correlate them with certain Ayurvedic diagnoses which is a good way for a practitioner to make a more risk-averse diagnosis. Utilizing AI to improve tongue diagnoses is not just a strong potential to increase the accuracy of diagnosis. However, there is an equal and ad-hoc democratization of expertise explanation becoming available for everyone, which enables Ayurvedic insights on a platter to all in sundry.

This union of ancient wisdom with the latest technology is of utmost importance, especially at a time when the world is waking up to personalized medicine and other holistic concepts of health. Amid rising global pressures on healthcare systems, cost-effective non-invasive diagnostics modalities are needed urgently to aid in the early detection and prevention of diverse diseases [9]. The present study suggests that utilizing algorithms/features like Image processing and AI in combination with tongue diagnostic techniques can be a potential mechanism to deal with this issue. This can lead to personalized solutions, in the context of Ayurveda, that are congruent with the Ayurvedic principles and characteristics, and provide large, real-time insight into the health of someone [10]. Therefore, combining tongue-based diagnostics with new technologies in healthcare improves it significantly. When used in combination with other diagnostics, such as blood tests, imaging studies, and a wide array of history of the patient, the tongue can be an incredibly useful tool to detect illnesses beforehand as it can help to provide the most comprehensive picture of a patient's well-being. This integrative approach supports the development of personalized treatment plans tailored to the individual's specific needs and conditions [6].

AI and imagery can be used to classify the condition of tongues, and this can be a significant addition to the larger field of integrative medical sciences that empowers the link between conventional and contemporary medical interventions. That partnership could result in end-to-end multi-diagnostics for health assessment, consecutively improving patient care. For the first time, the ability to perform such extensive analysis correctly from snaps and provide results via AI-based models is a great breakthrough for Ayurveda and the entire healthcare system. With the help of AI, tongue diagnosis could be the vanguard of complimentary computing in disease diagnosis in the years to come. AI has the power to enable earlier diagnosis, personalized treatment, and more effective ongoing monitoring, which is vital in improving the accuracy, availability, and comprehensiveness of diagnostics. The use of AI in tongue-based diagnostics as technology evolves could improve healthcare in both quality of results and patient recovery due to a more holistic approach to treatment.

12.2 TONGUE DIAGNOSIS IN AYURVEDIC TREATMENT

Tongue examination, as stated by Ayurvedic texts like "Charaka Samhita" and "Sushruta Samhita", has been long known about. Tongue descriptions and their relationship with health have been extensively described in this paper. Through time, Ayurvedic experts have examined the tongue visually to understand a patient's health and identify illnesses. In a tongue diagnosis, various aspects of the organ are looked at, which include color, shape, size, coating, or texture. Every characteristic is an indication of what is happening inside the body [4]. Pale-colored tongues indicate blood deprivation due to anemia or reduced blood volume, while reddish ones suggest excessive heat or inflammation. Enlarged or sunken sides of the tongue may relate to digestion problems or malnutrition. Coating presence, coloration, and thickness could be used to learn about the digestive system's status. For instance, a yellow coat on the tongue shows more Pitta, while a white-coated one means Ama (the toxins) in the digestive tract. Cracks or sores on the surface could be signs of dehydration or chronic ailments.

Research has demonstrated that diagnosis by observing people's tongues can determine whether they are suffering from any diseases without any pain being caused. The correlation between tongue properties and systemic diseases has also been proven through such studies, as shown in Table 12.1 [11, 12]. For instance, a study by Wu et al. (2016) found important associations between tongue indicators and metabolic syndrome components like obesity, hypertension, and dyslipidemia [13].

There have been recent studies into the validity of tongue diagnosis in Ayurveda. By the front of machine learning algorithms and the rapid evolution of imaging technologies, a new level of detailed tongue analysis can now be aimed for. More accurate objective tongue diagnoses with machine learning algorithms have been boldly promised by some, aided by advances in imaging technologies. The study completed by Wang et al. applied pattern recognition methods to the digital image of the tongue and developed a diagnostic support system for many diseases [14].

This is further compounded by incorporating other diagnostic tools including pulse diagnosis and clinical history facilitates the entirety of the diagnostic procedure with tongue reading. This integrative approach is in accordance with Ayurveda's attention to the individual treatment plans that ensure that therapies are conceived according to the individual constitution and health of the patient. Based on the

TABLE 12.1

The Results of Tongue Body Color and Clinical Variables Correlation Analyses [12]

Index	Sex (n=816)	Age (n=816)	DM (n=56)	HT (n=142)	HL (n=108)	Cancer (n=113)	CD (n=77)	AD (n=-53)	IBS (n=32)	Depression (n=38)	BMI (n=816)	SBP (n=816)	DBP (n=816)	PR (n=816)	BT (n=816)	Hb (n=816)	eGFR (n=816)	L* (n=816)	a* (n=816)	b* (n=816)
Sex (n=816)	-	0.09*	0.07	0	-0.04	0.08*	0	0.03	0	0.02	0.1*	-0.04	0.04	-0.05	0	0.28**	-0.05	0.18**	0.16**	-0.2**
Age (n=816)	0.07	-	0.06	0.15**	0.11**	0.18**	0.07	-0.13**	0	-0.05	-0.12**	0.34**	-0.11**	-0.02	-0.15**	-0.11**	-0.45**	-0.17**	-0.12**	0.11**
DM (n=56)	0.12**	0.15**	-	0.13**	0.04	-0.03	-0.04	0	-0.01	-0.02	0.09*	-0.03	-0.01	0.01	0	-0.06	-0.05	0.09	0.08	-0.01
HT (n=142)	0.36**	0.36**	0.36**	-	0.18**	0.0s9*	-0.04	-0.01	0.04	0	0.13**	0.13**	-0.02	-0.01	0	0.04	0	0	-0.03	-0.02
HL (n=108)	0.02	0.27**	0.11**	0.28**	-	-0.04	0.02	-0.01	-0.01	-0.05	0.05	0.06	-0.05	0.07	0.01	0.09*	-0.03	-0.01	-0.04	0.07
Caner (n=113)	0.04	0.26**	0.03	0.15**	0.03	-	-0.05	-0.02	-0.01	-0.04	-0.02	-0.04	0.02	0.04	0.04	-0.14**	-0.01	0.04	0.02	0.02
CD (n=77)	-0.03	0.04	-0.04	-0.04	0.01	-0.04	-	-0.05	0	0.08	0	-0.06	0.04	0.09	-0.05	-0.04	0.03	-0.01	0.04	0.01
AD (n=-53)	0.01	-0.21**	-0.03	-0.08	-0.07	-0.07	-0.05	-	-0.04	0	-0.03	0.07	-0.04	0.03	0.04	-0.01	0.05	-0.01	-0.01	-0.05
IBS (n=32)	0.01	-0.04	-0.03	0.01	-0.02	-0.02	0	-0.03	-	-0.03	-0.08*	-0.05	0.04	0.01	0	0.05	0.02	0	-0.05	-0.08
Depression (n=38)	0.02	-0.07	-0.03	-0.03	-0.06	-0.06	0.07	0.01	-0.03	-	-0.02	0.07	-0.04	-0.03	0.06	0.02	-0.03	0.05	0.01	0.01
BMI (n=816)	0.24**	0.07	0.16**	0.24**	0.12**	-0.01	-0.03	-0.02	-0.06	-0.01	-	0.16**	0.02	-0.03	-0.06	0.05	-0.08	0.08*	0.03	-0.21**
SBP (n=816)	0.14**	0.47**	0.09	0.35**	0.21**	0.09	-0.03	-0.05	-0.05	0.01	0.31**	-	0.68**	-0.05	0.04	-0.01	0.02	0	0.05	0

DBP (n=816)	0.17**	0.26**	0.05	0.23**	0.12**	0.04	0	-0.04	0	0	0.27**	0.74**	-	0.23**	0	0.14**	-0.06	0	-0.03	0.04
PR (n=816)	-0.03	0	0.01	0.02	0.06	0.05	0.08	0.03	0.01	-0.02	0.01	0.13**	0.25**	-	0.16**	-0.11**	0	0.04	0.07	-0.09*
BT (n=816)	-0.05	-0.19**	-0.03	-0.07	-0.05	0.01	-0.04	0.09*	0	0.06	-0.07	-0.04	0	0.18**	-	-0.11**	0	-0.02	0.02	-0.06
Hb (n=816)	0.38**	-0.07	0	0.08*	0.07	-0.15**	-0.04	0.01	0.05	0.03	0.22**	0.16**	0.23**	-0.06	-0.1	-	-0.03	-0.01	0.24**	-0. 2**
eGFR (n=816)	-0.11**	-0.58**	-0.14**	-0.24**	-0.19**	-0.15**	0.01	0.15**	0.04	0.02	-0.14**	-0.32**	-0.23**	-0.01	0.11**	-0.03	-	0.05	0.05	-0.01
L* (n=816)	0.05	-0.15**	0.06	-0.03	-0.03	0.02	-0.04	0.02	0.02	0.05	0.05	-0.09**	-0.58	0	0	-0.12**	0.1**	-	-0.52**	0.22**
a* (n=816)	0.13**	-0.06	0.02	-0.04	-0.03	-0.04	0.04	0	-0.06	0.01	0.01	0.03	0.04	0.02	0.2	0.27**	0.05	-0.48**	-	0.31**
b* (n=816)	-0.26**	0.09*	-0.02	-0.06	0.03	0.07	0.04	-0.07	-0.09	0	-0.27**	-0.9*	-0.17**	-0.08*	-0.05	0.27**	0	0.56	0.13**	-

For “*”, n=142, and for “**”, n=816.

findings from tongue diagnosis, ayurvedic practitioners suggest personal strategies for treatment such as dietary, herbal, panchakarma (detox procedures), lifestyle modifications, etc. [15, 16]. So if you get a thick white coating, that would lead to a detoxification program which eliminates the toxins, or if it looks red, it might need balancing Pitta with cooling herbs and stress management techniques.

Ayurvedic medicine cannot be prescribed without tongue diagnosis because it is a crucial part of it, as this approach gives important hints about one's health. By observing the characteristics of the tongue, medical practitioners can identify imbalances in doshas and create a unique treatment plan for each patient. Recent studies have proved that this ancient method is effective and could be used with modern diagnostic techniques. Ayurveda is increasingly becoming popular in holistic or integrative medicine as tongue diagnosis becomes more important in bridging traditional wisdom and contemporary healthcare.

12.3 DISEASE-SPECIFIC DIAGNOSES

12.3.1 Diabetes

Diabetes is a chronic disease with a high-fast prevalence. It is essential that complications are detected and treated early. A novel model was built based on the TCM tongue diagnosis and machine learning algorithm for the prediction. Using two datasets, 1512 subjects were recruited and trained. After the prediction, the performance of the model was evaluated by some of the metrics. Stacking 71% accurate, non-invasive, ResNet50 69% accurate results for the classical machine learning model showed that the prediction performance was significantly enhanced by incorporating tongue features in the study. For the detection of hyperglycemia and blood glucose in critical states, the optimal models of Stacking and ResNet50 have high precision, low false positive rates, and low misdiagnosis rates. The results of this study suggest that the tongue features do not change synchro-diachronically with the gradual progression of glucose metabolism from the normal to the impaired to the abnormal and the differential changes in the tongue. Features depict the abnormal glucose metabolism, and these results appear to be reasonable when the tongue diagnosis technique combines with the machine learning algorithm for predicting the risk of diabetes [17].

Diagnosis of diabetes from tongue image using a convolutional neural network consists of tongue image pre-processing after extracting color and texture features, tongue shape detection, followed by color intensity extraction for acne, and cracks detection. Researchers have used the five-layer VGG16 algorithm (three convolutional layers + two hidden layers) modified. This model is 98% based on health and diabetes tongue predictions [18].

The TFDA-1 tongue diagnosis instrument reveals the color, texture, and tongue coating ratio characteristics with tongue images of diabetic cases. Tongue images of diabetic patients were used to test the tongue diagnosis analysis system (TDAS) to analyze the distribution of tongue features. Clustering of these features was done using K-means and Self-organizing Maps (SOM) networks. Result indicated that the highest TB-a and TC-a features belong to Cluster 3 while the lowest TB-b and TC-b features are in Cluster 2 [19].

A substantial role is the effort by artificial intelligence to classify image labels, and this also helps to build new machine learning and deep learning methodologies. Such algorithms can be used for regression and classification like diabetes tongue, the features are extracted from the standard classification algorithms like K-Nearest Neighbors, Support Vector Machine, Decision tree, Logistic regression, and Convolution Neural Networks. Utilization of CNN in the proposed algorithm for dimensional reduction is proven to be more precise [20].

The introduction of a novel color descriptor that consists of clustering centers of color points from tongue images for representing colors. One of the descriptors is extended to RGB, HSV, LAB color spaces to mine rich color information. In this paper, a novel multiple color features fusion method was proposed, based on learning two projections to project multiple features to their corresponding shared and specific subspaces. The model integrates the discriminant effectively with the model by which it improves the accuracy of the diagnosis. The proposed method achieves an average accuracy of up to 93.38% on a clinical tongue dataset, suggesting the potential of the methodology for clinical DM diagnosis [21].

The researcher proposes a sequential method for preparing tongue images that bridge Chinese and Western medicine. It uses image processing methods to extract quantitative features, chromatic and textural scales, from images. Features such as edge and color intensity extraction are used to detect shapes and pimples/cracks, respectively. The Level Set Algorithm is important to correctly identify pixels associated with the two classes which describes superior segmentation results that the Level Set Algorithm produces. Mean and entropy values of all the subjects are compared with these to the normal and abnormal tongues [22].

Moreover, researchers also utilized ML algorithms based on ANN to detect diabetic conditions based on tongue features [23]. Zhang et al. have shown diagnostic approach based on tongue pictures in Traditional Chinese Medicine (TCM) is highly valuable, demonstrating the viability of digitalized tongue diagnosis [24].

12.3.2 Gastrointestinal Disorders

Gastrointestinal illnesses frequently cause changes in the tongue's structure. A deep neural network model was implemented to diagnose tongue cancer with 12,400 endoscopic images. The model had an area under the receiver operating characteristic curve. The study concluded that AI-based diagnosis presents huge potential in increasing early cancer detection and mitigating dependence on specialists [25].

In another study, a total of 27 participants were included, of which 19 were gastritis patients with cold or hot syndromes and 8 were healthy volunteers. Researchers further elaborated 123 and 258 species-level OTUs abundant in Chinese patients with cold/hot syndromes, as Cold Microbiota and Hot Microbiota, respectively. These findings mean that the microbiome of tongue coating is a new holistic biomarker for patient subtype development, supporting the diagnostic importance of the tongue in TCM [26].

This is a prospective evaluation of the feasibility of the Atrial and Transoral Diagnosis System (ATDS) in upper gastrointestinal disorders. Tongue images were taken from over 20 volunteer participants. Subjects were further subclassified into one of the following 4 pan endoscopy group categories: gastritis, peptic ulcer disease, gastroesophageal reflux disease (GORD), and normal. Analysis of nine large tongue features in total was done to evaluate the distinction of MRI features of the tongue [27].

In a cross-sectional study in China involving the China-Japan Friendship Hospital, inflammation and gastroesophageal reflux disease were the most common clinical features and were detected in 76.6%, followed by fissured tongue (34.3%). Regarding the distribution of ATFs, gender and age were statistically significant, with fissured tongue, red tongue, and yellowish, greasy tongue relatively prone to be observed in males, and purple tongue and ecchymotic tongue more common in females ($P<0.05$). Fissured tongue was an independent factor for upper gastrointestinal precancerous lesions (UGPLs), too. This study reinforces a likely association between fissured tongue and UGPLs and calls for a more extensive, multi-center, community-based investigation to validate these findings [28].

More than the normal amount of saliva and thicker fur on the tongue result in a diagnosis of gastroesophageal reflux disease (GERD) compared with those without GERD, as observed in a study at Kaohsiung Chang Gung Memorial Hospital in Taiwan. However, as the amount of saliva and tongue fur in the spleen-stomach area increased, the risk of GERD increased by 3.621 times and 1.019 times, respectively. After all, the study reveals that both saliva and tongue fur in the spleen-stomach area may be potential biomarkers of GERD risk as well as severity and that these biomarkers might be lag or non-invasive markers of GERD [29].

12.3.3 Cardiovascular Diseases

The tongue diagnosis is quite subjective and inconsistent. To solve this problem by using transfer learning, a new model called the SADTLTIADD (Simulated Annealing with Transfer Learning based Tongue Image Analysis for Disease Diagnosis) was proposed to enhance the quality of the input tongue images with preprocessing and it extracts useful features from the Enhanced tongue images by the feature extractor with EfficientNet. Their simulations demonstrated that PNET offers significantly better accuracy, reaching up to 99.30% [30].

This paper introduces an automated tongue inspection system that applies digital image processing to extract quantitative tongue features from tongue images. These are features (both observed and unobserved) and the diseases for which the extracted models are probabilistic graphical models named Bayesian networks. Process performance was tested on 455 patients and 13 commonly occurring diseases, using trained classifiers to forecast diagnostic assessment in 70 healthy volunteers [31].

A diagnostic signature based on tongue diagnostic parameters for the recognition of clopidogrel resistance was performed on 101 post-PCI patients with clopidogrel resistance, and a novel and reliable diagnostic signature comprised of tongue diagnostic parameters was established to identify the clopidogrel resistance diagnosis. Diagnostic signatures were created via univariate and multivariate logistic regression analysis (as receiver operating characteristic curve). The tongue diagnostic parameters-based signatures were significantly associated with clopidogrel resistance and harbored an area under the curve value of 0.819 [32].

Early screening is critical for preventing catastrophic incidents. Tongue hyperspectral imaging was used to evaluate HD patients with CHD in the early stages. The results revealed substantial differences between HD and HD-CHD hyperspectral data, indicating that hyperspectral imaging of the tongue may be used to screen HD patients for CHD complications [33]. Duan et.al. offer an approachable, practical, and non-invasive way to diagnose and screen for CHD on a wide scale. A potential useful marker for the diagnosis of CHD is tongue imaging data [33].

12.3.4 Nutritional Deficiencies

The study presents a smartphone application that is free and detects vitamin deficiencies in individuals by using artificial intelligence. The app can clearly identify what you might be missing in your body without even needing any blood, it does that via images of certain parts of your body, like an eye, lips, tongue, and nails. Then, applying its technology of nutritional micro-correction, writes a report guiding the choice of nutrient sources suitable to correct the deficiency it detected and to avoid any serious problems. Doctors can bring up the detection and accuracy of the bot by classifying and verifying visual data. It has the potential to outperform human medical condition diagnosis on a global scale (due to millions of individuals suffering needlessly from a preventable nutritional deficiency). It will also help medical professionals to diagnose with more accuracy [34].

12.4 IMAGE PROCESSING TECHNIQUES IN TONGUE DIAGNOSIS

Tongue images have been analyzed using various image processing techniques such as image segmentation, feature extraction, and pattern recognition algorithms. This begins by acquiring high-quality tongue images and pre-processing steps like noise reduction and color normalization to ensure consistency. High-resolution cameras capture clear images of the tongue, ensuring uniform lighting to avoid shadows and reflections that could distort the analysis. This involves several steps to enhance the image quality. Techniques like Gaussian blur or median filtering to remove noise. Adjusting brightness and contrast to standardize images for consistent analysis.

12.4.1 Segmentation

Image segmentation is an important technology in computer vision, which divides an image into various regions or segments to make the image simpler and facilitate easy identification. It is a common practice to find objects and boundaries in images using it. It can broadly be classified as either thresholding, edge-based segmentation, region-based segmentation, clustering-based segmentation, graph-based segmentation, or deep learning-based segmentation. It is used for thresholding the gray-scale image into binary components and then edge-based segmentation so it can be applied to locate the boundaries of different zones. Region-based segmentation nests pixels as their region-based attributes, clustering-based segmentation uses a clustering algorithm similar to K-means and Mean shift. Graph-based segmentation models the image as a graph and represents the similarity by edges between nodes. As a semi-automated segmentation approach, deep learning-based segmentation utilizes Convolutional Neural Networks (CNNs) along with other deep learning architectures to generate near-perfect segmentation maps. Medical imaging allows us to find out the defects in our body parts so we can cure in prior, traffic signs, etc. [35].

A new algorithm dubbed CGT proposes each pixel in an image its threshold (using the mean and the standard deviation of neighboring pixels grayscale values) and a unique threshold of the squared variance of neighbor pixels. It outputs the image border, like an edge detector in image processing. It was demonstrated that the algorithm contains precise edge boundaries in the images and pixel thresholds are quantifiable based on statistics calculated from nearby pixels [36].

In this paper, a variety of segmentation techniques that are used for medical images are discussed, which evidently focus on areas of the problem which are not solved yet. All algorithms can be improved. This excellent image processing quality makes LBM, which has real-time performance, adapted to a variety of circumstances, and easy fine-tuning mechanism, a popular new research area in image processing based on the predictions of the authors [37].

In this paper, researchers present an overview of the state-of-the-art image segmentation quality evaluation techniques, dealing with unsupervised and supervised methods. It talks about their use in natural, medical, and distant sensing picture evaluation and performs an empirical contrast of these methods. It also checks the veracity of traditional metrics for assessing remote sensing images and medical images [38].

Image segmentation is one of the most commonly used tasks to improve the results of diagnosis and analysis, especially in X-ray medical imaging. Researchers have presented medical image segmentation listing the benefits and pitfalls of each method. It also gives recommendations for future research on segmentation methods [39].

The accuracy of the diagnosis by using the tongue is important for the medical decision, and performing the segmentation of the tongue image is also essential. For example, deep learning methods often predict pixel points point-by-point for pixel-level segmentation, resulting in low-precision results. We also compare different models and loss functions to determine the model with the best performance. The red grid of the CNN is particularly useful for segmentation and in this work the paper tests a few methods to focus on the color traits of the original image. Researchers had proposed an improved encoder–decoder network model based on the backbone network of Resnet and borrows from the model of U-Net. We combine attention module from source image with the feature layer from the last up sampling in the U-Net. Experimental results show that the new algorithm is 2–3% better than the state-of-the-art one, so it is a better candidate for tongue segmentation task [40].

12.4.2 Feature Extraction

Feature extraction is an essential step in image processing to retrieve useful information from an image when required for analysis, classification, or image recognition. It is something very useful for Computer Vision applications like Object Detection, Facial Recognition, Image Retrieval, Scene Understanding, and so on. Basic image features like edges, corners, texture features, shape features, color features, key point descriptors, deep learning-based features, and frequency domain features are some of the key methods and techniques used in feature extraction. Edges represent the regions where the image intensities change dramatically, while corners are intersection points for edges. Examples of key point descriptors are Scale-Invariant Feature Transform (SIFT), Speeded-Up Robust Features (SURF), and Oriented FAST and Rotated BRIEF (ORB). Such features are Convolutional Neural Networks (CNNs), Transfer Learning and, Fourier Transform. Features, extraction methods and their performance in different scenarios especially in an application of a character recognition are discussed by researchers [41].

The study described in this article includes egg white protein thermal gelation image characteristics analysis and an attempt to extract external features under the optimal parameters. This benefits classic algorithms for image feature extraction as PCA and ICA and the way to improve them. Experiments and simulations are employed to research the recognition method of image recognition based on the egg white protein thermal gelation for the efficient recognition algorithm of image feature extraction under different solidification states and the accuracy of image under the multiple solidification states. This study has great reference value for the follow-up of high-efficiency experimental research [42].

Texture analysis using Gabor filters and wavelet transforms can identify surface patterns associated with doshas [43].

12.4.3 Pattern Recognition

Pattern recognition is all about identifying a character or object in an image giving different conditions with a large dataset of open source. The use of pattern recognition algorithms in machine learning and artificial intelligence is crucial, allowing systems to detect regularities, structures, and patterns in data. Some of the most common algorithms are Linear Regression, Logistic Regression, Support Vector Machines (SVM), Decision Trees, Random Forests, and Neural Networks. Examples of an unsupervised learning algorithm include K-Means Clustering, Principal Component Analysis (PCA), Independent Component Analysis (ICA), Gaussian Mixture Models (GMM), Semi-Supervised Learning, Reinforcement Learning, Dimensionality Reduction Techniques, Autoencoders, Anomaly Detection Algorithms, Instance-Based Learning Algorithms, Graph-Based Algorithms and Spectral Clustering. Supervised learning algorithms are used when the output is continuous or categorical such as Linear Regression, Logistic Regression, Support Vector Machines (SVM), Decision Trees and random forests, Neural networks, etc. For dimensionality reduction for visualization and efficient representation of data, unsupervised learning algorithms and related techniques are employed, KMeans Clustering, PCA (Principal Component Analysis), ICA (Independent Component Analysis), GMM (Gaussian Mixture Models), Semi-Supervised Learning, Reinforcement Learning, Dimensionality Reduction Techniques, Autoencoders.

ML algorithms, such as support vector machines (SVM) neural networks and DL models, classify the tongue images from the extracted features. Note: for simplicity, we say "trained on" without remarking on the immense labeling process behind all these thousands (and even more) labeled tongue pictures [44]. Algorithms like Canny or Sobel operators outline the tongue's shape. More advanced techniques like region growing or watershed segmentation to delineate specific areas of interest, such as the tongue's tip, body, and root.

12.5 METHODOLOGICAL ADVANCEMENTS IN TONGUE IMAGING

12.5.1 High-Resolution Imaging

With digital cameras and imaging devices that have reached a higher resolution, tongue diagnostics are now facilitated like never before. The surface of the tongue can be imaged in great detail with a modern camera and we can record it with great detail. These devices are equipped with such tools as tongue-imaging cameras that use specific lighting conditions and standardized views, helping reduce the impact of environmental factors on tongue photographs.

12.5.2 3D Imaging Techniques

Tongue diagnostics has acquired a new dimension with the application of 3D imaging technology. Generating precise, 3D models of the tongue enable clinicians to measure the surface topography and volume, revealing features such as swelling, texture changes, and mass abnormalities that cannot be visualized through 2D imaging. This technology is particularly well-suited for understanding changes across time, and how interventions may affect it.

12.5.3 Advanced Image Processing Techniques

With advanced image processing algorithms, even a slight change in the tongue could derive detailed features. Quantitative methods for the measurement of the tongue include image segmentation, edge detection, and texture analysis. These algorithms can identify things like the thickness of the coating on the tongue, the distribution of colors, or the presence of certain portions or spots on the tongue that are a symptom of some kind of medical issue.

12.5.4 Machine Learning and Pattern Recognition

Machine learning (ML) and pattern recognition make the analysis of tongue image more intelligent. Machine learning on bigger and bigger sets of tongue images, then, allows these algorithms to recognize patterns linked to certain diseases. As an example, various tongue diagnosis methods using convolutional neural networks (CNNs) achieve high accuracy in diagnosing diabetes, cardiovascular diseases, and gastrointestinal disorders.

12.5.5 AI-Based Diagnostic Systems

Taking advantage of the capabilities of AI-based diagnostic systems, we can integrate image processing with machine learning models and in turn offer automated and objective tongue diagnoses. Such systems can review images in real time and provide practitioners and patients with immediate results. Early identification of subtle changes, which can be easy to overlook to the human eye, can result in positive outcomes for patients if AI models are trained on diversified datasets.

12.5.6 Predictive Analytics

They also were developed to predict disease progression and the effects of treatment through the use of tongue image data with predictive analytics and AI. AI models can assess changes in longitudinal tongue image data and make predictions about future health states, thereby supporting proactive healthcare management. Especially useful for chronic diseases where early interventions can make all the difference in the world for a patient.

12.5.7 Integration between TCM and Western Medicine

This integration of tongue diagnosis with Western medical techniques has expanded the diagnostic scope. An example would be correlating tongue images with those of specific laboratory tests, imaging studies, and clinical examinations to gain a more holistic view of the patients' health. This multi-faceted version of knowledge improves diagnostics by tying the bridge between the ancient and the new school medicine.

12.5.8 Telemedicine and Remote Diagnostics

The introduction of telemedicine has conferred tongue diagnosis all over the world. Machine learning sent diagnostic feedback trends to both the patients and the doctor, along with high-quality images of the tongue from their smartphones that could then be uploaded to the doctor for analysis. Healthcare on the other hand has moved miles ahead and must thank AI-driven diagnostics tools in a major way to offer increased advantages to any type of remote consultancy to allow for more accessible and convenient healthcare.

12.5.9 Landmark Detection and Image Pre-processing

The second step we will tackle is studying various landmark detectors. It needs to be familiar with some of the simple image pre-processing methods like resizing, changing color spaces, etc., as well as other feature extraction techniques commonly deployed in object detection/recognition activities. The preprocessing forms the basis for the successful analysis of a tongue image. Commonly used methods include histogram equalization, image denoising, contrast enhancement, etc.

12.5.10 Ensemble Learning

Employing ensemble learning techniques that combine many models is an example of this and has also been used. Li et al. study maximizes each algorithm's benefit by using deep learning and standard machine learning algorithms based on tongue features. They build the non-invasive diabetic's risk prediction model with a features fusion algorithm, integrate possible characteristics with existing knowledge, and noninvasively identify prediabetics and diabetics [45].

12.6 APPLICATIONS AND CASE STUDIES

As we can see from some case studies the research has proven that there is may potential in tongue diagnosis by using image processing techniques [46]. Another study was published to demonstrate the classification of tongue images into categories carrying different dosha imbalances using SVM with an accuracy of more than 85% [47]. Another study by Tania et al. used the combination approach (texture and color features), which improved the diagnostic accuracy of diseases such as digestive disorders, stress, etc. to a greater extent [48].

Despite its promise, many predictive models helping designers optimize designs of spatial configurations based on human multi-modal interactions still exhibit deficiencies. The use cases mentioned in the previous sections have provided a good scope for challenges that lie ahead and need immediate attention. While the results are promising, several challenges still need to be addressed. However, the variability in intensity values of tongue images (caused by lighting conditions, image quality, individual differences, etc.) should be pre-processed and normalized. Furthermore, the requirement for substantial and diverse datasets in training machine learning models is vital to improving the universality of these diagnostic systems [49].

In a research the study included 270 adults in the age group of 21–40 years, to evaluate the lingual morphological features and to test the efficiency and reliability of lingual morphological structures as an aid for human identification. The shape registration specimens in terms of branch allotype, Longitudinal Medial Septum, and Lingual Apex type were kept in molded alginate. It was concluded that tongue impressions and photographic images are reliable methods for forensic dentistry identification, thereby providing proof of life and genetic individualization [50].

The tongue is one of a small handful of unique organs, which, like the nose, ears, and the iris, can be physically accessed and physically protruded, which is significant for applications concerning identity verification. Nevertheless, because of the nonexistence of 3D databases concerning tongue features, research on tongue features is very limited. This paper introduces a 3D tongue image database comprising geometric shapes and surface texture of 134 subjects intended as a new research resource for tongue [51].

Forensic odontology, a sub-branch of dentistry, depends on the identification of the oral structures for particular person, the distinct one is the tongue, its shape can provide useful geometric and texture physiological information. Identification was made by clinical examination, photos, and impressions to assess the morphology of the tongue. Thanks to the tofu-like nature of the human tongue, which takes the shape of whatever container it is living in, it can be a very personal part of our bodies and can actually help identify who we are, according to the researchers who used basswood mold of different tongues to conduct these 3D-rendered data points of varying tongues study [52].

When a biometric is physically or behaviorally unique to an individual, it can serve as a real-time identifier. The system provides a way to convert the user's data to digital data for the computer to interpret, by scanning their tongue-print for verification. There are several other biometrics authentication models as well supported like fingerprint, iris scan, digital signature, and voice recognition. But still, there are some serious constraints to this. Reddy et.al. have discussed different biometric techniques such as tongue scanning and how this issue has been surpassed [53].

The tongue is a very important internal organ. It helps identify each person. There are various systems based on biometrics such as fingerprints, iris scans, skin color, signature verification, voice recognition, and face recognition, etc. Sexual dimorphism of lingual impressions or tongue prints warrants their registration as secure personal identification. It focuses on the distinctiveness of tongue prints as a biometric system in comparison to the existing ones and, further elaborates on the collection and classification techniques of the tongue features [54].

This paper describes the distinctiveness of a human tongue, the minimally affected device, and how it enhances security for identification and authentication. The investigation of the person identification system procedure tongue print is presented, utilizing the Speeded Up Robust Factor (SURF), a local invariant attention point identifier and descriptor [55].

Three texture analysis methods, wavelet transform, Gabor filter, and spectral analysis were compared in the existing work for authentication of tongue print images. Features are extracted using 6 statistical measures and verified using k-Nearest Neighbor algorithm. The most accurate method is provided by wavelet analysis (92%), while it's the lowest for spectral images (75%). The relevant accuracy is highest for Gabor filter banks (83%). It is clear that wavelet-based features are superior over Gabor and spectral-based features [56].

Choras introduces a new modality approach for personal identification using tongue image. Pattern-matching tongues identify and verify users with the image of a tongue. The article uses steerable filters and the WLD (Weber Law Descriptors) for detecting textural features of the tongue. This can be combined with other demanding biometric characteristics to build multimodal biometric systems for use in authentication by law enforcement, where the systems perform considerably better than the systems using single-mode recognition [57].

The human tongue can be used for a combination of techniques of uniqueness identification, being a proof of identity due to its safety and difficulty of forgery. This gives geometric form and physiological footprint details that may be useful for purposes of identity authentication comparable to banks. Expanding these applications requires valid users or approving applicants from the admin end. The extraction procedure and the application of the inferred anatomical image in tongue databases and public systems are discussed [58].

The identification method proposed in this research is to use a tongue recognition approach. If you are in the habit of taking pictures of your tongue, you are at an advantage when it comes to confirming and correct identification of people. This paper extracts tongue features according to color and texture properties. The morphological characteristics of this can be utilized as a component of multimodal biometric systems combined with other more certain biometric characteristics for forensic uses [59].

12.7 AI/ML USE IN TONGUE IMAGE ANALYSIS FOR DISEASE DIAGNOSIS

The advent of artificial intelligence (AI) and machine learning (ML) has totally transformed the landscape of medical diagnostics. Tongue image examination plays a significant role in disease detection and is one of the novel applications for AI/ML out of the others. Traditional Chinese medicine has emphasized the importance of the tongue as a window to the body's health for centuries. It is re-emerging technology in medical science in the modern era and research is going on to take more clues by Artificial Intelligence (AI) and Machine Learning (ML) on board to refine its diagnosis with authentic and fast. In this paper, we will describe the methodologies, applications, benefits, challenges, and future scope of AI/ML in tongue image analysis which results in a popular tool for disease diagnosis.

12.7.1 Machine Learning Algorithms

The feature extraction method is used to extract basic features from the tongue images: Color; texture; shape and geometric features. For example, color features suggest the distribution and intensity of current disease state, and texture features can also identify tongue fissures or coatings. These traits are important predictors which are more susceptible to growing health problems. The extracted features are then used to perform a variety of ML algorithms. Some popular algorithms are listed in the following sections.

12.7.2 Support Vector Mechanics (SVMs)

SVMs are supervised learning models which are used for classification. It is a technique that, in the feature space (input space), tries to identify the hyperplane which helps segregate the classes well. The tongue image from patients with high quality will be collected and labeled with health conditions for SVM processing, by applying methods such as normalization, contrast enhancement, noise reduction, etc. Color, texture, and shape features are extracted by image processing algorithms. The model trained on a training dataset is evaluated on a different validation dataset to fine-tune parameters and finally tested on test dataset. Especially, diseases like diabetes, cardiovascular diseases, digestive disorders, and respiratory problems can be detected by recognizing tongue symptoms using SVM. Nonetheless, challenges associated with data quality, feature selection, computational costs and interpretability need to be overcome. In general, SVM can greatly improve disease detection in an automatic tongue diagnosis system.

12.7.3 Convolutional Neural Networks (CNNs)

It is a deep learning algorithm that can be used for analyzing visual imagery. They extract features from input images through convolutions and pooling operations. In tongue diagnosis, a large dataset of tongue images is collected, and labeled with the corresponding health conditions. Preprocessing steps include resizing, normalization, and augmentation. CNN architectures like AlexNet, VGGNet, ResNet, and Inception are designed to suit specific requirements. Labeled images are divided into training, validation, and test sets. The CNN's performance is assessed using metrics like accuracy, precision, recall, and F1 score. Once trained and validated, the CNN model can be integrated into a diagnostic system. The advantages of using CNNs in tongue diagnosis include automation, consistency, and early detection. Challenges include data quality, interpretability, generalization, and integration into clinical practice. Despite these challenges, CNNs hold significant promise for enhancing tongue diagnosis and disease detection.

12.7.4 K-Nearest Neighbors (KNN)

One of the machine learning algorithms that are usually used in medical diagnosing is the K-Nearest Neighbors (KNN) algorithm and for tongue diagnosis for disease detection. Finally, KNN is employed, by hobbling any tongue image dataset with its corresponding disease label, then prepossessing, then extracting, doing distances, nearest neighbors, and voting as majority dictate. Tongue diagnosis is employed in traditional Chinese Medicine (TCM) to diagnose diseases in detail by analyzing the tongue shape, color, texture, and coating. The labeled dataset is constructed after feature extraction using image processing techniques. Algorithm Trains on KNN Model and emulator picks an optimal k parameter to achieve this model The performance of this KNN is sensitive to the quality and relevance of the extracted features and is computationally very expensive. With the proper method, KNN can greatly help the accurate and efficient tongue-based disease diagnosis, instead of limitations.

12.7.5 Random Forests

In the domain of tongue diagnosis for disease detection, Random Forest is a machine learning technique for classification and regression tasks. This means sourcing high-quality photos of the tongue of patients with a variety of diseases (and health) and tagging each photo with the disease/health condition it belongs to. It includes responses to how to normalize, segment, and augment the data. The extracted features are used to train the Random Forests algorithm, with hyperparameter tuning fine-tuned. This model is evaluated with 10-fold cross-validation and performance metrics. Random Forests are robust, interpretable, accurate, and reliable machine learning model; therefore, Random Forests are best suited for the diagnosis of tongue images. Issues such as data quality, generalization, and ethical and privacy dilemmas. Nevertheless, Random Forests presents a very strong solution as a tool applicable in early disease detection, leading to a better patient and disease prognosis.

Recently, the development of Artificial Intelligence (AI) and Machine Learning (ML) in medical diagnostics has made a breakthrough, and tongue image analysis is not an exception which works tremendously [60–62]. The tongue is not only a vital human organ but also a key to discovering various diseases. The color, size, and surface cover structure provide functional diagnosis information(anchor). Researchers have provided insight/glimpse regarding the recent uses, approaches, and algorithms implemented through AI and ML to enhance disease detection using tongue image analysis [50].

Tongue diagnosis, a technique from Traditional Chinese Medicine (TCM), has been a process of disease detection and, ultimately, insight into clinical care [63]. As you can see, AI & ML have been used to accomplish the same. A study by Li et al. developed a tongue image segmentation and classification system based on Convolutional Neural Networks (CNNs)[64]. The results show that this system can accurately distinguish between healthy subjects and gastritis patients, which suggests AI technology has promising prospects in diagnosing TCM.

12.8 CONCLUSION

Tongue image analysis, when combined with AI and ML, is thus a hot frontier in disease diagnosis. Research has proven that it can accurately diagnose diseases like diabetes, gastrointestinal, or Cardiovascular. Even so, it is necessary to develop more improvements to better cope with the difficulties still found and enjoy all of the advantages this non-invasive diagnostic approach offers.

Imaging technologies are now able to provide good-quality images of the tongue allowing visual examination under standardized lighting conditions and large-resolution cameras with properly documented protocols for detailed analysis. Reliable and accurate feature extraction is important in determining better diagnostic outcomes and as such preprocessing techniques such as noise reduction, contrast enhancement, and segmentation are necessary. It extracts strong features to better represent the color, texture, shape, and coating of the tongue, which can be associated with diseases. These meaningful features are extracted by methods such as color space transformation, texture analysis, or geometric analysis on the images for preparing machine learning models. It has recently been demonstrated to be very successful in classifying tongue images with Machine Learning algorithms, especially Convolutional Neural Networks (CNNs) and effective models, e.g., Support Vector Machines (SVMs), Random Forests, and k-Nearest Neighbors (k-NN), have been applied in these tasks. In recent years, the use of ensemble methods and hybrid models has further improved the accuracy and robustness of disease detection. In recent years, and even centuries ago, diseases such as diabetes, anemia, jaundice, oral cancer, gastrointestinal disorders, and several other health problems were detectable with the visual appearance of the tongue. They have the capability to aid medical professionals by providing them with second opinions, help in avoiding diagnostic errors, and allow early diagnosis of diseases. As it becomes more feasible for tongue image analysis systems to be integrated into clinical practice, patients can capture images of their tongues from home to allow for remote monitoring and early interventions. In this way, democratization of diagnostic tools not only improves healthcare accessibility but largely affects underserved regions.

Even though AI diagnostics have progressed greatly over the years, many obstacles to overcome. Some are related to the data quality and variability resulting in noise and artifacts whereas others are associated with the acquisition protocols needing standardization. The Model performance in different subsets of population (genomic, ethic, or lifestyle) can change sequences from different datasets. Interpretability and explainability are also critical for realizing provider and patient trust. These components are also paramount in addressing regulatory and ethical dimensions for the privacy of patients, data security, and ethical principles governing AI. Model performance, limitations, and potential biases should be transparently reported for compliance of regulatory and ethical practices. Integration with existing Telco networks means relying on standard interfaces and appropriate methods for integration. However, in the aggregate, AI-based diagnostics will remain as part of the solution for the betterment of patient care.

There are several possible directions of growth and improvement in the future of AI and ML in tongue image analysis to detect diseases. By synthesizing tongue image analysis with other diagnostic modalities invasive blood tests, genomic data, past medical exams, etc., multimodal data integration can broaden the scope of improved diagnostic authenticity. Adaptive and performance improvement can be granted using continuous learning systems, ones that every new data can be used to feed the models and also the feedback from HCPs and patients. The worldwide health projects can become a response to healthcare inequality to be used by AI-based tongue image analysis and offer healthcare benefits in underprivileged areas. These AI systems enable personalized medicine by customizing recommendations on diagnosis and treatment according to patient characteristics. Collaboration of research and open data are needed to further the field to innovate faster and develop stronger AI models. Shared standards and best practices can also help manage ethical and regulatory challenges with more effective coordination.

In the future, we should attempt to integrate multivocal data in AyuSoft, perhaps by running a pulse diagnosis and asking the patient for their history. Suppose this could improve our diagnoses' accuracy and/or reliability over the past decade. In that case, major advances in deep learning approaches—particularly convolutional neural networks (CNNs)—have raised great hope for automating feature extraction and achieving more accurate classification.

Incorporating image-processing techniques in Ayurveda shows major changes and developments in the classical medical system with advanced steps. Systems Approaches in Automation Technologies (SAAT) technologies modernize the Ayurveda diagnostic practice by augmenting, rather than replacing, the practitioner's diagnosis and treatment. More research and development are required to overcome the current challenges and take maximum advantage of image processing in achieving holistic health care. However, using these advanced techniques presents several challenges. These include establishing standardized protocols for image acquisition and processing to ensure consistency across different devices and conditions and ensuring that the algorithms can handle variations in lighting, tongue position, and other factors. It is also important to conduct extensive clinical trials to validate the accuracy and reliability of these techniques.

REFERENCES

1. A. K. Abdullah, S. L. Mohammed, A. Al-Naji, and M. S. Alsabah, "Tongue color analysis and diseases detection based on a computer vision system," *J Techniq*, vol. 5, no. 1, pp. 22–37, Mar. 2023, doi: 10.51173/jt.v5i1.868
2. B. Zhang, X. Wang, J. You, and D. Zhang, "Tongue color analysis for medical application," *Evid-Based Complement Altern Med*, vol. 2013, pp. 1–11, 2013, doi: 10.1155/2013/264742
3. J. Xie, C. Jing, Z. Zhang, J. Xu, Y. Duan, and D. Xu, "Digital tongue image analyses for health assessment," *Med Rev*, vol. 1, no. 2, pp. 172–198, Dec. 2021, doi: 10.1515/mr-2021-0018
4. D. Miryala, P. Parvataneni, and G. Aliperi, "Computer aided image enhancement of tongue for diagnosis in ayurvedic medical treatment," *Appl Med Inform*, vol. 34, pp. 46–56, 2014, [Online]. Available: https://api.semanticscholar.org/CorpusID:56821253
5. Y. Omura, "Accurate localization of organ representation areas of the tongue, using the bi-digital o-ring test: Its clinical application, and re-evaluation of classical oriental tongue diagnosis – part i," *Acupunct Electro-Therapeut Res*, vol. 16, no. 1, pp. 27–43, Jan. 1991, doi: 10.3727/036012991816358062
6. L. Yuan et al., "Development of a tongue image-based machine learning tool for the diagnosis of gastric cancer: A prospective multicentre clinical cohort study," *E Clin Med*, vol. 57, p. 101834, Mar. 2023, doi: 10.1016/j.eclinm.2023.101834
7. M. Segawa et al., "Objective evaluation of tongue diagnosis ability using a tongue diagnosis e-learning/e-assessment system based on a standardized tongue image database," *Front Med Technol*, vol. 5, Mar. 2023, doi: 10.3389/fmedt.2023.1050909
8. B. Tiryaki, K. Torenek-Agirman, O. Miloglu, B. Korkmaz, İ. Y. Ozbek, and E. A. Oral, "Artificial intelligence in tongue diagnosis: Classification of tongue lesions and normal tongue images using deep convolutional neural network," *BMC Med Imaging*, vol. 24, no. 1, p. 59, Mar. 2024, doi: 10.1186/s12880-024-01234-3
9. A. Haleem, M. Javaid, R. Pratap Singh, and R. Suman, "Exploring the revolution in healthcare systems through the applications of digital twin technology," *Biomed Technol*, vol. 4, pp. 28–38, Dec. 2023, doi: 10.1016/j.bmt.2023.02.001
10. T. Jiang et al., "Deep learning multi-label tongue image analysis and its application in a population undergoing routine medical checkup," *Evid Based Complement Alternat Med*, vol. 2022, pp. 1–12, Sep. 2022, doi: 10.1155/2022/3384209
11. B. Bordoni, B. Morabito, R. Mitrano, M. Simonelli, and A. Toccafondi, "The anatomical relationships of the tongue with the body system," *Cureus*, Dec. 2018, doi: 10.7759/cureus.3695
12. T. Kawanabe et al., "Correlation between tongue body colour, as quantified by machine learning, and clinical indices," *Adv Integr Med*, vol. 7, no. 1, pp. 8–13, Mar. 2020, doi: 10.1016/j.aimed.2019.01.005
13. T.-C. Lee, L.-C. Lo, and F.-C. Wu, "Traditional Chinese medicine for metabolic syndrome via TCM pattern differentiation: Tongue diagnosis for predictor," *Evid Based Complement Alternat Med*, vol. 2016, pp. 1–8, 2016, doi: 10.1155/2016/1971295
14. K. Wang, D. Zhang, N. Li, and B. Pang, "Tongue diagnosis based on biometric pattern recognition technology," in *Pattern Recogn*, 2001, pp. 575–598. doi: 10.1142/9789812386533_0021
15. V. Kurande, A. E. Bilgrau, R. Waagepetersen, E. Toft, and R. Prasad, "Interrater reliability of diagnostic methods in traditional Indian ayurvedic medicine," *Evid Based Complement Alternat Med*, vol. 2013, pp. 1–12, 2013, doi: 10.1155/2013/658275

16. S. P. Vinjamury, M. Vinjamury, S. Sucharitakul, and I. Ziegler, "Panchakarma: Ayurvedic detoxification and allied therapies—Is there any evidence?," in *Evidence-Based Practice in Complementary and Alternative Medicine*, Berlin, Heidelberg: Springer Berlin Heidelberg, 2012, pp. 113–137. doi: 10.1007/978-3-642-24565-7_7
17. J. Li et al., "Establishment of noninvasive diabetes risk prediction model based on tongue features and machine learning techniques," *Int J Med Inform*, vol. 149, p. 104429, May 2021, doi: 10.1016/j.ijmedinf.2021.104429
18. R Bharani, K. T. Manishaa, and D. Jaisurya, "Diabetes mellitus diagnosis based on tongue images using machine learning," in *2023 9th International Conference on Advanced Computing and Communication Systems (ICACCS)*, IEEE, Mar. 2023, pp. 1614–1618. doi: 10.1109/ICACCS57279.2023.10112849
19. J. Li et al., "Research of the distribution of tongue features of diabetic population based on unsupervised learning technology," *Evid Based Complement Alternat Med*, vol. 2022, pp. 1–14, Jul. 2022, doi: 10.1155/2022/7684714
20. M. Bharathi, D. Prasad, T. Venkatakrishnamoorthy, and M. Dharani, "Diabetes diagnostic method based on tongue image classification using machine learning algorithms," *J Pharm Negat Results*, vol. 13, no. 4, pp. 1247–1250, 2022.
21. N. Zhang, Z. Jiang, J. Li, and D. Zhang, "Multiple color representation and fusion for diabetes mellitus diagnosis based on back tongue images," *Comput Biol Med*, vol. 155, p. 106652, Mar. 2023, doi: 10.1016/j.compbiomed.2023.106652
22. B. Sridhar, C. A. Kumar, and P. Anjaneyulu, "Detection of diabetes using tongue image analysis," 2023, p. 030073. doi: 10.1063/5.0113319
23. E. Srividhya and A. M. Kumaravel, "Diabetic detection using tongue images based on ANNCl assification," *Int J Eng Adv Technol*, vol. 9, no. 1, pp. 2704–2710, Oct. 2019, doi: 10.35940/ijeat.A9750.109119
24. J. Zhang et al., "Diagnostic method of diabetes based on support vector machine and tongue images," *Biomed Res Int*, vol. 2017, pp. 1–9, 2017, doi: 10.1155/2017/7961494
25. J. Heo et al., "Deep learning model for tongue cancer diagnosis using endoscopic images," *Sci Rep*, vol. 12, no. 1, p. 6281, Apr. 2022, doi: 10.1038/s41598-022-10287-9
26. B. Jiang et al., "Integrating next-generation sequencing and traditional tongue diagnosis to determine tongue coating microbiome," *Sci Rep*, vol. 2, no. 1, p. 936, Dec. 2012, doi: 10.1038/srep00936
27. T.-C. Wu et al., "Tongue diagnosis indices for upper gastrointestinal disorders," *Medicine*, vol. 97, no. 2, p. e9607, Jan. 2018, doi: 10.1097/MD.0000000000009607
28. S. Liu et al., "The relationship between abnormal tongue features and non-malignant upper gastrointestinal disorders: A hospital-based cross-sectional study," *Eur J Integr Med*, vol. 47, p. 101379, Oct. 2021, doi: 10.1016/j.eujim.2021.101379
29. T.-C. Wu et al., "Tongue diagnosis indices for gastroesophageal reflux disease," *Medicine*, vol. 99, no. 29, p. e20471, Jul. 2020, doi: 10.1097/MD.0000000000020471
30. S. Sivasubramaniam and S. P. Balamurugan, "Simulated annealing with deep learning based tongue image analysis for heart disease diagnosis," *Intell Autom Soft Comput*, vol. 37, no. 1, pp. 111–126, 2023, doi: 10.32604/iasc.2023.035199
31. B. Pang, D. Zhang, N. Li, and K. Wang, "Computerized tongue diagnosis based on Bayesian networks," *IEEE Trans Biomed Eng*, vol. 51, no. 10, pp. 1803–1810, Oct. 2004, doi: 10.1109/TBME.2004.831534
32. B. Liang, R. Li, J. Lu, X.-J. Tian, and N. Gu, "Tongue diagnostic parameters-based diagnostic signature in coronary artery disease patients with clopidogrel resistance after percutaneous coronary intervention," *Explore*, vol. 19, no. 4, pp. 528–535, Jul. 2023, doi: 10.1016/j.explore.2022.10.018

33. M. Liu and Y.-M. Wang, "Study on screening of hypertension complicated with coronary heart disease based on tongue hyperspectral imaging," *Spectrosc Spectr Anal*, vol. 42, no. 2, pp. 512–516, 2022.
34. M. Supritha, S Theeksha, and K. H. Asha "A comprehensive approach to vitamin deficiency detection through image analysis of skin, tongue, eyes and nail images using convolutional neural networks," *Int J Adv Res Sci Commun Technol*, pp. 709–715, Feb. 2024, doi: 10.48175/IJARSCT-15394
35. S. Prabu and J. M. Gnanasekar, "A study on image segmentation method for image processing," 2021. doi: 10.3233/APC210223
36. S. Zhu, X. Xia, Q. Zhang, and K. Belloulata, "An image segmentation algorithm in image processing based on threshold segmentation," in *2007 Third International IEEE Conference on Signal-Image Technologies and Internet-Based System*, IEEE, Dec 2007, pp. 673–678. doi: 10.1109/SITIS.2007.116
37. K. K. D. Ramesh, G. Kumar, K. Swapna, D. Datta, and S. Rajest, "A review of medical image segmentation algorithms," *EAI Endorsed Trans Pervasive Heal Technol*, p. 169184, Jul. 2018, doi: 10.4108/eai.12-4-2021.169184
38. Z. Wang, E. Wang, and Y. Zhu, "Image segmentation evaluation: A survey of methods," *Artif Intell Rev*, vol. 53, no. 8, pp. 5637–5674, Dec. 2020, doi: 10.1007/s10462-020-09830-9
39. W. A. Mustafa, N. M. Salleh, S. Z. S. Idrus, M. A. Jamlos, and M. N. K. H. Rohani, "Overview of segmentation x-ray medical images using image processing technique," *J Phys Conf Ser*, vol. 1529, no. 4, p. 042017, Apr. 2020, doi: 10.1088/1742-6596/1529/4/042017
40. C. Tian, Y. Liu, M. Li, and C. Fen, "Tongue image segmentation algorithm based on deep convolutional neural network and attention mechanism," *J Intell Fuzzy Syst*, vol. 45, no. 1, pp. 1473–1480, Jul. 2023, doi: 10.3233/JIFS-221411
41. G. Kumar and P. K. Bhatia, "A detailed review of feature extraction in image processing systems," in *2014 Fourth International Conference on Advanced Computing & Communication Technologies*, IEEE, Feb. 2014, pp. 5–12. doi: 10.1109/ACCT.2014.74
42. X. Liu and C. Zhao, "Research on image feature extraction algorithm of the egg and egg white protein thermal gelation based on PCA/ICA," *Comput Intell Neurosci*, vol. 2022, pp. 1–11, Mar. 2022, doi: 10.1155/2022/1266332
43. A. Kaur and S. Gupta, "Texture classification based on Gabor wavelet," *Int J Res Comput Sci*, vol. 2, no. 4, pp. 39–44, Jul. 2012, doi: 10.7815/ijorcs.24.2012.038
44. Z. Feng and X. Hua, "Pattern recognition and its application in image processing," *J Phys Conf Ser*, vol. 1518, no. 1, p. 012071, Apr. 2020, doi: 10.1088/1742-6596/1518/1/012071
45. J. Li et al., "A tongue features fusion approach to predicting prediabetes and diabetes with machine learning," *J Biomed Inform*, vol. 115, p. 103693, Mar. 2021, doi: 10.1016/j.jbi.2021.103693
46. S. Dulam, V. Ramesh, and M. Ganesan, "Tongue image analysis for Covid-19 diagnosis and disease detection," *Int J Adv Trends Comput Sci Eng*, vol. 9, no. 5, pp. 7924–7928, Oct. 2020, doi: 10.30534/ijatcse/2020/145952020
47. S. Jain, "'Ayurvedic doshas identification using face and body image features' – A review," *Int J Adv Res Comput Sci*, vol. 12, no. 3, pp. 19–22, Jun. 2021, doi: 10.26483/ijarcs.v12i3.6741
48. M. H. Tania, K. Lwin, and M. A. Hossain, "Advances in automated tongue diagnosis techniques," *Integr Med Res*, vol. 8, no. 1, pp. 42–56, Mar. 2019, doi: 10.1016/j.imr.2018.03.001

49. V. Bhatnagar and P. P. Bansod, "Challenges and solutions in automated tongue diagnosis techniques: A review," *Crit Rev Biomed Eng*, vol. 50, no. 1, pp. 47–63, 2022, doi: 10.1615/CritRevBiomedEng.2022044392
50. C. L. Stefanescu, M. F. Popa, and L. S. Candea, "Preliminary study on the tongue-based forensic identification," *Romanian J Legal Med*, vol. 22, no. 4, pp. 263–266, Dec. 2014, doi: 10.4323/rjlm.2014.263
51. Z. Liu, J. Yan, D. Zhang, and Q. Tang, "A tongue-print image database for recognition," in *ICMLC 2007: Proceedings of the Sixth International Conference on Machine Learning and Cybernetics: Hong Kong*, IEEE, Aug. 2007, pp. 2235–2238.
52. A. Johnson, "A morphological study of tongue and its role in forensics odontology," *J Forensic Sci Crim Investig*, vol. 7, no. 5, Feb. 2018, doi: 10.19080/JFSCI.2018.07.555723
53. M. V. Reddy, R. Kiranmai, and N. V. Kumar, "Tongue scanning as a biometric tool for improvising the security in identification," 2017. [Online]. Available: https://api.semanticscholar.org/CorpusID:212486754
54. T. Radhika, N. Jeddy, and S. Nithya, "Tongue prints: A novel biometric and potential forensic tool," *J Forensic Dent Sci*, vol. 8, no. 3, p. 117, 2016, doi: 10.4103/0975-1475.195119
55. M. Vibhooti, "Speeded up robust factor for tongue biometrics- person identification method," *i-manager's J Pattern Recogn*, vol. 3, no. 2, p. 24, 2016, doi: 10.26634/jpr.3.2.8265
56. S. Lahmiri, "Recognition of tongueprint textures for personal authentication: A wavelet approach," *J Adv Inf Technol*, vol. 3, no. 3, Aug. 2012, 10.4304/jait.3.3.168-175
57. R. S. Choras, "Biometric identification through tongue texture measurements," 2016. [Online]. Available: https://api.semanticscholar.org/CorpusID:10465087
58. A. Paulose, P. S. Fazeela, N. T. Jacob, and V. S. Babu, "Biometric applications of tongue images," *Int J Eng Trends Technol*, vol. 31, no. 2, pp. 69–72, Jan. 2016, doi: 10.14445/22315381/IJETT-V31P213
59. R. S. Choraś, "Automatic tongue recognition based on color and textural features," 2017, pp. 16–26. doi: 10.1007/978-3-319-47274-4_2
60. Y. Kumar, A. Koul, R. Singla, and M. F. Ijaz, "Artificial intelligence in disease diagnosis: A systematic literature review, synthesizing framework and future research agenda," *J Ambient Intell Humaniz Comput*, vol. 14, no. 7, pp. 8459–8486, Jul. 2023, doi: 10.1007/s12652-021-03612-z
61. N. Ghaffar Nia, E. Kaplanoglu, and A. Nasab, "Evaluation of artificial intelligence techniques in disease diagnosis and prediction," *Discover Artif Intell*, vol. 3, no. 1, p. 5, Jan. 2023, doi: 10.1007/s44163-023-00049-5
62. M. Mirbabaie, S. Stieglitz, and N. R. J. Frick, "Artificial intelligence in disease diagnostics: A critical review and classification on the current state of research guiding future direction," *Health Technol (Berl)*, vol. 11, no. 4, pp. 693–731, Jul. 2021, doi: 10.1007/s12553-021-00555-5
63. J. K. Anastasi, M. Chang, J. Quinn, and B. Capili, "Tongue inspection in TCM: Observations in a study sample of patients living with HIV," *Med Acupunct*, vol. 26, no. 1, pp. 15–22, Feb. 2014, doi: 10.1089/acu.2013.1011
64. J. Li, B. Xu, X. Ban, P. Tai, and B. Ma, "A tongue image segmentation method based on enhanced HSV convolutional neural network," 2017, pp. 252–260. doi: 10.1007/978-3-319-66805-5_32

Index

Pages in **bold** refer to tables.

A

AI algorithms, 76, 98, 117, 129, 196–200, 203, 225, 227, 237
artificial intelligence, 12–20, 22, 36–39, 45, 91, 92, 94–99, 101, 104, 117, 119, 123, 127, 128, 131, 147, 154, 191, 196, 203, 206–210, 212, 218, 228, 233–235, 249, 250, 255, 274, 279, 281, 283, 288, 295
artificial neural networks, **47**, **48**, 115, 225, 261
Automated rehabilitation devices, 73

B

bioanalytical tool, 198
Biomedical imaging sensors, 55
biomedical monitoring, 141, 143
biometric devices, 141
Bluetooth technology, 155

C

Cardiovascular Disease, 153
Clinical Decision Support Systems, 204
COVID-19, 13, 14, 19, 50, 76, 84, 89, 90, 96, 106, 107, 121, 135, 143, 146, 147, 205, 212, 231, 243–245, 249, 250, 252, 253, 265, 266, 270, 271

D

Data acquisition systems, 56
dedicated systems, 4
Deep Learning, 5, 6, 13, 124–129, 131–133, 211, 261, 264, 271
deep learning algo- rithms, 261
defibrillators, 4, 43, 45, 49, 141, 142, 191, 259
digital surgery, 228, 234

E

electromagnetic sensor, 260
Electronic Health Record, 141
electronic health records, 6, 26, 36, 73, 75, 80, 97, 217
electronic medical record, 36, 42

G

gastroesophageal reflux disease, 211, 227, 234, 280, 293
Generative Adversarial Networks, 264

H

healthcare institutions, 23, 28, 29, 30, 237
Hospital Information System, 9
Hyperspectral imaging, 112

I

imaging equipment, 43, 83, 103, 106, 137, 190, 255
implantable medical devices, 43, 45
INTERNET OF MEDICAL THINGS, 11, 15, 16, 18, 37, 85, 198, 250, 267
Internet of Things, 13, 17, 22, 40, 44, **48**, 86, 88, 89, 90, 101, 117, 119, 130, 131, 134, 135, 149, 191, 207, 246, 267, 271

M

mammography, 101, 114, 115, 116, 123
medical devices, 6–9, 12, 13, 28, 31, 33, 37–39, 41, 43–45, 49–72, 74–78, 80, 85, 87, 89, 92–95, 100, 101, 103, 104, 114, 118–120, 122, 136, 137, 141–144, 146, 148, 151, 152, 155, 193, 206, 249, 259
Medical imaging, 100, 101, 130, 282
medical imaging systems, 35, 60
MEDICAL IMPLANTS, 5, 6
medical thermography, 114
metabolic bariatric surgery, 212, 218, 228
metadata, 176, 181
Microcontrollers, 5, 21, 52, 254
Microprocessors, 21, 52, 271
ML algorithms, **46**, **47**, 115, 197, 199, 238, 239, 241, 242, 244–247, 261, 263, 265, 266, 279, 283, 288
modern monitoring machines, 190

O

Obesity, 10, 211, 225, 226, 230, 270

P

patient monitoring, 1, 2, 5, 14–16, 23–26, 31–33, 37, 40, 43, 45, 50, 51, 53, 55, 75, 76, 81, 96, 98, 119, 135, 136, 138, 141, 142, 143, 191, 203, 205, 232
Patient monitoring devices, 5
Primary Health Centers, 153
quality management systems, 32, 68, 93

R

Radiology, **47**, 60, 73, 89, 91, 95, 101, 102, 114
Regulatory bodies, 31, 50, 65–68
Regulatory compliance, 31, 32, 66
Regulatory frameworks, 65–67, 206
Rehabilitation, 9, 59, 73, 96, 191
Remote patient management, 23, 24, 27
Remote patient monitoring, 50
Robotic surgery, **46**, 73
Robotic-assisted surgery, 43, 56

S

Security Concerns, 28
Sensor technology, 11
Supervised learning, 238, 283

T

telecommunications, 124, 125, 126
telemedicine, 2, 3, 13, 14, 17, 23, 24, 25, 37, 75, 76, 89, 96, 103, 133, 135, 138, 141, 142, 167, 187, 205, 212, 218, 221, 231, 233, 285
Telemedicine, 13, 26, 75, 76, 130, 138, 147, 212, 285
telemonitoring platform, 216, 232
therapeutic devices, 45, 49

W

wearable devices, 12, 25, 33, 35, 38, 49, 52, 75, 76, 89, 95, 119, 136, 137, 154, 205, 221, 261
Wearable Health Devices, 5, 6, 34
Wearable health systems, 34, 42
wearable sensors, 18, 55, 74, 76, 87, 90, 136, 138, 203, 212, 261